Name _____ Da _____

Last   First   Middle

Directions for Marking Answers

- Use a black lead pencil (No. 2 or softer). Do NOT use pen or a pencil with hard lead.
- Make each mark heavy and black enough to completely obliterate the letter within the circle. Marks should fill the circles.
- Erase clearly any answer you wish to change.
- Make no stray marks on this answer sheet.
- Mark one and only one answer for each question. Multiple answers will be counted as wrong.

Example

WRONG   Ⓐ Ⓑ̸ Ⓒ Ⓓ Ⓔ
WRONG   Ⓐ ⓧ Ⓒ Ⓓ Ⓔ
WRONG   Ⓐ Ⓑ Ⓒ Ⓓ Ⓔ
RIGHT   Ⓐ Ⓑ Ⓒ ● Ⓔ

1 Ⓐ Ⓑ Ⓒ Ⓓ Ⓔ   26 Ⓐ Ⓑ Ⓒ Ⓓ Ⓔ   51 Ⓐ Ⓑ Ⓒ Ⓓ Ⓔ   76 Ⓐ Ⓑ Ⓒ Ⓓ Ⓔ
2 Ⓐ Ⓑ Ⓒ Ⓓ Ⓔ   27 Ⓐ Ⓑ Ⓒ Ⓓ Ⓔ   52 Ⓐ Ⓑ Ⓒ Ⓓ Ⓔ   77 Ⓐ Ⓑ Ⓒ Ⓓ Ⓔ
3 Ⓐ Ⓑ Ⓒ Ⓓ Ⓔ   28 Ⓐ Ⓑ Ⓒ Ⓓ Ⓔ   53 Ⓐ Ⓑ Ⓒ Ⓓ Ⓔ   78 Ⓐ Ⓑ Ⓒ Ⓓ Ⓔ
4 Ⓐ Ⓑ Ⓒ Ⓓ Ⓔ   29 Ⓐ Ⓑ Ⓒ Ⓓ Ⓔ   54 Ⓐ Ⓑ Ⓒ Ⓓ Ⓔ   79 Ⓐ Ⓑ Ⓒ Ⓓ Ⓔ
5 Ⓐ Ⓑ Ⓒ Ⓓ Ⓔ   30 Ⓐ Ⓑ Ⓒ Ⓓ Ⓔ   55 Ⓐ Ⓑ Ⓒ Ⓓ Ⓔ   80 Ⓐ Ⓑ Ⓒ Ⓓ Ⓔ
6 Ⓐ Ⓑ Ⓒ Ⓓ Ⓔ   31 Ⓐ Ⓑ Ⓒ Ⓓ Ⓔ   56 Ⓐ Ⓑ Ⓒ Ⓓ Ⓔ   81 Ⓐ Ⓑ Ⓒ Ⓓ Ⓔ
7 Ⓐ Ⓑ Ⓒ Ⓓ Ⓔ   32 Ⓐ Ⓑ Ⓒ Ⓓ Ⓔ   57 Ⓐ Ⓑ Ⓒ Ⓓ Ⓔ   82 Ⓐ Ⓑ Ⓒ Ⓓ Ⓔ
8 Ⓐ Ⓑ Ⓒ Ⓓ Ⓔ   33 Ⓐ Ⓑ Ⓒ Ⓓ Ⓔ   58 Ⓐ Ⓑ Ⓒ Ⓓ Ⓔ   83 Ⓐ Ⓑ Ⓒ Ⓓ Ⓔ
9 Ⓐ Ⓑ Ⓒ Ⓓ Ⓔ   34 Ⓐ Ⓑ Ⓒ Ⓓ Ⓔ   59 Ⓐ Ⓑ Ⓒ Ⓓ Ⓔ   84 Ⓐ Ⓑ Ⓒ Ⓓ Ⓔ
10 Ⓐ Ⓑ Ⓒ Ⓓ Ⓔ   35 Ⓐ Ⓑ Ⓒ Ⓓ Ⓔ   60 Ⓐ Ⓑ Ⓒ Ⓓ Ⓔ   85 Ⓐ Ⓑ Ⓒ Ⓓ Ⓔ
11 Ⓐ Ⓑ Ⓒ Ⓓ Ⓔ   36 Ⓐ Ⓑ Ⓒ Ⓓ Ⓔ   61 Ⓐ Ⓑ Ⓒ Ⓓ Ⓔ   86 Ⓐ Ⓑ Ⓒ Ⓓ Ⓔ
12 Ⓐ Ⓑ Ⓒ Ⓓ Ⓔ   37 Ⓐ Ⓑ Ⓒ Ⓓ Ⓔ   62 Ⓐ Ⓑ Ⓒ Ⓓ Ⓔ   87 Ⓐ Ⓑ Ⓒ Ⓓ Ⓔ
13 Ⓐ Ⓑ Ⓒ Ⓓ Ⓔ   38 Ⓐ Ⓑ Ⓒ Ⓓ Ⓔ   63 Ⓐ Ⓑ Ⓒ Ⓓ Ⓔ   88 Ⓐ Ⓑ Ⓒ Ⓓ Ⓔ
14 Ⓐ Ⓑ Ⓒ Ⓓ Ⓔ   39 Ⓐ Ⓑ Ⓒ Ⓓ Ⓔ   64 Ⓐ Ⓑ Ⓒ Ⓓ Ⓔ   89 Ⓐ Ⓑ Ⓒ Ⓓ Ⓔ
15 Ⓐ Ⓑ Ⓒ Ⓓ Ⓔ   40 Ⓐ Ⓑ Ⓒ Ⓓ Ⓔ   65 Ⓐ Ⓑ Ⓒ Ⓓ Ⓔ   90 Ⓐ Ⓑ Ⓒ Ⓓ Ⓔ
16 Ⓐ Ⓑ Ⓒ Ⓓ Ⓔ   41 Ⓐ Ⓑ Ⓒ Ⓓ Ⓔ   66 Ⓐ Ⓑ Ⓒ Ⓓ Ⓔ   91 Ⓐ Ⓑ Ⓒ Ⓓ Ⓔ
17 Ⓐ Ⓑ Ⓒ Ⓓ Ⓔ   42 Ⓐ Ⓑ Ⓒ Ⓓ Ⓔ   67 Ⓐ Ⓑ Ⓒ Ⓓ Ⓔ   92 Ⓐ Ⓑ Ⓒ Ⓓ Ⓔ
18 Ⓐ Ⓑ Ⓒ Ⓓ Ⓔ   43 Ⓐ Ⓑ Ⓒ Ⓓ Ⓔ   68 Ⓐ Ⓑ Ⓒ Ⓓ Ⓔ   93 Ⓐ Ⓑ Ⓒ Ⓓ Ⓔ
19 Ⓐ Ⓑ Ⓒ Ⓓ Ⓔ   44 Ⓐ Ⓑ Ⓒ Ⓓ Ⓔ   69 Ⓐ Ⓑ Ⓒ Ⓓ Ⓔ   94 Ⓐ Ⓑ Ⓒ Ⓓ Ⓔ
20 Ⓐ Ⓑ Ⓒ Ⓓ Ⓔ   45 Ⓐ Ⓑ Ⓒ Ⓓ Ⓔ   70 Ⓐ Ⓑ Ⓒ Ⓓ Ⓔ   95 Ⓐ Ⓑ Ⓒ Ⓓ Ⓔ
21 Ⓐ Ⓑ Ⓒ Ⓓ Ⓔ   46 Ⓐ Ⓑ Ⓒ Ⓓ Ⓔ   71 Ⓐ Ⓑ Ⓒ Ⓓ Ⓔ   96 Ⓐ Ⓑ Ⓒ Ⓓ Ⓔ
22 Ⓐ Ⓑ Ⓒ Ⓓ Ⓔ   47 Ⓐ Ⓑ Ⓒ Ⓓ Ⓔ   72 Ⓐ Ⓑ Ⓒ Ⓓ Ⓔ   97 Ⓐ Ⓑ Ⓒ Ⓓ Ⓔ
23 Ⓐ Ⓑ Ⓒ Ⓓ Ⓔ   48 Ⓐ Ⓑ Ⓒ Ⓓ Ⓔ   73 Ⓐ Ⓑ Ⓒ Ⓓ Ⓔ   98 Ⓐ Ⓑ Ⓒ Ⓓ Ⓔ
24 Ⓐ Ⓑ Ⓒ Ⓓ Ⓔ   49 Ⓐ Ⓑ Ⓒ Ⓓ Ⓔ   74 Ⓐ Ⓑ Ⓒ Ⓓ Ⓔ   99 Ⓐ Ⓑ Ⓒ Ⓓ Ⓔ
25 Ⓐ Ⓑ Ⓒ Ⓓ Ⓔ   50 Ⓐ Ⓑ Ⓒ Ⓓ Ⓔ   75 Ⓐ Ⓑ Ⓒ Ⓓ Ⓔ   100 Ⓐ Ⓑ Ⓒ Ⓓ Ⓔ

Name _____ **Date** _____

Last   First   Middle

Directions for Marking Answers

- Use a black lead pencil (No. 2 or softer). Do NOT use pen or a pencil with hard lead.
- Make each mark heavy and black enough to completely obliterate the letter within the circle. Marks should fill the circles.
- Erase clearly any answer you wish to change.
- Make no stray marks on this answer sheet.
- Mark one and only one answer for each question. Multiple answers will be counted as wrong.

Example

WRONG Ⓐ Ⓑ Ⓒ Ⓓ Ⓔ
WRONG Ⓐ Ⓑ Ⓒ Ⓓ Ⓔ
WRONG Ⓐ Ⓑ Ⓒ Ⓓ Ⓔ
RIGHT Ⓐ Ⓑ Ⓒ ● Ⓔ

101 Ⓐ Ⓑ Ⓒ Ⓓ Ⓔ	126 Ⓐ Ⓑ Ⓒ Ⓓ Ⓔ	151 Ⓐ Ⓑ Ⓒ Ⓓ Ⓔ	176 Ⓐ Ⓑ Ⓒ Ⓓ Ⓔ
102 Ⓐ Ⓑ Ⓒ Ⓓ Ⓔ	127 Ⓐ Ⓑ Ⓒ Ⓓ Ⓔ	152 Ⓐ Ⓑ Ⓒ Ⓓ Ⓔ	177 Ⓐ Ⓑ Ⓒ Ⓓ Ⓔ
103 Ⓐ Ⓑ Ⓒ Ⓓ Ⓔ	128 Ⓐ Ⓑ Ⓒ Ⓓ Ⓔ	153 Ⓐ Ⓑ Ⓒ Ⓓ Ⓔ	178 Ⓐ Ⓑ Ⓒ Ⓓ Ⓔ
104 Ⓐ Ⓑ Ⓒ Ⓓ Ⓔ	129 Ⓐ Ⓑ Ⓒ Ⓓ Ⓔ	154 Ⓐ Ⓑ Ⓒ Ⓓ Ⓔ	179 Ⓐ Ⓑ Ⓒ Ⓓ Ⓔ
105 Ⓐ Ⓑ Ⓒ Ⓓ Ⓔ	130 Ⓐ Ⓑ Ⓒ Ⓓ Ⓔ	155 Ⓐ Ⓑ Ⓒ Ⓓ Ⓔ	180 Ⓐ Ⓑ Ⓒ Ⓓ Ⓔ
106 Ⓐ Ⓑ Ⓒ Ⓓ Ⓔ	131 Ⓐ Ⓑ Ⓒ Ⓓ Ⓔ	156 Ⓐ Ⓑ Ⓒ Ⓓ Ⓔ	181 Ⓐ Ⓑ Ⓒ Ⓓ Ⓔ
107 Ⓐ Ⓑ Ⓒ Ⓓ Ⓔ	132 Ⓐ Ⓑ Ⓒ Ⓓ Ⓔ	157 Ⓐ Ⓑ Ⓒ Ⓓ Ⓔ	182 Ⓐ Ⓑ Ⓒ Ⓓ Ⓔ
108 Ⓐ Ⓑ Ⓒ Ⓓ Ⓔ	133 Ⓐ Ⓑ Ⓒ Ⓓ Ⓔ	158 Ⓐ Ⓑ Ⓒ Ⓓ Ⓔ	183 Ⓐ Ⓑ Ⓒ Ⓓ Ⓔ
109 Ⓐ Ⓑ Ⓒ Ⓓ Ⓔ	134 Ⓐ Ⓑ Ⓒ Ⓓ Ⓔ	159 Ⓐ Ⓑ Ⓒ Ⓓ Ⓔ	184 Ⓐ Ⓑ Ⓒ Ⓓ Ⓔ
110 Ⓐ Ⓑ Ⓒ Ⓓ Ⓔ	135 Ⓐ Ⓑ Ⓒ Ⓓ Ⓔ	160 Ⓐ Ⓑ Ⓒ Ⓓ Ⓔ	185 Ⓐ Ⓑ Ⓒ Ⓓ Ⓔ
111 Ⓐ Ⓑ Ⓒ Ⓓ Ⓔ	136 Ⓐ Ⓑ Ⓒ Ⓓ Ⓔ	161 Ⓐ Ⓑ Ⓒ Ⓓ Ⓔ	186 Ⓐ Ⓑ Ⓒ Ⓓ Ⓔ
112 Ⓐ Ⓑ Ⓒ Ⓓ Ⓔ	137 Ⓐ Ⓑ Ⓒ Ⓓ Ⓔ	162 Ⓐ Ⓑ Ⓒ Ⓓ Ⓔ	187 Ⓐ Ⓑ Ⓒ Ⓓ Ⓔ
113 Ⓐ Ⓑ Ⓒ Ⓓ Ⓔ	138 Ⓐ Ⓑ Ⓒ Ⓓ Ⓔ	163 Ⓐ Ⓑ Ⓒ Ⓓ Ⓔ	188 Ⓐ Ⓑ Ⓒ Ⓓ Ⓔ
114 Ⓐ Ⓑ Ⓒ Ⓓ Ⓔ	139 Ⓐ Ⓑ Ⓒ Ⓓ Ⓔ	164 Ⓐ Ⓑ Ⓒ Ⓓ Ⓔ	189 Ⓐ Ⓑ Ⓒ Ⓓ Ⓔ
115 Ⓐ Ⓑ Ⓒ Ⓓ Ⓔ	140 Ⓐ Ⓑ Ⓒ Ⓓ Ⓔ	165 Ⓐ Ⓑ Ⓒ Ⓓ Ⓔ	190 Ⓐ Ⓑ Ⓒ Ⓓ Ⓔ
116 Ⓐ Ⓑ Ⓒ Ⓓ Ⓔ	141 Ⓐ Ⓑ Ⓒ Ⓓ Ⓔ	166 Ⓐ Ⓑ Ⓒ Ⓓ Ⓔ	191 Ⓐ Ⓑ Ⓒ Ⓓ Ⓔ
117 Ⓐ Ⓑ Ⓒ Ⓓ Ⓔ	142 Ⓐ Ⓑ Ⓒ Ⓓ Ⓔ	167 Ⓐ Ⓑ Ⓒ Ⓓ Ⓔ	192 Ⓐ Ⓑ Ⓒ Ⓓ Ⓔ
118 Ⓐ Ⓑ Ⓒ Ⓓ Ⓔ	143 Ⓐ Ⓑ Ⓒ Ⓓ Ⓔ	168 Ⓐ Ⓑ Ⓒ Ⓓ Ⓔ	193 Ⓐ Ⓑ Ⓒ Ⓓ Ⓔ
119 Ⓐ Ⓑ Ⓒ Ⓓ Ⓔ	144 Ⓐ Ⓑ Ⓒ Ⓓ Ⓔ	169 Ⓐ Ⓑ Ⓒ Ⓓ Ⓔ	194 Ⓐ Ⓑ Ⓒ Ⓓ Ⓔ
120 Ⓐ Ⓑ Ⓒ Ⓓ Ⓔ	145 Ⓐ Ⓑ Ⓒ Ⓓ Ⓔ	170 Ⓐ Ⓑ Ⓒ Ⓓ Ⓔ	195 Ⓐ Ⓑ Ⓒ Ⓓ Ⓔ
121 Ⓐ Ⓑ Ⓒ Ⓓ Ⓔ	146 Ⓐ Ⓑ Ⓒ Ⓓ Ⓔ	171 Ⓐ Ⓑ Ⓒ Ⓓ Ⓔ	196 Ⓐ Ⓑ Ⓒ Ⓓ Ⓔ
122 Ⓐ Ⓑ Ⓒ Ⓓ Ⓔ	147 Ⓐ Ⓑ Ⓒ Ⓓ Ⓔ	172 Ⓐ Ⓑ Ⓒ Ⓓ Ⓔ	197 Ⓐ Ⓑ Ⓒ Ⓓ Ⓔ
123 Ⓐ Ⓑ Ⓒ Ⓓ Ⓔ	148 Ⓐ Ⓑ Ⓒ Ⓓ Ⓔ	173 Ⓐ Ⓑ Ⓒ Ⓓ Ⓔ	198 Ⓐ Ⓑ Ⓒ Ⓓ Ⓔ
124 Ⓐ Ⓑ Ⓒ Ⓓ Ⓔ	149 Ⓐ Ⓑ Ⓒ Ⓓ Ⓔ	174 Ⓐ Ⓑ Ⓒ Ⓓ Ⓔ	199 Ⓐ Ⓑ Ⓒ Ⓓ Ⓔ
125 Ⓐ Ⓑ Ⓒ Ⓓ Ⓔ	150 Ⓐ Ⓑ Ⓒ Ⓓ Ⓔ	175 Ⓐ Ⓑ Ⓒ Ⓓ Ⓔ	200 Ⓐ Ⓑ Ⓒ Ⓓ Ⓔ

Name _____ **Date** _____

Last   First   Middle

Directions for Marking Answers

- Use a black lead pencil (No. 2 or softer). Do NOT use pen or a pencil with hard lead.
- Make each mark heavy and black enough to completely obliterate the letter within the circle. Marks should fill the circles.
- Erase clearly any answer you wish to change.
- Make no stray marks on this answer sheet.
- Mark one and only one answer for each question. Multiple answers will be counted as wrong.

Example

WRONG ⒶⒷ̸ⒸⒹⒺ
WRONG ⒶⓍⒸⒹⒺ
WRONG ⒶⒷⒸ̲ⒹⒺ
RIGHT   ⒶⒷⒸ●Ⓔ

201 ⒶⒷⒸⒹⒺ	226 ⒶⒷⒸⒹⒺ	251 ⒶⒷⒸⒹⒺ	276 ⒶⒷⒸⒹⒺ
202 ⒶⒷⒸⒹⒺ	227 ⒶⒷⒸⒹⒺ	252 ⒶⒷⒸⒹⒺ	277 ⒶⒷⒸⒹⒺ
203 ⒶⒷⒸⒹⒺ	228 ⒶⒷⒸⒹⒺ	253 ⒶⒷⒸⒹⒺ	278 ⒶⒷⒸⒹⒺ
204 ⒶⒷⒸⒹⒺ	229 ⒶⒷⒸⒹⒺ	254 ⒶⒷⒸⒹⒺ	279 ⒶⒷⒸⒹⒺ
205 ⒶⒷⒸⒹⒺ	230 ⒶⒷⒸⒹⒺ	255 ⒶⒷⒸⒹⒺ	280 ⒶⒷⒸⒹⒺ
206 ⒶⒷⒸⒹⒺ	231 ⒶⒷⒸⒹⒺ	256 ⒶⒷⒸⒹⒺ	281 ⒶⒷⒸⒹⒺ
207 ⒶⒷⒸⒹⒺ	232 ⒶⒷⒸⒹⒺ	257 ⒶⒷⒸⒹⒺ	282 ⒶⒷⒸⒹⒺ
208 ⒶⒷⒸⒹⒺ	233 ⒶⒷⒸⒹⒺ	258 ⒶⒷⒸⒹⒺ	283 ⒶⒷⒸⒹⒺ
209 ⒶⒷⒸⒹⒺ	234 ⒶⒷⒸⒹⒺ	259 ⒶⒷⒸⒹⒺ	284 ⒶⒷⒸⒹⒺ
210 ⒶⒷⒸⒹⒺ	235 ⒶⒷⒸⒹⒺ	260 ⒶⒷⒸⒹⒺ	285 ⒶⒷⒸⒹⒺ
211 ⒶⒷⒸⒹⒺ	236 ⒶⒷⒸⒹⒺ	261 ⒶⒷⒸⒹⒺ	286 ⒶⒷⒸⒹⒺ
212 ⒶⒷⒸⒹⒺ	237 ⒶⒷⒸⒹⒺ	262 ⒶⒷⒸⒹⒺ	287 ⒶⒷⒸⒹⒺ
213 ⒶⒷⒸⒹⒺ	238 ⒶⒷⒸⒹⒺ	263 ⒶⒷⒸⒹⒺ	288 ⒶⒷⒸⒹⒺ
214 ⒶⒷⒸⒹⒺ	239 ⒶⒷⒸⒹⒺ	264 ⒶⒷⒸⒹⒺ	289 ⒶⒷⒸⒹⒺ
215 ⒶⒷⒸⒹⒺ	240 ⒶⒷⒸⒹⒺ	265 ⒶⒷⒸⒹⒺ	290 ⒶⒷⒸⒹⒺ
216 ⒶⒷⒸⒹⒺ	241 ⒶⒷⒸⒹⒺ	266 ⒶⒷⒸⒹⒺ	291 ⒶⒷⒸⒹⒺ
217 ⒶⒷⒸⒹⒺ	242 ⒶⒷⒸⒹⒺ	267 ⒶⒷⒸⒹⒺ	292 ⒶⒷⒸⒹⒺ
218 ⒶⒷⒸⒹⒺ	243 ⒶⒷⒸⒹⒺ	268 ⒶⒷⒸⒹⒺ	293 ⒶⒷⒸⒹⒺ
219 ⒶⒷⒸⒹⒺ	244 ⒶⒷⒸⒹⒺ	269 ⒶⒷⒸⒹⒺ	294 ⒶⒷⒸⒹⒺ
220 ⒶⒷⒸⒹⒺ	245 ⒶⒷⒸⒹⒺ	270 ⒶⒷⒸⒹⒺ	295 ⒶⒷⒸⒹⒺ
221 ⒶⒷⒸⒹⒺ	246 ⒶⒷⒸⒹⒺ	271 ⒶⒷⒸⒹⒺ	296 ⒶⒷⒸⒹⒺ
222 ⒶⒷⒸⒹⒺ	247 ⒶⒷⒸⒹⒺ	272 ⒶⒷⒸⒹⒺ	297 ⒶⒷⒸⒹⒺ
223 ⒶⒷⒸⒹⒺ	248 ⒶⒷⒸⒹⒺ	273 ⒶⒷⒸⒹⒺ	298 ⒶⒷⒸⒹⒺ
224 ⒶⒷⒸⒹⒺ	249 ⒶⒷⒸⒹⒺ	274 ⒶⒷⒸⒹⒺ	299 ⒶⒷⒸⒹⒺ
225 ⒶⒷⒸⒹⒺ	250 ⒶⒷⒸⒹⒺ	275 ⒶⒷⒸⒹⒺ	300 ⒶⒷⒸⒹⒺ

The Medical Assisting Examination Guide
A Comprehensive Review for Certification
Edition 2

KAREN LANE, CMA-AC
The Johns Hopkins University, Neuroscience Critical Care Division,
Baltimore, Maryland

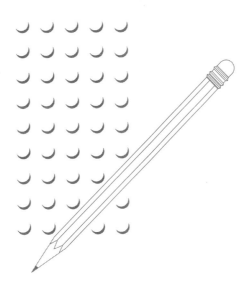

 F. A. DAVIS COMPANY • Philadelphia

F. A. Davis Company
1915 Arch Street
Philadelphia, PA 19103

Printed in the United States of America

Last digit indicates print number: 10 9 8 7 6 5

Publisher, Allied Health: Jean-François Vilain
Developmental Editor: Crystal Spraggins
Production Editor: Glenn L. Fechner
Cover Designer: Steven R. Morrone

As new scientific information becomes available through basic and clinical research, recommended treatments and drug therapies undergo changes. The author and publisher have done everything possible to make this book accurate, up to date, and in accord with accepted standards at the time of publication. The author, editors, and publisher are not responsible for errors or omissions or for consequences from application of the book, and make no warranty, expressed or implied, in regard to the contents of the book. Any practice described in this book should be applied by the reader in accordance with professional standards of care used in regard to the unique circumstances that may apply in each situation. The reader is advised always to check product information (package inserts) for changes and new information regarding dose and contraindications before administering any drug. Caution is especially urged when using new or infrequently ordered drugs.

Contents

Foreword

John Wooden, architect of one of the greatest college basketball programs in history, once said, "Failure to prepare is preparing to fail." By using this book, you will be preparing to succeed. This book is meant to assist you in studying for your medical assistant certification examination. As you study this book, you are embarking on a journey. With hard work and study, you will arrive at your destination—becoming a credentialed medical assistant.

Using this book will assist you as you take this next step toward professionalism: earning a credential. There are many reasons to be a credentialed medical assistant, and it will become more important in the coming years. Medical assisting is being challenged on many fronts. Legally, many questions are being asked concerning just what tasks medical assistants can perform on the job. Educationally, debates are stirring concerning credentialing versus licensure and registration versus education, and professionally, perceptions are changing about our role in health care. Our flexibility and training enables us to perform administrative and clinical procedures, which makes us the ideal candidate for any position in a physician's office. It also makes our occupation difficult to define.

The awarding of a credential is the process by which an association grants recognition to an individual who has met certain predetermined qualifications. This can be done by acceptable performance on a qualifying examination. The credential you receive, after successfully challenging your examination, provides you with proof of competency. It also is a benchmark for physicians and other potential employees judging your competence.

What will your credential mean to you? Will being a certified medical assistant or a registered medical assistant mean more recognition from physicians, medical group managers, other employers, or even within the allied health professions? Certainly, it will show a deep commitment to your chosen profession, and hopefully, other rewards and benefits will follow.

We must join together to let the medical and allied health professions know what a credentialed medical assistant is, and have our voices heard. In order to enhance our professionalism and obtain the recognition credentialed medical assistants deserve, we must continually educate our patients, our employers, and the public about who we are. To this end, I challenge each of you to do three things:

1. When asked who you are and what you do, use your credential proudly. "My name is Barbara Parker, and I am a certified medical assistant." Your patients and others with whom you work will come to see you not as the "girl" in the office or the "receptionist" or the "nurse" but as the credentialed person you are.
2. Demonstrate current competence by participating in continuing education activities. The CMA and RMA credentials have mandatory requirements for the revalidation of competence every five years. This can be attained through documented continuing education or by reexamination. If the credential you obtain is to have continued meaning, you must be able to demonstrate continued competence. This will set you apart from many of your peers.

3. Become involved in a professional association that is established to meet the needs of practicing medical assistants. Investigate the different ones, and choose the one that best meets your needs. It is by uniting with other medical assistants that we ensure the continued recognition we so justly deserve.

Good luck in your quest to become a credentialed medical assistant. When you receive your pin, wear it proudly, knowing that you are "the best you can be." Continue to strive for excellence, and remember the words of Vince Lombardi:

> "The quality of a person's life is in direct proportion to their commitment to excellence, regardless of their chosen field of endeavor."

Barbara Parker, CMA-AC
Immediate Past President, AAMA
Silverdale, WA, 1990

Preface to the Second Edition

New and Expanded Content

The second edition fulfills two primary aims: to introduce more test items sufficiently important to be part of the medical assistant's knowledge base (i.e., without the aid of references) in the workplace and to parallel, as closely as possible, the test items on actual examinations. This edition adds two new examination simulations and updates the original simulations, giving the reader a total of 1500 review items. The new edition eliminates the use of K-type questions, because the actual certification examinations no longer contain this style of test question. New review items have been chosen based on their continued relevance to current practice, and items that remain esoteric or rarely used by the medical assistant in the outpatient medical facility continue to be excluded.

In the tradition of the first edition, each new or revised simulation begins with information from the related sciences (anatomy and physiology, medical terminology, legal dimensions of practice, and the art of health care). Part II of each simulation continues with reviews of basic administrative procedures, including up-to-date test items on the newest regulations in health care (Occupational Safety and Health Administration procedures, Medicare coding procedures, to name a few), all very important and timely subjects. The final section of each simulation provides a review of basic patient care procedures, laboratory and diagnostic test performance, patient education, and special precautions for patients undergoing treatments or tests. Items concerning patient education for specific prescriptions are limited to the newest list of the 50 most commonly prescribed drugs. The second edition includes items to test the candidate's knowledge of actions, side effects, dosage calculation, and administration techniques. These items are limited to the pharmaceutical products frequently used in the outpatient setting.

The purpose of a good examination review book is to assess the technical knowledge and skills of the examination candidate. In keeping with this philosophy, new and revised items measure either basic knowledge (making it possible for the medical assistant to deal with new situations or problems) or the important areas of technical knowledge and skill by concentrating on medical assistants as a distinct group to be evaluated. The simulations allow the medical assistant to self-evaluate his or her ability to synthesize and evaluate medical data, formulate plans for patient action, and compose medical documentation, all within humanitarian, safe, and legal parameters.

New References

For the second edition, a secondary project was establishing subject scope guidelines and compiling a list of recommended books to accompany the new edition. As a result, the book no longer attempts to include as large a sphere of literature as in the first edition. When the budget is tight, it is important to purchase reference books wisely. New to the second edition is a more complete reference source for verification of each correct answer. Every item specifies at least one complete reference source (author, title, edition, year of publication, and page number) for the correct answer.

Actual certification examination test items are based on references from selected lists of books recommended for medical assistants. Therefore, these same types of books that support accredited educational programs or are geared specifically for the development of the medical assisting student are used solely as reference guides in this review book. Other literature of the health professions considered autonomous (medicine, nursing, pharmacy, etc.) is excluded, as is nonmedical literature that otherwise might be included in general education courses independent of a medical assisting curriculum.

A small yet comprehensive book collection is important and necessary for successful preparation. The references included in the appendix support the successful preparation of medical assisting certification. The list covers anatomy and terminology, legal dimensions of medical assisting practice, and the psychosocial and cognitive aspects related to human growth and development and patient-medical assistant interaction.

Besides two comprehensive administrative and clinical reference works and a recommended medical dictionary, a number of single-topic textbooks is selected for the review of laboratory and diagnostic testing, diseases of the human body, and the administration of medications. Additional single-topic references have been chosen for coding terminology, medical transcription and writing style, English grammar, and basic computer applications. Because of OSHA (Occupational Safety and Health Administration) legal complexities, government publication brochures have been chosen in two instances.

Each reference is uncomplicated, direct in its approach, and related to actual on-the-job performance. As a rule, the selected books focus specifically on medical assisting or are an integral part of the medical assisting discipline. Emphasis is on current materials, predominantly F.A. Davis publications, although works by other publishers have been included. All the books chosen have been published since 1988; 80% since 1990. New editions of two pre-1990 books are scheduled for 1995. Only one (style manual) is dated prior to 1988, but it is a classic. "New" does not necessarily mean "better" in its case.

These books are readily available for purchase or in academic libraries supporting medical assisting programs. The author has recommended these books because they are authoritative in the medical assisting field, well organized, effectively indexed, readable, and in use by medical assisting educators, but this list should not be considered as a required item-by-item standard. Selection lists tend to be somewhat outdated by the time they appear in print, and this list will not prove an exception. It can, however, provide a basis for developing a medical assisting collection, not only for certification preparation but as an ongoing source of reference throughout career development.

Karen Lane

Preface to the First Edition

This review is for medical assistants who are candidates for the Certified Medical Assistant (CMA) Examination, which is offered by the American Association of Medical Assistants, and the Registered Medical Assistant (RMA) Examination, which is offered by the American Medical Technologists Association.

Medical assisting practice encompasses a wide range of subject matter, and the functions of a medical assistant may differ, depending on the employer and the type of health care facility. Because of this diversity, no review could totally examine the concepts of all the principles and activities involved in the medical assistant's job. Therefore, the questions in this book have been strategically chosen to parallel the wide range of knowledge and practices being measured in both medical assisting examinations. Items in this review may contain practices not accepted or used in all facilities, but they have been included for the benefit of the medical assistant "generalist" who must be prepared for all aspects of a medical assisting examination.

Although every topic and issue cannot be covered in one volume, the organization of the review is topic-oriented, lending a sense of continuity and meaning to the thought and study process; yet it is designed to resemble, as closely as possible, the actual experience of writing (sitting for) the examinations.

The review items are selected to signal areas of strengths and weaknesses. Do not be discouraged if you discover a weakness in an area. The review is designed to do this. It is your partner in preparing you for the examination. So jump right in. Use your knowledge and practice strengths as indicators for those areas where you need not spend preparation time. Use incorrectly answered items to earmark topic areas where time should be spent for learning and reviewing.

This book can serve as a valuable tool for practitioners and students. It hopefully will be used for other review purposes. It can be used by students who are preparing for externship and final exams or by students who wish to challenge examinations for advanced school standing or credit. It can be used by medical assistants who are designing medical-assisting continuing education, both at the job site and throughout the various levels of association membership. Inactive medical assistants, who wish to return to medical assisting practice, will also find the review useful for self-evaluation.

Above all, use the review in the spirit of continued professional growth and for the delivery of high quality care to the patients you serve. And enjoy!

Karen Lane

Acknowledgments

The author sincerely thanks the following reviewers for their valuable contributions and assistance in preparing this review manual:

Teressa H. Buran, MST, CMA-C, Medical Assisting Program Director, Broome Community College, Binghamton, New York

Brenda M. Foster, MS, Medical Assisting Program Director, East Tennessee State University, Elizabethton, Tennessee

Rodney E. Frothingham, MD, Practitioner and Vice-Chairman, Curriculum Review Board, American Association of Medical Assistants Endowment, Greenville, Mississippi

Norman D. Lindley, MD, Practitioner and Physician Liaison, American Association of Medical Assistants Board of Trustees, Alamogordo, New Mexico

Carole J. Miller, RMA, Director, The Bryman School, Glendale, Arizona

Virginia E. Shunk, RN, CMA, Medical Assisting Program Director, Lehigh County Community College, Schnecksville, Pennsylvania

Introduction

The purpose of medical assisting credentialing is to determine minimum competency for the safe practice of medical assisting. No examination can test all knowledge related to medical assisting. Therefore, each national examination includes as much material as appropriate to meet the objectives of safe and competent medical assisting practice. Likewise, this is the purpose of this review manual.

Design of the Review

It is well known that medical assistants may be well prepared for writing the credentialing examinations but answer items incorrectly because they are unfamiliar with taking a test or unfamiliar with the way test items are written. This review offers the opportunity to practice taking objective-item examinations that resemble the credentialing examinations.

This review is divided into five examinations of 300 items each. Each examination comes with three complete answer sheets, so you may take each examination up to three times without marking the answers on the book pages. This permits you to review for your credentialing examination on at least 15 separate testing occasions, either individually or in study groups. You may further simulate the actual examination by timing your reviews. Or, you may choose to use the book item-by-item, totally as a study guide.

Each examination is subdivided into the three main areas of medical assisting practice: general medical knowledge (anatomy and physiology, medical terminology, psychology, and law and ethics); administrative medical assisting; and clinical and laboratory medical assisting. You may wish to stop after each of the test subdivisions to study a single area.

Within each of the subdivisions, topics are generally grouped together. Occasionally, they may be randomly sequenced. For example, within the Administrative section, an item on insurance may follow an item on bookkeeping. This random ordering within each subdivision parallels the actual examination experience. Hopefully, this technique will be just one of the many in this review manual to help you successfully write the actual examination.

References and Study Sources

The manual contains references for the test items. Although each item is referenced to a particular source, the bibliography is intended as recommended reading only. Some references will verify correct answers; others will suggest concepts for understanding the answers. A referenced source does not indicate that the topic will be found only in that source.

There are many excellent texts for medical assistants to use. The selections used in this review are references that are particular to medical assisting, relevant to current practice, and easy to access. In general, they are broad in scope and depth. Occasionally, when general medical assisting texts are not specific enough, topic-specific sources are recommended. The references and study aids are listed under Appendix A.

Subject Matter of the Review

The review is designed to measure universal knowledge that is both frequently performed by the medical assistant and critical for safe performance on the job. The items are relevant to current practice and considered sufficiently specific to problems encountered where differentiation between a correct technique and a mistake is important.

The items are specifically designed to assess the skills needed by the medical assistant. As much as possible, theory is presented in the format of application. This does not preclude items that measure basic knowledge and that enable the medical assistant to analyze and assess new situations. The review items attempt, as much as possible, to integrate concepts from the basic sciences to administrative situations, office management, diet therapy, pharmacology, clinical situations, and patient interaction. Some items are memory items where you recall learned information. Other items are reasoning items where you use learned information to interpret or solve situations.

Items are written to help you measure your knowledge of concepts and skills in a general overview. For instance, there may be only three or four A & P items about the eye. If you can select the correct answer for each item and understand why the distracters are incorrect, then you can generally assume your information base on the A & P of the eye is sound. If you must return to a reference for information, then take the time to review the information in its entirety. If you incorrectly answer an item in the review, there are probably more questions on the topic that you will not remember or understand. Of course, only you know your limitations, and no review can guarantee that you will master all of the necessary material, or that some other piece of information won't be asked on the national examinations.

Answer Sheets and Answers

Answer sheets are provided for each of the three examinations. They resemble the answer sheets used for the CMA and RMA examinations. The examinee should use pencil and completely blacken the circle on the answer sheet that corresponds to the answer chosen for the item. The review also includes the correct answer and rationale for each item.

Using the Examination Guide

- Use the prepared test items in this book to help you study, not as a replacement for study.
- Take a practice test before you begin to study, as a pretest.
- Use the test results to help you determine your strengths and weaknesses.
- Begin reviewing areas of known weakness first. This will allow time for additional review again before the examination.
- Ask yourself questions about incorrect selections and make notes of key concepts or facts about which you feel uncertain.
- Begin 2 to 3 months before the examination, and take each test at least once.
- Take each test more than once so that you can measure your improvement.

Review Planning

- Plan to begin your review well in advance of the examination. Cramming for an examination is unwise. Choose the technique that works best for you. You might review your texts and classroom materials first, then practice the examinations. You may wish to use your reference sources in conjunction with the review. Or, you may wish to take each examination first, then use your notes and references for further study.

- Avoid looking at the answers and rationales until you have completed the test. Mark any incorrect items on your answer sheet and use the incorrect items for study guidance.

- Time yourself. Try to complete 60 questions per hour. Read carefully and think logically. Leave items you cannot answer until you have completed the test. Then go back and try to answer those left blank. Sometimes other questions will lead you back to the correct train of thought necessary to answer a skipped item.

- Read items carefully. Look for key words, such as "except," "least," "not," and "contraindicated." Missing these key words and assuming you know what the item is asking can often lead to incorrect answers for the wrong reason—not paying attention.

- Do not look for cues for correct answers, such as a pattern of correct answers, or an option length as an indicator of a correct response. Answers are randomly selected and are rearranged by computer.

- Do not try to memorize any items as they appear in this review, or in any other. It is unlikely that you will see any item written exactly alike on the actual examinations or among the various review sources. It is better to learn the concept behind a test item. Then, you will own the information rather than have memorized it.

- Analyze your incorrect responses. Did you choose the incorrect response because you did not read the question properly or understand the question? Or, is it because you do not have knowledge of the subject matter?

- Use the tests seriously. Set aside the proper amount of time in the proper setting. Do not allow distractions during the testing situation.

Hints for Writing the CMA or RMA Examinations

- Know the location of your examination, the exact time of the examination, the length of the examination, and who is administering the examination. Make a practice run to know where you are going and how much time it will take you to get there. Leave early enough to account for traffic jams or other unforeseen problems.

- Relax. Practice relaxation techniques to reduce tension and anxiety. Use the day before the examination to relax and enjoy yourself in a special activity. Have a good night's sleep before the examination and eat a nourishing breakfast.

- Wear comfortable clothing and bring a sweater or jacket to the examination, in case the room is uncomfortably cool.

- Do not burden yourself by taking books and papers to the examination. You will not be allowed to take them into the examination room, and last minute cramming is never wise. This is your time to relax, remember?

- Approach the examination with confidence. It is very likely that you will not answer every question correctly on the examination. Do not get upset over items you do not know or remember. A positive attitude will allow you to think freely and to do a good job of responding to all of the items that you do know.

- Listen carefully to the examination directions, and ask questions if you do not understand all of the procedures. You must take two #2 pencils with you to the examination. You will be given an answer sheet and a sealed examination book. Read the test book instructions carefully before beginning the examination.

- Every item answered correctly is scored as one point. There are no extra scoring penalties for an incorrect response that may or may not result from guessing. It is better to guess than to leave an item blank.

- Do not make stray marks on your answer sheets. If you want to mark items to return to them, do so directly in your examination booklet. Do not waste time artfully darkening the circles on the answer sheet. Fill in the circles neatly and darkly. Erase completely any changes.

- Read all responses to an item before choosing one. You may miss the best answer. Eliminate the obviously incorrect distractors first, then concentrate on the plausible option or options.

- Do not try to read in tricks to test items. Use only the information given in the item and do not try to make assumptions beyond the item information.

- When you have completed the examination, review your work, if there is still time. However, beware of changing first answers. Your first response is usually the correct response. You may, however, discover and have time to change an obvious mistake.

The CMA Examination Items

Correctly speaking, a "test question" is termed an item. Each item has two parts: the stem and the response options. The stem presents a problem and is stated either as an incomplete sentence or as a question. The options contain the correct answer option and incorrect options. The incorrect options are called distractors. The review contains the 2 item types most commonly encountered in the Certified Medical Assisting Examinations:

1. The **A-type** is the traditional and most frequently used multiple-choice format. It consists of a stem and a series of five lettered response options. The examinee is required to select the **one best** answer. Distractors will be plausible; they may even be partially correct, but there will be only one best choice.

Traditional A-type Pattern

A. v
B. w
C. x
D. y
E. z
   Ex: Of the following U.S, presidents, whose administration has been stigmatized as one of the most corrupt in U.S. history?

A. Washington
B. Lincoln
C. Harding
D. Eisenhower
E. Reagan

Answer: C. The Harding administration was exposed in the Teapot Dome scandal and other lesser scandals; as a result, his administration has been stigmatized as one of the most corrupt in U.S. history.

Mutually Exclusive A-type Pattern

A. x only
B. y only
C. both x and y
D. z only
E. both x and z
   Ex: Of the following U.S. presidential administrations, those that have been stigmatized with scandal include:

A. Harding
B. Washington
C. Harding and Washington

    D. Nixon
    E. Harding and Nixon

Answer: E. The Harding Teapot Dome scandal and the Nixon Watergate scandal have left both administrations with the stigma of scandal.

"EXCEPT" A-type Pattern

. . . each of the following is true EXCEPT:

A. v
B. w
C. x
D. y
E. z

    Ex: Of the following U.S. presidents, each was a Republican EXCEPT:

A. Washington
B. Lincoln
C. Harding
D. Nixon
E. Reagan

Answer: A. George Washington was a member of the Federalist party.

    2. The **B-type** item is a matching item and consists of a header followed by a series of two or three statements or phrases. The header may be a diagram or a set of related diseases, tests, or drugs. The examinee must select from the diagram or set the letter that matches the statement or phrase. Each numbered item within a set counts as one scoring unit. For example:

B-type Pattern

    Ex: A. Washington   B. Lincoln   C. Harding   D. Nixon   E. Reagan

    1. The first president of the United States
    2. Assassinated while in office
    3. Resigned while in office

Answer #1.: A. Washington was the first U.S. president.
Answer #2.: B. Lincoln was assassinated in 1865, while serving his second term.
Answer #3.: D. Nixon resigned, while serving his second term.

General Information about the CMA Examination

The CMA Examination is competency-based. Competence is determined by the DACUM Analysis of the Medical Assisting Profession. The examination is norm-referenced. The successful examinee is required to prove competence within a range of competency that is determined by the performance of the entire testing group for each examination.

    Each CMA Examination contains 300 test items. The number of items is equally distributed among three main divisions: General, Administrative Procedures, and Clinical Procedures. The divisions are broken down into categories and subcategories. The number of items is equally distributed among the three divisions. Outline details are available in a booklet entitled: *A Candidate's Guide to the AAMA Certification Examination.*

    For specific information, see "Applying for the CMA National Examination."

Applying for the CMA National Examination

The Certified Medical Assistant (CMA) Examination is offered by the American Association of Medical Assistants Certifying Board, a nationally recognized, nonprofit certifying body. The National Board of Medical Examiners (NBME), a nonprofit corporation engaged in medical test development and research, assists the AAMA in the development of the examinations and provides test administration services. The CMA is awarded to candidates who pass the Certification Examination.

To be eligible, a medical assistant must:

1. Be a student or recent graduate of a program accredited by the Committee on Allied Health Education and Accreditation (CAHEA). Students must have completed their formal training, including externship, by the end of the month in which they wish to be examined. Recent graduates must have graduated no more than 11 months before the date of the examination.
2. Be a graduate of a CAHEA accredited program.
3. Be a medical assisting instructor in a postsecondary institution approved by a nationally recognized accrediting agency.
4. Have been employed as a medical assistant/allied health professional for at least 12 months of full-time or 24 months of part-time work, under the supervision of a licensed health care practitioner.

Testing is conducted on the last Friday in January and the last Friday in June. The examinations are offered at approximately 100 test centers throughout the United States.

Examination results are usually available within 8 to 10 weeks following the administration. Each candidate receives a letter and scores from the AAMA office. Unsuccessful candidates are informed of specific areas of weakness to help them to prepare for retesting. Membership in the AAMA is not a requirement for CMA Examination eligibility.

See Appendix B for the CMA Application sample.

For additional information and application instructions, contact:

AAMA Certifying Board
20 North Wacker Drive, Suite 1575
Chicago, IL 60606
(312) 899-1500

The RMA (AMT) Examination Items

Correctly speaking, a "test question" is termed an item. Each item has two parts: the stem and the response options. The stem presents a problem and is stated either as an incomplete sentence or as a question. The options contain the correct answer option and incorrect options. The incorrect options are called distractors.

The traditional **A-type** test item issued as the examination format. It consists of a stem and a series of four lettered response options. The examinee is required to select the **one best** answer. Distractors will be plausible; they may even be partially correct, but there will be only one best choice.

Traditional A-type Pattern

A. v
B. w
C. x
D. y
E. z

> **Ex:** Of the following U.S. presidents, whose administration has been stigmatized as the most corrupt in U.S. history?

A. Washington
B. Lincoln
C. Harding
D. Eisenhower
E. Reagan

Answer: C. The Harding administration was exposed in the Teapot Dome scandal and other lesser scandals; as a result, his administration has been stigmatized as one of the most corrupt in U.S. history.

General Information about the RMA Examination

The RMA Examination is competency-based and criterion-referenced. Criterion-referenced means a test is not scored "on the curve": the successful examinee is required to perform within a range that is predetermined by the testing agency.

Criterion-referenced examinations do not use the group performance as standard. They use an external, predetermined standard (criterion) to determine whether an individual score is in a range to demonstrate competence in the occupation. Each examination has a predetermined minimum pass level (mpl).

Each RMA Examination contains 200 test items. The examination separates the test items into three divisions: general medical assisting knowledge, administrative medical assisting, and clinical medical assisting. The three divisions are then broken down into numerous sub-category topics. Outline details are available in a booklet entitled: *Registered Medical Assistant Certification Examination Overview.*

For specific information, see "Applying for the RMA National Examination."

Applying for the RMA (AMT) National Examination

The Registered Medical Assistant (RMA) Certification Examination is offered by the American Medical Technologists (AMT), a nationally recognized and nonprofit certifying body for medical assistants who meet the eligibility requirements and who can prove their competency to perform entry level skills through written examination. The RMA (AMT) is awarded to candidates who pass the Certification Examination.

To be eligible, a medical assistant must:

1. Be a graduate of a medical assisting program accredited by the Accrediting Bureau of Health Education Schools (ABHES).
2. Be a graduate of a medical assistant program accredited by a regional accrediting commission.
3. Have formal medical services training in the United States Armed Forces.
4. Be a graduate of a medical assistant program accredited by a nationally recognized accrediting agency other than ABHES and have been employed as a medical assistant for a minimum of 1 year.
5. Have been employed as a medical assistant for a minimum of 5 years (not more than 2 of which may have been as an instructor in a postsecondary medical assisting program).

Testing is available throughout the year. The RMA offers examination administrations at one location in each state three times per year (March, June, and November), and it provides additional examination administrations at ABHES accredited school locations, when a sufficient number of candidates apply for the examination.

Examination results are usually available within 6 to 8 weeks following the administration. Each candidate will receive a letter and scores from the AMT office. Unsuccessful candidates are informed of specific areas of weakness to help in preparation for retesting. Membership in the AMT is not a requirement for RMA Examination eligibility.

See Appendix C for the RMA Application sample.

For additional information and application instructions, contact:

Registered Medical Assistants
710 Higgins Road
Park Ridge, IL 60068-5765
(708) 823-5169

RMA (AMT) Continuing Education*

A Professional Improvement Program Through Continuing Education

American Medical Technologists (AMT), in cooperation with the AMT Institute for Education (AMTIE), has developed a continuing education (CE) program and recording system: A Professional Improvement Program Through Continuing Education. The program will assist AMT registrants in maintaining an annual record of their participation in CE activities relating to their certification a job responsibility. A report indicating participation in CE activities attests to employers, third-party payers, regulators, and certifying agencies that AMT registrants consider education and evaluation as being essential to maintaining individual competency in the workplace. This mechanism will enable AMT registrants to grow and prosper as professionals in an ever-expanding and complex health care delivery system. The program allows the AMT registrant to gauge the quality, appropriateness, and utility of CE activity in maintaining ongoing professional/job-related competencies.

Essentials of the Program

1. An annual report is issued to each AMT registrant participant.
2. Categories of credit:
    1) Category I—All CE programs related to the registrant's initial certification and job responsibility. This includes programs that issue college credits.
    2) Category II—Professional growth and other CE programs not related to Category I.
3. All credits will be recorded in clock hours. In the case of college credits, 1 semester hour will be equivalent to 15 clock hours of credit. One quarter-hour of credit will be equivalent to 10 clock hours of credit.
4. A standard is assigned to each category of credit as determined by the AMT Board of Directors on recommendation of the AMT Education. Qualifications and Standards Committee for each allied health discipline AMT certifies. The standard is as follows for Category I credits:

MT/MLT	15 clock hours/year
RMA	15 clock hours/year
RDA	10 clock hours/year
RPT	5 clock hours/year

Please note: No standard is assigned to Category II credits earned. (See #6.)
5. AMT member participation is measured against the above standard. If the clock hours one earns match or exceed the set standard, the individual is in compliance with the program.

*Courtesy of American Medical Technologists, Park Ridge, Illinois.

6. While no standard is applied to Category II it is important that a record of participation in CE be maintained for all AMT registrants. The latter will indicate to the employer and third-party payers the AMT registrant's interest in a broad spectrum of education programs to enhance his or her certification and job-related competencies.

7. Only credits earned during the current calendar year will be accepted for credit in that year's report. **NO EXCEPTIONS.** (Calendar year is January 1 to December 31.)

8. A period of 30 days after the December 31 close of the calendar year will be allowed for submission of credit information for the past year. Credits received by AMTIE after the 30-day period will be returned to sender. **PLEASE NOTE:** Such credits cannot be applied to the new recording year.

9. All AMT registrants submitting programs for credit will be issued a report in March of credits recorded for the previous year.

10. Reminders for submitting credits will be printed in *AMT EVENTS.*

11. Exceeding the annual clock hour standard established for your category of certification enhances the individual's record.

AMT Registrants Meeting or Exceeding the Set Standard

1. The annual report can be duplicated and given to registrants' employer to be included in the individual's personnel file.

2. A certificate verifying compliance with the standard will be issued.

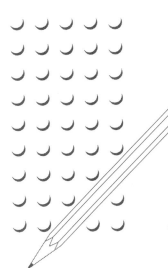

Sample Examination Simulation 1

- The following pages contain 300 test items.

- The examination is divided into:

  Part 1—General Medical Knowledge
  Part 2—Administrative Procedures
  Part 3—Clinical Procedures

- Answer sheets are provided for your use.

- The answer key immediately follows the test items and includes references with page numbers.

- References and suggested readings are at the end of the book.

Name _____ Date _____

Last   First   Middle

Directions for Marking Answers

- Use a black lead pencil (No. 2 or softer). Do NOT use pen or a pencil with hard lead.
- Make each mark heavy and black enough to completely obliterate the letter within the circle. Marks should fill the circles.
- Erase clearly any answer you wish to change.
- Make no stray marks on this answer sheet.
- Mark one and only one answer for each question. Multiple answers will be counted as wrong.

Example

WRONG Ⓐ ⊘ Ⓒ Ⓓ Ⓔ

WRONG Ⓐ ⊗ Ⓒ Ⓓ Ⓔ

WRONG Ⓐ Ⓑ ◎ Ⓓ Ⓔ

RIGHT Ⓐ Ⓑ Ⓒ ● Ⓔ

1 Ⓐ Ⓑ Ⓒ Ⓓ Ⓔ	26 Ⓐ Ⓑ Ⓒ Ⓓ Ⓔ	51 Ⓐ Ⓑ Ⓒ Ⓓ Ⓔ	76 Ⓐ Ⓑ Ⓒ Ⓓ Ⓔ
2 Ⓐ Ⓑ Ⓒ Ⓓ Ⓔ	27 Ⓐ Ⓑ Ⓒ Ⓓ Ⓔ	52 Ⓐ Ⓑ Ⓒ Ⓓ Ⓔ	77 Ⓐ Ⓑ Ⓒ Ⓓ Ⓔ
3 Ⓐ Ⓑ Ⓒ Ⓓ Ⓔ	28 Ⓐ Ⓑ Ⓒ Ⓓ Ⓔ	53 Ⓐ Ⓑ Ⓒ Ⓓ Ⓔ	78 Ⓐ Ⓑ Ⓒ Ⓓ Ⓔ
4 Ⓐ Ⓑ Ⓒ Ⓓ Ⓔ	29 Ⓐ Ⓑ Ⓒ Ⓓ Ⓔ	54 Ⓐ Ⓑ Ⓒ Ⓓ Ⓔ	79 Ⓐ Ⓑ Ⓒ Ⓓ Ⓔ
5 Ⓐ Ⓑ Ⓒ Ⓓ Ⓔ	30 Ⓐ Ⓑ Ⓒ Ⓓ Ⓔ	55 Ⓐ Ⓑ Ⓒ Ⓓ Ⓔ	80 Ⓐ Ⓑ Ⓒ Ⓓ Ⓔ
6 Ⓐ Ⓑ Ⓒ Ⓓ Ⓔ	31 Ⓐ Ⓑ Ⓒ Ⓓ Ⓔ	56 Ⓐ Ⓑ Ⓒ Ⓓ Ⓔ	81 Ⓐ Ⓑ Ⓒ Ⓓ Ⓔ
7 Ⓐ Ⓑ Ⓒ Ⓓ Ⓔ	32 Ⓐ Ⓑ Ⓒ Ⓓ Ⓔ	57 Ⓐ Ⓑ Ⓒ Ⓓ Ⓔ	82 Ⓐ Ⓑ Ⓒ Ⓓ Ⓔ
8 Ⓐ Ⓑ Ⓒ Ⓓ Ⓔ	33 Ⓐ Ⓑ Ⓒ Ⓓ Ⓔ	58 Ⓐ Ⓑ Ⓒ Ⓓ Ⓔ	83 Ⓐ Ⓑ Ⓒ Ⓓ Ⓔ
9 Ⓐ Ⓑ Ⓒ Ⓓ Ⓔ	34 Ⓐ Ⓑ Ⓒ Ⓓ Ⓔ	59 Ⓐ Ⓑ Ⓒ Ⓓ Ⓔ	84 Ⓐ Ⓑ Ⓒ Ⓓ Ⓔ
10 Ⓐ Ⓑ Ⓒ Ⓓ Ⓔ	35 Ⓐ Ⓑ Ⓒ Ⓓ Ⓔ	60 Ⓐ Ⓑ Ⓒ Ⓓ Ⓔ	85 Ⓐ Ⓑ Ⓒ Ⓓ Ⓔ
11 Ⓐ Ⓑ Ⓒ Ⓓ Ⓔ	36 Ⓐ Ⓑ Ⓒ Ⓓ Ⓔ	61 Ⓐ Ⓑ Ⓒ Ⓓ Ⓔ	86 Ⓐ Ⓑ Ⓒ Ⓓ Ⓔ
12 Ⓐ Ⓑ Ⓒ Ⓓ Ⓔ	37 Ⓐ Ⓑ Ⓒ Ⓓ Ⓔ	62 Ⓐ Ⓑ Ⓒ Ⓓ Ⓔ	87 Ⓐ Ⓑ Ⓒ Ⓓ Ⓔ
13 Ⓐ Ⓑ Ⓒ Ⓓ Ⓔ	38 Ⓐ Ⓑ Ⓒ Ⓓ Ⓔ	63 Ⓐ Ⓑ Ⓒ Ⓓ Ⓔ	88 Ⓐ Ⓑ Ⓒ Ⓓ Ⓔ
14 Ⓐ Ⓑ Ⓒ Ⓓ Ⓔ	39 Ⓐ Ⓑ Ⓒ Ⓓ Ⓔ	64 Ⓐ Ⓑ Ⓒ Ⓓ Ⓔ	89 Ⓐ Ⓑ Ⓒ Ⓓ Ⓔ
15 Ⓐ Ⓑ Ⓒ Ⓓ Ⓔ	40 Ⓐ Ⓑ Ⓒ Ⓓ Ⓔ	65 Ⓐ Ⓑ Ⓒ Ⓓ Ⓔ	90 Ⓐ Ⓑ Ⓒ Ⓓ Ⓔ
16 Ⓐ Ⓑ Ⓒ Ⓓ Ⓔ	41 Ⓐ Ⓑ Ⓒ Ⓓ Ⓔ	66 Ⓐ Ⓑ Ⓒ Ⓓ Ⓔ	91 Ⓐ Ⓑ Ⓒ Ⓓ Ⓔ
17 Ⓐ Ⓑ Ⓒ Ⓓ Ⓔ	42 Ⓐ Ⓑ Ⓒ Ⓓ Ⓔ	67 Ⓐ Ⓑ Ⓒ Ⓓ Ⓔ	92 Ⓐ Ⓑ Ⓒ Ⓓ Ⓔ
18 Ⓐ Ⓑ Ⓒ Ⓓ Ⓔ	43 Ⓐ Ⓑ Ⓒ Ⓓ Ⓔ	68 Ⓐ Ⓑ Ⓒ Ⓓ Ⓔ	93 Ⓐ Ⓑ Ⓒ Ⓓ Ⓔ
19 Ⓐ Ⓑ Ⓒ Ⓓ Ⓔ	44 Ⓐ Ⓑ Ⓒ Ⓓ Ⓔ	69 Ⓐ Ⓑ Ⓒ Ⓓ Ⓔ	94 Ⓐ Ⓑ Ⓒ Ⓓ Ⓔ
20 Ⓐ Ⓑ Ⓒ Ⓓ Ⓔ	45 Ⓐ Ⓑ Ⓒ Ⓓ Ⓔ	70 Ⓐ Ⓑ Ⓒ Ⓓ Ⓔ	95 Ⓐ Ⓑ Ⓒ Ⓓ Ⓔ
21 Ⓐ Ⓑ Ⓒ Ⓓ Ⓔ	46 Ⓐ Ⓑ Ⓒ Ⓓ Ⓔ	71 Ⓐ Ⓑ Ⓒ Ⓓ Ⓔ	96 Ⓐ Ⓑ Ⓒ Ⓓ Ⓔ
22 Ⓐ Ⓑ Ⓒ Ⓓ Ⓔ	47 Ⓐ Ⓑ Ⓒ Ⓓ Ⓔ	72 Ⓐ Ⓑ Ⓒ Ⓓ Ⓔ	97 Ⓐ Ⓑ Ⓒ Ⓓ Ⓔ
23 Ⓐ Ⓑ Ⓒ Ⓓ Ⓔ	48 Ⓐ Ⓑ Ⓒ Ⓓ Ⓔ	73 Ⓐ Ⓑ Ⓒ Ⓓ Ⓔ	98 Ⓐ Ⓑ Ⓒ Ⓓ Ⓔ
24 Ⓐ Ⓑ Ⓒ Ⓓ Ⓔ	49 Ⓐ Ⓑ Ⓒ Ⓓ Ⓔ	74 Ⓐ Ⓑ Ⓒ Ⓓ Ⓔ	99 Ⓐ Ⓑ Ⓒ Ⓓ Ⓔ
25 Ⓐ Ⓑ Ⓒ Ⓓ Ⓔ	50 Ⓐ Ⓑ Ⓒ Ⓓ Ⓔ	75 Ⓐ Ⓑ Ⓒ Ⓓ Ⓔ	100 Ⓐ Ⓑ Ⓒ Ⓓ Ⓔ

Directions for Marking Answers

- Use a black lead pencil (No. 2 or softer). Do NOT use pen or a pencil with hard lead.
- Make each mark heavy and black enough to completely obliterate the letter within the circle. Marks should fill the circles.
- Erase clearly any answer you wish to change.
- Make no stray marks on this answer sheet.
- Mark one and only one answer for each question. Multiple answers will be counted as wrong.

Example

WRONG Ⓐ Ⓑ Ⓒ Ⓓ Ⓔ
WRONG Ⓐ Ⓑ Ⓒ Ⓓ Ⓔ
WRONG Ⓐ Ⓑ Ⓒ Ⓓ Ⓔ
RIGHT Ⓐ Ⓑ Ⓒ ● Ⓔ

101 Ⓐ Ⓑ Ⓒ Ⓓ Ⓔ	126 Ⓐ Ⓑ Ⓒ Ⓓ Ⓔ	151 Ⓐ Ⓑ Ⓒ Ⓓ Ⓔ	176 Ⓐ Ⓑ Ⓒ Ⓓ Ⓔ
102 Ⓐ Ⓑ Ⓒ Ⓓ Ⓔ	127 Ⓐ Ⓑ Ⓒ Ⓓ Ⓔ	152 Ⓐ Ⓑ Ⓒ Ⓓ Ⓔ	177 Ⓐ Ⓑ Ⓒ Ⓓ Ⓔ
103 Ⓐ Ⓑ Ⓒ Ⓓ Ⓔ	128 Ⓐ Ⓑ Ⓒ Ⓓ Ⓔ	153 Ⓐ Ⓑ Ⓒ Ⓓ Ⓔ	178 Ⓐ Ⓑ Ⓒ Ⓓ Ⓔ
104 Ⓐ Ⓑ Ⓒ Ⓓ Ⓔ	129 Ⓐ Ⓑ Ⓒ Ⓓ Ⓔ	154 Ⓐ Ⓑ Ⓒ Ⓓ Ⓔ	179 Ⓐ Ⓑ Ⓒ Ⓓ Ⓔ
105 Ⓐ Ⓑ Ⓒ Ⓓ Ⓔ	130 Ⓐ Ⓑ Ⓒ Ⓓ Ⓔ	155 Ⓐ Ⓑ Ⓒ Ⓓ Ⓔ	180 Ⓐ Ⓑ Ⓒ Ⓓ Ⓔ
106 Ⓐ Ⓑ Ⓒ Ⓓ Ⓔ	131 Ⓐ Ⓑ Ⓒ Ⓓ Ⓔ	156 Ⓐ Ⓑ Ⓒ Ⓓ Ⓔ	181 Ⓐ Ⓑ Ⓒ Ⓓ Ⓔ
107 Ⓐ Ⓑ Ⓒ Ⓓ Ⓔ	132 Ⓐ Ⓑ Ⓒ Ⓓ Ⓔ	157 Ⓐ Ⓑ Ⓒ Ⓓ Ⓔ	182 Ⓐ Ⓑ Ⓒ Ⓓ Ⓔ
108 Ⓐ Ⓑ Ⓒ Ⓓ Ⓔ	133 Ⓐ Ⓑ Ⓒ Ⓓ Ⓔ	158 Ⓐ Ⓑ Ⓒ Ⓓ Ⓔ	183 Ⓐ Ⓑ Ⓒ Ⓓ Ⓔ
109 Ⓐ Ⓑ Ⓒ Ⓓ Ⓔ	134 Ⓐ Ⓑ Ⓒ Ⓓ Ⓔ	159 Ⓐ Ⓑ Ⓒ Ⓓ Ⓔ	184 Ⓐ Ⓑ Ⓒ Ⓓ Ⓔ
110 Ⓐ Ⓑ Ⓒ Ⓓ Ⓔ	135 Ⓐ Ⓑ Ⓒ Ⓓ Ⓔ	160 Ⓐ Ⓑ Ⓒ Ⓓ Ⓔ	185 Ⓐ Ⓑ Ⓒ Ⓓ Ⓔ
111 Ⓐ Ⓑ Ⓒ Ⓓ Ⓔ	136 Ⓐ Ⓑ Ⓒ Ⓓ Ⓔ	161 Ⓐ Ⓑ Ⓒ Ⓓ Ⓔ	186 Ⓐ Ⓑ Ⓒ Ⓓ Ⓔ
112 Ⓐ Ⓑ Ⓒ Ⓓ Ⓔ	137 Ⓐ Ⓑ Ⓒ Ⓓ Ⓔ	162 Ⓐ Ⓑ Ⓒ Ⓓ Ⓔ	187 Ⓐ Ⓑ Ⓒ Ⓓ Ⓔ
113 Ⓐ Ⓑ Ⓒ Ⓓ Ⓔ	138 Ⓐ Ⓑ Ⓒ Ⓓ Ⓔ	163 Ⓐ Ⓑ Ⓒ Ⓓ Ⓔ	188 Ⓐ Ⓑ Ⓒ Ⓓ Ⓔ
114 Ⓐ Ⓑ Ⓒ Ⓓ Ⓔ	139 Ⓐ Ⓑ Ⓒ Ⓓ Ⓔ	164 Ⓐ Ⓑ Ⓒ Ⓓ Ⓔ	189 Ⓐ Ⓑ Ⓒ Ⓓ Ⓔ
115 Ⓐ Ⓑ Ⓒ Ⓓ Ⓔ	140 Ⓐ Ⓑ Ⓒ Ⓓ Ⓔ	165 Ⓐ Ⓑ Ⓒ Ⓓ Ⓔ	190 Ⓐ Ⓑ Ⓒ Ⓓ Ⓔ
116 Ⓐ Ⓑ Ⓒ Ⓓ Ⓔ	141 Ⓐ Ⓑ Ⓒ Ⓓ Ⓔ	166 Ⓐ Ⓑ Ⓒ Ⓓ Ⓔ	191 Ⓐ Ⓑ Ⓒ Ⓓ Ⓔ
117 Ⓐ Ⓑ Ⓒ Ⓓ Ⓔ	142 Ⓐ Ⓑ Ⓒ Ⓓ Ⓔ	167 Ⓐ Ⓑ Ⓒ Ⓓ Ⓔ	192 Ⓐ Ⓑ Ⓒ Ⓓ Ⓔ
118 Ⓐ Ⓑ Ⓒ Ⓓ Ⓔ	143 Ⓐ Ⓑ Ⓒ Ⓓ Ⓔ	168 Ⓐ Ⓑ Ⓒ Ⓓ Ⓔ	193 Ⓐ Ⓑ Ⓒ Ⓓ Ⓔ
119 Ⓐ Ⓑ Ⓒ Ⓓ Ⓔ	144 Ⓐ Ⓑ Ⓒ Ⓓ Ⓔ	169 Ⓐ Ⓑ Ⓒ Ⓓ Ⓔ	194 Ⓐ Ⓑ Ⓒ Ⓓ Ⓔ
120 Ⓐ Ⓑ Ⓒ Ⓓ Ⓔ	145 Ⓐ Ⓑ Ⓒ Ⓓ Ⓔ	170 Ⓐ Ⓑ Ⓒ Ⓓ Ⓔ	195 Ⓐ Ⓑ Ⓒ Ⓓ Ⓔ
121 Ⓐ Ⓑ Ⓒ Ⓓ Ⓔ	146 Ⓐ Ⓑ Ⓒ Ⓓ Ⓔ	171 Ⓐ Ⓑ Ⓒ Ⓓ Ⓔ	196 Ⓐ Ⓑ Ⓒ Ⓓ Ⓔ
122 Ⓐ Ⓑ Ⓒ Ⓓ Ⓔ	147 Ⓐ Ⓑ Ⓒ Ⓓ Ⓔ	172 Ⓐ Ⓑ Ⓒ Ⓓ Ⓔ	197 Ⓐ Ⓑ Ⓒ Ⓓ Ⓔ
123 Ⓐ Ⓑ Ⓒ Ⓓ Ⓔ	148 Ⓐ Ⓑ Ⓒ Ⓓ Ⓔ	173 Ⓐ Ⓑ Ⓒ Ⓓ Ⓔ	198 Ⓐ Ⓑ Ⓒ Ⓓ Ⓔ
124 Ⓐ Ⓑ Ⓒ Ⓓ Ⓔ	149 Ⓐ Ⓑ Ⓒ Ⓓ Ⓔ	174 Ⓐ Ⓑ Ⓒ Ⓓ Ⓔ	199 Ⓐ Ⓑ Ⓒ Ⓓ Ⓔ
125 Ⓐ Ⓑ Ⓒ Ⓓ Ⓔ	150 Ⓐ Ⓑ Ⓒ Ⓓ Ⓔ	175 Ⓐ Ⓑ Ⓒ Ⓓ Ⓔ	200 Ⓐ Ⓑ Ⓒ Ⓓ Ⓔ

Name _____ **Date** _____
Last   First   Middle

Directions for Marking Answers

- Use a black lead pencil (No. 2 or softer). Do NOT use pen or a pencil with hard lead.
- Make each mark heavy and black enough to completely obliterate the letter within the circle. Marks should fill the circles.
- Erase clearly any answer you wish to change.
- Make no stray marks on this answer sheet.
- Mark one and only one answer for each question. Multiple answers will be counted as wrong.

Example

WRONG Ⓐ Ⓑ Ⓒ Ⓓ Ⓔ
WRONG Ⓐ Ⓧ Ⓒ Ⓓ Ⓔ
WRONG Ⓐ Ⓑ Ⓒ Ⓓ Ⓔ
RIGHT Ⓐ Ⓑ Ⓒ ● Ⓔ

201 Ⓐ Ⓑ Ⓒ Ⓓ Ⓔ   226 Ⓐ Ⓑ Ⓒ Ⓓ Ⓔ   251 Ⓐ Ⓑ Ⓒ Ⓓ Ⓔ   276 Ⓐ Ⓑ Ⓒ Ⓓ Ⓔ
202 Ⓐ Ⓑ Ⓒ Ⓓ Ⓔ   227 Ⓐ Ⓑ Ⓒ Ⓓ Ⓔ   252 Ⓐ Ⓑ Ⓒ Ⓓ Ⓔ   277 Ⓐ Ⓑ Ⓒ Ⓓ Ⓔ
203 Ⓐ Ⓑ Ⓒ Ⓓ Ⓔ   228 Ⓐ Ⓑ Ⓒ Ⓓ Ⓔ   253 Ⓐ Ⓑ Ⓒ Ⓓ Ⓔ   278 Ⓐ Ⓑ Ⓒ Ⓓ Ⓔ
204 Ⓐ Ⓑ Ⓒ Ⓓ Ⓔ   229 Ⓐ Ⓑ Ⓒ Ⓓ Ⓔ   254 Ⓐ Ⓑ Ⓒ Ⓓ Ⓔ   279 Ⓐ Ⓑ Ⓒ Ⓓ Ⓔ
205 Ⓐ Ⓑ Ⓒ Ⓓ Ⓔ   230 Ⓐ Ⓑ Ⓒ Ⓓ Ⓔ   255 Ⓐ Ⓑ Ⓒ Ⓓ Ⓔ   280 Ⓐ Ⓑ Ⓒ Ⓓ Ⓔ
206 Ⓐ Ⓑ Ⓒ Ⓓ Ⓔ   231 Ⓐ Ⓑ Ⓒ Ⓓ Ⓔ   256 Ⓐ Ⓑ Ⓒ Ⓓ Ⓔ   281 Ⓐ Ⓑ Ⓒ Ⓓ Ⓔ
207 Ⓐ Ⓑ Ⓒ Ⓓ Ⓔ   232 Ⓐ Ⓑ Ⓒ Ⓓ Ⓔ   257 Ⓐ Ⓑ Ⓒ Ⓓ Ⓔ   282 Ⓐ Ⓑ Ⓒ Ⓓ Ⓔ
208 Ⓐ Ⓑ Ⓒ Ⓓ Ⓔ   233 Ⓐ Ⓑ Ⓒ Ⓓ Ⓔ   258 Ⓐ Ⓑ Ⓒ Ⓓ Ⓔ   283 Ⓐ Ⓑ Ⓒ Ⓓ Ⓔ
209 Ⓐ Ⓑ Ⓒ Ⓓ Ⓔ   234 Ⓐ Ⓑ Ⓒ Ⓓ Ⓔ   259 Ⓐ Ⓑ Ⓒ Ⓓ Ⓔ   284 Ⓐ Ⓑ Ⓒ Ⓓ Ⓔ
210 Ⓐ Ⓑ Ⓒ Ⓓ Ⓔ   235 Ⓐ Ⓑ Ⓒ Ⓓ Ⓔ   260 Ⓐ Ⓑ Ⓒ Ⓓ Ⓔ   285 Ⓐ Ⓑ Ⓒ Ⓓ Ⓔ
211 Ⓐ Ⓑ Ⓒ Ⓓ Ⓔ   236 Ⓐ Ⓑ Ⓒ Ⓓ Ⓔ   261 Ⓐ Ⓑ Ⓒ Ⓓ Ⓔ   286 Ⓐ Ⓑ Ⓒ Ⓓ Ⓔ
212 Ⓐ Ⓑ Ⓒ Ⓓ Ⓔ   237 Ⓐ Ⓑ Ⓒ Ⓓ Ⓔ   262 Ⓐ Ⓑ Ⓒ Ⓓ Ⓔ   287 Ⓐ Ⓑ Ⓒ Ⓓ Ⓔ
213 Ⓐ Ⓑ Ⓒ Ⓓ Ⓔ   238 Ⓐ Ⓑ Ⓒ Ⓓ Ⓔ   263 Ⓐ Ⓑ Ⓒ Ⓓ Ⓔ   288 Ⓐ Ⓑ Ⓒ Ⓓ Ⓔ
214 Ⓐ Ⓑ Ⓒ Ⓓ Ⓔ   239 Ⓐ Ⓑ Ⓒ Ⓓ Ⓔ   264 Ⓐ Ⓑ Ⓒ Ⓓ Ⓔ   289 Ⓐ Ⓑ Ⓒ Ⓓ Ⓔ
215 Ⓐ Ⓑ Ⓒ Ⓓ Ⓔ   240 Ⓐ Ⓑ Ⓒ Ⓓ Ⓔ   265 Ⓐ Ⓑ Ⓒ Ⓓ Ⓔ   290 Ⓐ Ⓑ Ⓒ Ⓓ Ⓔ
216 Ⓐ Ⓑ Ⓒ Ⓓ Ⓔ   241 Ⓐ Ⓑ Ⓒ Ⓓ Ⓔ   266 Ⓐ Ⓑ Ⓒ Ⓓ Ⓔ   291 Ⓐ Ⓑ Ⓒ Ⓓ Ⓔ
217 Ⓐ Ⓑ Ⓒ Ⓓ Ⓔ   242 Ⓐ Ⓑ Ⓒ Ⓓ Ⓔ   267 Ⓐ Ⓑ Ⓒ Ⓓ Ⓔ   292 Ⓐ Ⓑ Ⓒ Ⓓ Ⓔ
218 Ⓐ Ⓑ Ⓒ Ⓓ Ⓔ   243 Ⓐ Ⓑ Ⓒ Ⓓ Ⓔ   268 Ⓐ Ⓑ Ⓒ Ⓓ Ⓔ   293 Ⓐ Ⓑ Ⓒ Ⓓ Ⓔ
219 Ⓐ Ⓑ Ⓒ Ⓓ Ⓔ   244 Ⓐ Ⓑ Ⓒ Ⓓ Ⓔ   269 Ⓐ Ⓑ Ⓒ Ⓓ Ⓔ   294 Ⓐ Ⓑ Ⓒ Ⓓ Ⓔ
220 Ⓐ Ⓑ Ⓒ Ⓓ Ⓔ   245 Ⓐ Ⓑ Ⓒ Ⓓ Ⓔ   270 Ⓐ Ⓑ Ⓒ Ⓓ Ⓔ   295 Ⓐ Ⓑ Ⓒ Ⓓ Ⓔ
221 Ⓐ Ⓑ Ⓒ Ⓓ Ⓔ   246 Ⓐ Ⓑ Ⓒ Ⓓ Ⓔ   271 Ⓐ Ⓑ Ⓒ Ⓓ Ⓔ   296 Ⓐ Ⓑ Ⓒ Ⓓ Ⓔ
222 Ⓐ Ⓑ Ⓒ Ⓓ Ⓔ   247 Ⓐ Ⓑ Ⓒ Ⓓ Ⓔ   272 Ⓐ Ⓑ Ⓒ Ⓓ Ⓔ   297 Ⓐ Ⓑ Ⓒ Ⓓ Ⓔ
223 Ⓐ Ⓑ Ⓒ Ⓓ Ⓔ   248 Ⓐ Ⓑ Ⓒ Ⓓ Ⓔ   273 Ⓐ Ⓑ Ⓒ Ⓓ Ⓔ   298 Ⓐ Ⓑ Ⓒ Ⓓ Ⓔ
224 Ⓐ Ⓑ Ⓒ Ⓓ Ⓔ   249 Ⓐ Ⓑ Ⓒ Ⓓ Ⓔ   274 Ⓐ Ⓑ Ⓒ Ⓓ Ⓔ   299 Ⓐ Ⓑ Ⓒ Ⓓ Ⓔ
225 Ⓐ Ⓑ Ⓒ Ⓓ Ⓔ   250 Ⓐ Ⓑ Ⓒ Ⓓ Ⓔ   275 Ⓐ Ⓑ Ⓒ Ⓓ Ⓔ   300 Ⓐ Ⓑ Ⓒ Ⓓ Ⓔ

Name _____ **Date** _____

Last   First   Middle

Directions for Marking Answers

- Use a black lead pencil (No. 2 or softer). Do NOT use pen or a pencil with hard lead.
- Make each mark heavy and black enough to completely obliterate the letter within the circle. Marks should fill the circles.
- Erase clearly any answer you wish to change.
- Make no stray marks on this answer sheet.
- Mark one and only one answer for each question. Multiple answers will be counted as wrong.

Example

WRONG   Ⓐ Ⓑ̸ Ⓒ Ⓓ Ⓔ

WRONG   Ⓐ Ⓑ̶ Ⓒ Ⓓ Ⓔ

WRONG   Ⓐ Ⓑ ⓒ⃝ Ⓓ Ⓔ

RIGHT   Ⓐ Ⓑ Ⓒ ● Ⓔ

1 Ⓐ Ⓑ Ⓒ Ⓓ Ⓔ	26 Ⓐ Ⓑ Ⓒ Ⓓ Ⓔ	51 Ⓐ Ⓑ Ⓒ Ⓓ Ⓔ	76 Ⓐ Ⓑ Ⓒ Ⓓ Ⓔ
2 Ⓐ Ⓑ Ⓒ Ⓓ Ⓔ	27 Ⓐ Ⓑ Ⓒ Ⓓ Ⓔ	52 Ⓐ Ⓑ Ⓒ Ⓓ Ⓔ	77 Ⓐ Ⓑ Ⓒ Ⓓ Ⓔ
3 Ⓐ Ⓑ Ⓒ Ⓓ Ⓔ	28 Ⓐ Ⓑ Ⓒ Ⓓ Ⓔ	53 Ⓐ Ⓑ Ⓒ Ⓓ Ⓔ	78 Ⓐ Ⓑ Ⓒ Ⓓ Ⓔ
4 Ⓐ Ⓑ Ⓒ Ⓓ Ⓔ	29 Ⓐ Ⓑ Ⓒ Ⓓ Ⓔ	54 Ⓐ Ⓑ Ⓒ Ⓓ Ⓔ	79 Ⓐ Ⓑ Ⓒ Ⓓ Ⓔ
5 Ⓐ Ⓑ Ⓒ Ⓓ Ⓔ	30 Ⓐ Ⓑ Ⓒ Ⓓ Ⓔ	55 Ⓐ Ⓑ Ⓒ Ⓓ Ⓔ	80 Ⓐ Ⓑ Ⓒ Ⓓ Ⓔ
6 Ⓐ Ⓑ Ⓒ Ⓓ Ⓔ	31 Ⓐ Ⓑ Ⓒ Ⓓ Ⓔ	56 Ⓐ Ⓑ Ⓒ Ⓓ Ⓔ	81 Ⓐ Ⓑ Ⓒ Ⓓ Ⓔ
7 Ⓐ Ⓑ Ⓒ Ⓓ Ⓔ	32 Ⓐ Ⓑ Ⓒ Ⓓ Ⓔ	57 Ⓐ Ⓑ Ⓒ Ⓓ Ⓔ	82 Ⓐ Ⓑ Ⓒ Ⓓ Ⓔ
8 Ⓐ Ⓑ Ⓒ Ⓓ Ⓔ	33 Ⓐ Ⓑ Ⓒ Ⓓ Ⓔ	58 Ⓐ Ⓑ Ⓒ Ⓓ Ⓔ	83 Ⓐ Ⓑ Ⓒ Ⓓ Ⓔ
9 Ⓐ Ⓑ Ⓒ Ⓓ Ⓔ	34 Ⓐ Ⓑ Ⓒ Ⓓ Ⓔ	59 Ⓐ Ⓑ Ⓒ Ⓓ Ⓔ	84 Ⓐ Ⓑ Ⓒ Ⓓ Ⓔ
10 Ⓐ Ⓑ Ⓒ Ⓓ Ⓔ	35 Ⓐ Ⓑ Ⓒ Ⓓ Ⓔ	60 Ⓐ Ⓑ Ⓒ Ⓓ Ⓔ	85 Ⓐ Ⓑ Ⓒ Ⓓ Ⓔ
11 Ⓐ Ⓑ Ⓒ Ⓓ Ⓔ	36 Ⓐ Ⓑ Ⓒ Ⓓ Ⓔ	61 Ⓐ Ⓑ Ⓒ Ⓓ Ⓔ	86 Ⓐ Ⓑ Ⓒ Ⓓ Ⓔ
12 Ⓐ Ⓑ Ⓒ Ⓓ Ⓔ	37 Ⓐ Ⓑ Ⓒ Ⓓ Ⓔ	62 Ⓐ Ⓑ Ⓒ Ⓓ Ⓔ	87 Ⓐ Ⓑ Ⓒ Ⓓ Ⓔ
13 Ⓐ Ⓑ Ⓒ Ⓓ Ⓔ	38 Ⓐ Ⓑ Ⓒ Ⓓ Ⓔ	63 Ⓐ Ⓑ Ⓒ Ⓓ Ⓔ	88 Ⓐ Ⓑ Ⓒ Ⓓ Ⓔ
14 Ⓐ Ⓑ Ⓒ Ⓓ Ⓔ	39 Ⓐ Ⓑ Ⓒ Ⓓ Ⓔ	64 Ⓐ Ⓑ Ⓒ Ⓓ Ⓔ	89 Ⓐ Ⓑ Ⓒ Ⓓ Ⓔ
15 Ⓐ Ⓑ Ⓒ Ⓓ Ⓔ	40 Ⓐ Ⓑ Ⓒ Ⓓ Ⓔ	65 Ⓐ Ⓑ Ⓒ Ⓓ Ⓔ	90 Ⓐ Ⓑ Ⓒ Ⓓ Ⓔ
16 Ⓐ Ⓑ Ⓒ Ⓓ Ⓔ	41 Ⓐ Ⓑ Ⓒ Ⓓ Ⓔ	66 Ⓐ Ⓑ Ⓒ Ⓓ Ⓔ	91 Ⓐ Ⓑ Ⓒ Ⓓ Ⓔ
17 Ⓐ Ⓑ Ⓒ Ⓓ Ⓔ	42 Ⓐ Ⓑ Ⓒ Ⓓ Ⓔ	67 Ⓐ Ⓑ Ⓒ Ⓓ Ⓔ	92 Ⓐ Ⓑ Ⓒ Ⓓ Ⓔ
18 Ⓐ Ⓑ Ⓒ Ⓓ Ⓔ	43 Ⓐ Ⓑ Ⓒ Ⓓ Ⓔ	68 Ⓐ Ⓑ Ⓒ Ⓓ Ⓔ	93 Ⓐ Ⓑ Ⓒ Ⓓ Ⓔ
19 Ⓐ Ⓑ Ⓒ Ⓓ Ⓔ	44 Ⓐ Ⓑ Ⓒ Ⓓ Ⓔ	69 Ⓐ Ⓑ Ⓒ Ⓓ Ⓔ	94 Ⓐ Ⓑ Ⓒ Ⓓ Ⓔ
20 Ⓐ Ⓑ Ⓒ Ⓓ Ⓔ	45 Ⓐ Ⓑ Ⓒ Ⓓ Ⓔ	70 Ⓐ Ⓑ Ⓒ Ⓓ Ⓔ	95 Ⓐ Ⓑ Ⓒ Ⓓ Ⓔ
21 Ⓐ Ⓑ Ⓒ Ⓓ Ⓔ	46 Ⓐ Ⓑ Ⓒ Ⓓ Ⓔ	71 Ⓐ Ⓑ Ⓒ Ⓓ Ⓔ	96 Ⓐ Ⓑ Ⓒ Ⓓ Ⓔ
22 Ⓐ Ⓑ Ⓒ Ⓓ Ⓔ	47 Ⓐ Ⓑ Ⓒ Ⓓ Ⓔ	72 Ⓐ Ⓑ Ⓒ Ⓓ Ⓔ	97 Ⓐ Ⓑ Ⓒ Ⓓ Ⓔ
23 Ⓐ Ⓑ Ⓒ Ⓓ Ⓔ	48 Ⓐ Ⓑ Ⓒ Ⓓ Ⓔ	73 Ⓐ Ⓑ Ⓒ Ⓓ Ⓔ	98 Ⓐ Ⓑ Ⓒ Ⓓ Ⓔ
24 Ⓐ Ⓑ Ⓒ Ⓓ Ⓔ	49 Ⓐ Ⓑ Ⓒ Ⓓ Ⓔ	74 Ⓐ Ⓑ Ⓒ Ⓓ Ⓔ	99 Ⓐ Ⓑ Ⓒ Ⓓ Ⓔ
25 Ⓐ Ⓑ Ⓒ Ⓓ Ⓔ	50 Ⓐ Ⓑ Ⓒ Ⓓ Ⓔ	75 Ⓐ Ⓑ Ⓒ Ⓓ Ⓔ	100 Ⓐ Ⓑ Ⓒ Ⓓ Ⓔ

Name _____ **Date** _____

| Last | First | Middle |

101 Ⓐ Ⓑ Ⓒ Ⓓ Ⓔ   126 Ⓐ Ⓑ Ⓒ Ⓓ Ⓔ   151 Ⓐ Ⓑ Ⓒ Ⓓ Ⓔ   176 Ⓐ Ⓑ Ⓒ Ⓓ Ⓔ

102 Ⓐ Ⓑ Ⓒ Ⓓ Ⓔ   127 Ⓐ Ⓑ Ⓒ Ⓓ Ⓔ   152 Ⓐ Ⓑ Ⓒ Ⓓ Ⓔ   177 Ⓐ Ⓑ Ⓒ Ⓓ Ⓔ

103 Ⓐ Ⓑ Ⓒ Ⓓ Ⓔ   128 Ⓐ Ⓑ Ⓒ Ⓓ Ⓔ   153 Ⓐ Ⓑ Ⓒ Ⓓ Ⓔ   178 Ⓐ Ⓑ Ⓒ Ⓓ Ⓔ

104 Ⓐ Ⓑ Ⓒ Ⓓ Ⓔ   129 Ⓐ Ⓑ Ⓒ Ⓓ Ⓔ   154 Ⓐ Ⓑ Ⓒ Ⓓ Ⓔ   179 Ⓐ Ⓑ Ⓒ Ⓓ Ⓔ

105 Ⓐ Ⓑ Ⓒ Ⓓ Ⓔ   130 Ⓐ Ⓑ Ⓒ Ⓓ Ⓔ   155 Ⓐ Ⓑ Ⓒ Ⓓ Ⓔ   180 Ⓐ Ⓑ Ⓒ Ⓓ Ⓔ

106 Ⓐ Ⓑ Ⓒ Ⓓ Ⓔ   131 Ⓐ Ⓑ Ⓒ Ⓓ Ⓔ   156 Ⓐ Ⓑ Ⓒ Ⓓ Ⓔ   181 Ⓐ Ⓑ Ⓒ Ⓓ Ⓔ

107 Ⓐ Ⓑ Ⓒ Ⓓ Ⓔ   132 Ⓐ Ⓑ Ⓒ Ⓓ Ⓔ   157 Ⓐ Ⓑ Ⓒ Ⓓ Ⓔ   182 Ⓐ Ⓑ Ⓒ Ⓓ Ⓔ

108 Ⓐ Ⓑ Ⓒ Ⓓ Ⓔ   133 Ⓐ Ⓑ Ⓒ Ⓓ Ⓔ   158 Ⓐ Ⓑ Ⓒ Ⓓ Ⓔ   183 Ⓐ Ⓑ Ⓒ Ⓓ Ⓔ

109 Ⓐ Ⓑ Ⓒ Ⓓ Ⓔ   134 Ⓐ Ⓑ Ⓒ Ⓓ Ⓔ   159 Ⓐ Ⓑ Ⓒ Ⓓ Ⓔ   184 Ⓐ Ⓑ Ⓒ Ⓓ Ⓔ

110 Ⓐ Ⓑ Ⓒ Ⓓ Ⓔ   135 Ⓐ Ⓑ Ⓒ Ⓓ Ⓔ   160 Ⓐ Ⓑ Ⓒ Ⓓ Ⓔ   185 Ⓐ Ⓑ Ⓒ Ⓓ Ⓔ

111 Ⓐ Ⓑ Ⓒ Ⓓ Ⓔ   136 Ⓐ Ⓑ Ⓒ Ⓓ Ⓔ   161 Ⓐ Ⓑ Ⓒ Ⓓ Ⓔ   186 Ⓐ Ⓑ Ⓒ Ⓓ Ⓔ

112 Ⓐ Ⓑ Ⓒ Ⓓ Ⓔ   137 Ⓐ Ⓑ Ⓒ Ⓓ Ⓔ   162 Ⓐ Ⓑ Ⓒ Ⓓ Ⓔ   187 Ⓐ Ⓑ Ⓒ Ⓓ Ⓔ

113 Ⓐ Ⓑ Ⓒ Ⓓ Ⓔ   138 Ⓐ Ⓑ Ⓒ Ⓓ Ⓔ   163 Ⓐ Ⓑ Ⓒ Ⓓ Ⓔ   188 Ⓐ Ⓑ Ⓒ Ⓓ Ⓔ

114 Ⓐ Ⓑ Ⓒ Ⓓ Ⓔ   139 Ⓐ Ⓑ Ⓒ Ⓓ Ⓔ   164 Ⓐ Ⓑ Ⓒ Ⓓ Ⓔ   189 Ⓐ Ⓑ Ⓒ Ⓓ Ⓔ

115 Ⓐ Ⓑ Ⓒ Ⓓ Ⓔ   140 Ⓐ Ⓑ Ⓒ Ⓓ Ⓔ   165 Ⓐ Ⓑ Ⓒ Ⓓ Ⓔ   190 Ⓐ Ⓑ Ⓒ Ⓓ Ⓔ

116 Ⓐ Ⓑ Ⓒ Ⓓ Ⓔ   141 Ⓐ Ⓑ Ⓒ Ⓓ Ⓔ   166 Ⓐ Ⓑ Ⓒ Ⓓ Ⓔ   191 Ⓐ Ⓑ Ⓒ Ⓓ Ⓔ

117 Ⓐ Ⓑ Ⓒ Ⓓ Ⓔ   142 Ⓐ Ⓑ Ⓒ Ⓓ Ⓔ   167 Ⓐ Ⓑ Ⓒ Ⓓ Ⓔ   192 Ⓐ Ⓑ Ⓒ Ⓓ Ⓔ

118 Ⓐ Ⓑ Ⓒ Ⓓ Ⓔ   143 Ⓐ Ⓑ Ⓒ Ⓓ Ⓔ   168 Ⓐ Ⓑ Ⓒ Ⓓ Ⓔ   193 Ⓐ Ⓑ Ⓒ Ⓓ Ⓔ

119 Ⓐ Ⓑ Ⓒ Ⓓ Ⓔ   144 Ⓐ Ⓑ Ⓒ Ⓓ Ⓔ   169 Ⓐ Ⓑ Ⓒ Ⓓ Ⓔ   194 Ⓐ Ⓑ Ⓒ Ⓓ Ⓔ

120 Ⓐ Ⓑ Ⓒ Ⓓ Ⓔ   145 Ⓐ Ⓑ Ⓒ Ⓓ Ⓔ   170 Ⓐ Ⓑ Ⓒ Ⓓ Ⓔ   195 Ⓐ Ⓑ Ⓒ Ⓓ Ⓔ

121 Ⓐ Ⓑ Ⓒ Ⓓ Ⓔ   146 Ⓐ Ⓑ Ⓒ Ⓓ Ⓔ   171 Ⓐ Ⓑ Ⓒ Ⓓ Ⓔ   196 Ⓐ Ⓑ Ⓒ Ⓓ Ⓔ

122 Ⓐ Ⓑ Ⓒ Ⓓ Ⓔ   147 Ⓐ Ⓑ Ⓒ Ⓓ Ⓔ   172 Ⓐ Ⓑ Ⓒ Ⓓ Ⓔ   197 Ⓐ Ⓑ Ⓒ Ⓓ Ⓔ

123 Ⓐ Ⓑ Ⓒ Ⓓ Ⓔ   148 Ⓐ Ⓑ Ⓒ Ⓓ Ⓔ   173 Ⓐ Ⓑ Ⓒ Ⓓ Ⓔ   198 Ⓐ Ⓑ Ⓒ Ⓓ Ⓔ

124 Ⓐ Ⓑ Ⓒ Ⓓ Ⓔ   149 Ⓐ Ⓑ Ⓒ Ⓓ Ⓔ   174 Ⓐ Ⓑ Ⓒ Ⓓ Ⓔ   199 Ⓐ Ⓑ Ⓒ Ⓓ Ⓔ

125 Ⓐ Ⓑ Ⓒ Ⓓ Ⓔ   150 Ⓐ Ⓑ Ⓒ Ⓓ Ⓔ   175 Ⓐ Ⓑ Ⓒ Ⓓ Ⓔ   200 Ⓐ Ⓑ Ⓒ Ⓓ Ⓔ

201 Ⓐ Ⓑ Ⓒ Ⓓ Ⓔ	226 Ⓐ Ⓑ Ⓒ Ⓓ Ⓔ	251 Ⓐ Ⓑ Ⓒ Ⓓ Ⓔ	276 Ⓐ Ⓑ Ⓒ Ⓓ Ⓔ
202 Ⓐ Ⓑ Ⓒ Ⓓ Ⓔ	227 Ⓐ Ⓑ Ⓒ Ⓓ Ⓔ	252 Ⓐ Ⓑ Ⓒ Ⓓ Ⓔ	277 Ⓐ Ⓑ Ⓒ Ⓓ Ⓔ
203 Ⓐ Ⓑ Ⓒ Ⓓ Ⓔ	228 Ⓐ Ⓑ Ⓒ Ⓓ Ⓔ	253 Ⓐ Ⓑ Ⓒ Ⓓ Ⓔ	278 Ⓐ Ⓑ Ⓒ Ⓓ Ⓔ
204 Ⓐ Ⓑ Ⓒ Ⓓ Ⓔ	229 Ⓐ Ⓑ Ⓒ Ⓓ Ⓔ	254 Ⓐ Ⓑ Ⓒ Ⓓ Ⓔ	279 Ⓐ Ⓑ Ⓒ Ⓓ Ⓔ
205 Ⓐ Ⓑ Ⓒ Ⓓ Ⓔ	230 Ⓐ Ⓑ Ⓒ Ⓓ Ⓔ	255 Ⓐ Ⓑ Ⓒ Ⓓ Ⓔ	280 Ⓐ Ⓑ Ⓒ Ⓓ Ⓔ
206 Ⓐ Ⓑ Ⓒ Ⓓ Ⓔ	231 Ⓐ Ⓑ Ⓒ Ⓓ Ⓔ	256 Ⓐ Ⓑ Ⓒ Ⓓ Ⓔ	281 Ⓐ Ⓑ Ⓒ Ⓓ Ⓔ
207 Ⓐ Ⓑ Ⓒ Ⓓ Ⓔ	232 Ⓐ Ⓑ Ⓒ Ⓓ Ⓔ	257 Ⓐ Ⓑ Ⓒ Ⓓ Ⓔ	282 Ⓐ Ⓑ Ⓒ Ⓓ Ⓔ
208 Ⓐ Ⓑ Ⓒ Ⓓ Ⓔ	233 Ⓐ Ⓑ Ⓒ Ⓓ Ⓔ	258 Ⓐ Ⓑ Ⓒ Ⓓ Ⓔ	283 Ⓐ Ⓑ Ⓒ Ⓓ Ⓔ
209 Ⓐ Ⓑ Ⓒ Ⓓ Ⓔ	234 Ⓐ Ⓑ Ⓒ Ⓓ Ⓔ	259 Ⓐ Ⓑ Ⓒ Ⓓ Ⓔ	284 Ⓐ Ⓑ Ⓒ Ⓓ Ⓔ
210 Ⓐ Ⓑ Ⓒ Ⓓ Ⓔ	235 Ⓐ Ⓑ Ⓒ Ⓓ Ⓔ	260 Ⓐ Ⓑ Ⓒ Ⓓ Ⓔ	285 Ⓐ Ⓑ Ⓒ Ⓓ Ⓔ
211 Ⓐ Ⓑ Ⓒ Ⓓ Ⓔ	236 Ⓐ Ⓑ Ⓒ Ⓓ Ⓔ	261 Ⓐ Ⓑ Ⓒ Ⓓ Ⓔ	286 Ⓐ Ⓑ Ⓒ Ⓓ Ⓔ
212 Ⓐ Ⓑ Ⓒ Ⓓ Ⓔ	237 Ⓐ Ⓑ Ⓒ Ⓓ Ⓔ	262 Ⓐ Ⓑ Ⓒ Ⓓ Ⓔ	287 Ⓐ Ⓑ Ⓒ Ⓓ Ⓔ
213 Ⓐ Ⓑ Ⓒ Ⓓ Ⓔ	238 Ⓐ Ⓑ Ⓒ Ⓓ Ⓔ	263 Ⓐ Ⓑ Ⓒ Ⓓ Ⓔ	288 Ⓐ Ⓑ Ⓒ Ⓓ Ⓔ
214 Ⓐ Ⓑ Ⓒ Ⓓ Ⓔ	239 Ⓐ Ⓑ Ⓒ Ⓓ Ⓔ	264 Ⓐ Ⓑ Ⓒ Ⓓ Ⓔ	289 Ⓐ Ⓑ Ⓒ Ⓓ Ⓔ
215 Ⓐ Ⓑ Ⓒ Ⓓ Ⓔ	240 Ⓐ Ⓑ Ⓒ Ⓓ Ⓔ	265 Ⓐ Ⓑ Ⓒ Ⓓ Ⓔ	290 Ⓐ Ⓑ Ⓒ Ⓓ Ⓔ
216 Ⓐ Ⓑ Ⓒ Ⓓ Ⓔ	241 Ⓐ Ⓑ Ⓒ Ⓓ Ⓔ	266 Ⓐ Ⓑ Ⓒ Ⓓ Ⓔ	291 Ⓐ Ⓑ Ⓒ Ⓓ Ⓔ
217 Ⓐ Ⓑ Ⓒ Ⓓ Ⓔ	242 Ⓐ Ⓑ Ⓒ Ⓓ Ⓔ	267 Ⓐ Ⓑ Ⓒ Ⓓ Ⓔ	292 Ⓐ Ⓑ Ⓒ Ⓓ Ⓔ
218 Ⓐ Ⓑ Ⓒ Ⓓ Ⓔ	243 Ⓐ Ⓑ Ⓒ Ⓓ Ⓔ	268 Ⓐ Ⓑ Ⓒ Ⓓ Ⓔ	293 Ⓐ Ⓑ Ⓒ Ⓓ Ⓔ
219 Ⓐ Ⓑ Ⓒ Ⓓ Ⓔ	244 Ⓐ Ⓑ Ⓒ Ⓓ Ⓔ	269 Ⓐ Ⓑ Ⓒ Ⓓ Ⓔ	294 Ⓐ Ⓑ Ⓒ Ⓓ Ⓔ
220 Ⓐ Ⓑ Ⓒ Ⓓ Ⓔ	245 Ⓐ Ⓑ Ⓒ Ⓓ Ⓔ	270 Ⓐ Ⓑ Ⓒ Ⓓ Ⓔ	295 Ⓐ Ⓑ Ⓒ Ⓓ Ⓔ
221 Ⓐ Ⓑ Ⓒ Ⓓ Ⓔ	246 Ⓐ Ⓑ Ⓒ Ⓓ Ⓔ	271 Ⓐ Ⓑ Ⓒ Ⓓ Ⓔ	296 Ⓐ Ⓑ Ⓒ Ⓓ Ⓔ
222 Ⓐ Ⓑ Ⓒ Ⓓ Ⓔ	247 Ⓐ Ⓑ Ⓒ Ⓓ Ⓔ	272 Ⓐ Ⓑ Ⓒ Ⓓ Ⓔ	297 Ⓐ Ⓑ Ⓒ Ⓓ Ⓔ
223 Ⓐ Ⓑ Ⓒ Ⓓ Ⓔ	248 Ⓐ Ⓑ Ⓒ Ⓓ Ⓔ	273 Ⓐ Ⓑ Ⓒ Ⓓ Ⓔ	298 Ⓐ Ⓑ Ⓒ Ⓓ Ⓔ
224 Ⓐ Ⓑ Ⓒ Ⓓ Ⓔ	249 Ⓐ Ⓑ Ⓒ Ⓓ Ⓔ	274 Ⓐ Ⓑ Ⓒ Ⓓ Ⓔ	299 Ⓐ Ⓑ Ⓒ Ⓓ Ⓔ
225 Ⓐ Ⓑ Ⓒ Ⓓ Ⓔ	250 Ⓐ Ⓑ Ⓒ Ⓓ Ⓔ	275 Ⓐ Ⓑ Ⓒ Ⓓ Ⓔ	300 Ⓐ Ⓑ Ⓒ Ⓓ Ⓔ

SIMULATION TEST 1

Part 1—General Medical Knowledge

Directions: *Each of the following questions or incomplete statements precedes five suggested answers or completions. Select the ONE answer or completion that is BEST in each case, and fill in the circle containing the corresponding letter on the answer sheet.*

1. With which of the following conditions do we associate shivering and chills?
   A. pyrexia
   B. hypothermia
   C. both A and B
   D. diaphoresis
   E. both A and D

2. A nonspecific test for the heterophile antibody present in patients with infectious mononucleosis is
   A. monocyte count
   B. differential leukocyte count
   C. erythrocyte sedimentation rate
   D. latex fixation
   E. Monospot

3. In which structure is urine formation considered complete?
   A. proximal tubule
   B. loop of Henle
   C. collecting tubule
   D. ureter
   E. bladder

4. In male sterilization, the structure that is dissected and excised is the
   A. seminiferous tubule
   B. duct of the epididymis
   C. ejaculatory duct
   D. vas deferens
   E. urethra

5. Intracellular and extracellular fluids contain electrolytes that
   A. conduct electrical currents
   B. are decomposed by the passage of an electrical current
   C. both A and B
   D. oxidize carbohydrates into CO_2 and H_2O
   E. both A and D

6. Disposable airway equipment reduces the risk of disease transmission through saliva. Which of the following organisms is linked to transmission in saliva?
   A. HIV virus
   B. herpes simplex virus
   C. hepatitis B virus
   D. *Neisseria gonorrhoeae*
   E. hepatitis A virus

7. Compared with adults, children have which of the following?
   A. lesser distribution of interstitial fluid
   B. greater distribution of dry weight
   C. lesser distribution of intracellular fluid
   D. a slower metabolism
   E. faster rates of pulse and respiration

8. During the menstrual cycle, the growth of the endometrium is in direct response to
   A. follicle-stimulating hormone
   B. luteinizing hormone
   C. estrogen
   D. progesterone
   E. human chorionic gonadotropin

9. Which of the following infections is a bacterial infection?
   A. herpes simplex
   B. condyloma acuminatum
   C. candida infections
   D. *Trichomonas vaginalis*
   E. *Haemophilus* vaginitis

10. There is a correlation between the risk of developing cervical cancer and
    A. the number of male sexual partners
    B. the age of menarche
    C. both A and B
    D. prior infection by human papilloma virus (HPV)
    E. both A and D

11. The most frequently reported sexually transmitted disease in the United States is
    A. gonorrhea
    B. syphilis
    C. trichomoniasis
    D. chlamydia infections
    E. acquired immunodeficiency syndrome

12. Diseases once again on the rise and considered "not now eradicable" include
    A. poliomyelitis
    B. smallpox
    C. both A and B
    D. tuberculosis
    E. both A and D

13. The last product to be produced in the coagulation sequence is
    A. prothrombin
    B. thrombin
    C. calcium
    D. fibrin
    E. fibrinogen

14. Sites of an ectopic pregnancy include the
    A. fallopian tubes
    B. cervical os
    C. both A and B
    D. abdominal cavity
    E. both A and D

15. In which of the following conditions is the concentration of cholesterol in the blood below normal?
    A. untreated diabetes mellitus
    B. bile duct obstruction
    C. both A and B
    D. hyperthyroidism
    E. both A and D

16. Which of the following information does the hematocrit provide?
    A. red blood cell volume available to transport oxygen
    B. approximate size of an average red blood cell
    C. amount of hemoglobin in an average red blood cell
    D. number of circulating red blood cells
    E. concentration of hemoglobin per unit volume of red blood cells

17. Renal calculi are most often associated with
    A. hypocalcemia
    B. hypercalcemia
    C. hypernatremia
    D. hyponatremia
    E. hyperkalemia

18. The universal donor blood type is
    A. A negative
    B. A positive
    C. AB positive
    D. O negative
    E. O positive

19. A fibrous, structural protein in the connective tissue that includes skin, bone, ligaments, and cartilage is
    A. albumin
    B. collagen
    C. fibrin
    D. fibrinogen
    E. immunoglobulin

20. The macroscopic structure that carries urine to the bladder is the
    A. urethra
    B. ureter
    C. renal tubule
    D. nephron
    E. glomerulus

21. Yellow-brown urine caused by diminished liver function usually contains
    A. hemoglobin
    B. red blood cells
    C. white blood cells
    D. bilirubin
    E. phenylketones

22. Bilirubin is changed to urobilinogen when
    A. red blood cells lyse and release hemoglobin
    B. bilirubin attaches to albumen in the blood
    C. free bilirubin enters the liver
    D. bilirubin is absorbed by the kidneys
    E. bilirubin enters and is excreted through the intestines ✓

23. Plantar warts or verrucae are caused by
    A. several fungal species
    B. handling certain reptiles
    C. papilloma viruses ✓
    D. poor hygiene
    E. pressure or friction from ill-fitting shoes

24. Insulin regulates blood glucose by
    A. breaking down carbohydrates in the liver
    B. enabling glucose transportation from the blood to the cells
    C. enabling glucose transportation from the cells to the blood
    D. raising the concentration of blood sugar
    E. enabling glucose absorption through the intestines ✓

25. Pediculosis is a skin infestation by
    A. redbugs
    B. fleas
    C. lice ✓
    D. itch mites
    E. ticks

26. The liquid portion of coagulated blood is termed
    A. whole blood
    B. serum ✓
    C. plasma
    D. buffy coat
    E. complement

27. Language in the Durable Power of Attorney for Health Care document
    A. contains instruction regarding use of life-sustaining procedures
    B. permits deliberate acts or omission to end life
    C. prohibits another person to make decisions in terminal conditions ✓
    D. states it is not in effect if the patient is able to make medical decisions
    E. designates which physician(s) can make decisions in terminal illnesses

28. Under federal regulations, all states are required to regulate
    A. the performance of venipuncture
    B. laboratory testing ✓
    C. physical therapy
    D. radiography
    E. the administration of injections

29. According to federal wage and hour regulations, employees must receive overtime pay for
    A. holidays
    B. a 45-hour week ✓
    C. a 9-hour day
    D. a 6-day week
    E. evenings and weekends

30. Certain procedures cannot be performed by medical assistants in all 50 states. These procedures include
    A. piercing human tissue with needles
    B. erythrocyte sedimentation rate estimations
    C. both A and B
    D. exposing patients to ionizing radiation
    E. both A and D ✓

31. In which situation does an employer have the right to access an employee's medical record?
    A. pre-employment examination, paid for by the employer ✓
    B. a company that is self-insured
    C. alcohol or drug abuse testing
    D. pre-employment investigation regarding disability history
    E. employee request for alcohol or drug treatment

32. Under federal regulations, DEA licenses must be renewed
    A. when a physician receives prescribing privileges at a new hospital
    B. every year ✓
    C. both A and B
    D. when a new practice is opened or a medical facility moves ✓
    E. both A and D

33. The medical assistant notes that it is 1.5 months before the posted DEA certificate expires. The medical assistant knows that
    A. the renewal application is due any day
    B. the renewal application will arrive on the expiration date
    C. there is a 45-day grace period after the expiration date to renew
    D. there is a 60-day grace period after the expiration date to renew
    ✓E. it is the responsibility of the physician to notify the DEA that the renewal application has not arrived

34. In informed consent, the medical assistant's signature as witness signifies that the medical assistant
    A. prepared the consent forms
    Ⓑ verified the signature of the patient
    C. verified the signature of the physician
    ✓D. participated in the discussion with the patient and the physician
    E. explained the medical treatment to the patient

35. A patient requesting access to his or her medical record is entitled under federal regulations to receive medical information
    A. if the physician deems it necessary
    ✓B. after paying a fee to have the record duplicated
    C. with a court order
    D. using an appointed attorney as an intermediary
    Ⓔ within a specified time on demand

36. A medical facility employee who can work under the supervision of the physician or can function alone is
    A. licensed practical nurse
    B. medical assistant
    C. medical laboratory technician
    ✓D. nurse practitioner
    E. certified or registered medical assistant

37. An established patient wishes to pay for the medical expenses of an adult sister. To be binding, this arrangement must be
    A. typed on the patient's ledger card
    B. entered on the patient's medical record
    C. approved by the physician's signature
    D. typed on a separate ledger card with the third party's name and address on it
    ✓E. typed on a separate form with the third party's signature

38. Which of the following omissions could result in patient charges of abandonment?
    ✓A. failing to return a telephone call within a reasonable time
    B. use of a nonsterile instrument during a dressing change
    C. mistakenly sending a patient account to a collection agency
    D. treating a patient via the telephone
    E. leaving a patient chart open for another patient to see

39. A medical assistant who makes a derogatory statement about the practices of another medical group to a new patient is liable under the tort of
    A. battery
    B. assault
    ✓C. defamation
    D. invasion of privacy
    E. malpractice

40. Which statute of limitations should determine the decision to keep a medical record indefinitely?
    A. occurrence of a negligence
    B. end of a course of treatment
    Ⓒ discovery of a negligence
    D. age of majority
    ✓E. end of the physician-patient relationship

41. Which of the following is true concerning professional liability insurance coverage for the medical assistant?
    A. Employment in an HMO guarantees professional liability coverage for all employees.
    ✓B. Many employers carry professional liability insurance only on themselves.
    C. An employer's liability insurance automatically covers all employees.
    D. An employer's liability insurance policy must include the name of every full-time employee.
    E. Patients sue the physicians and not the employees, making employee insurance unnecessary.

42. A patient who has not been seen in 1 year calls and requests a refill for Percodan (schedule II). The physician is out of town and another physician is on call. The medical assistant should
    A. approve a refill of the original prescription
    B. approve a refill in an amount limited to when the attending physician returns
    C. approve a refill under the name of the on-call physician
    D. refer the patient to the physician who is on call
    E. refuse to OK the refill, then make an appointment for the patient to see the attending physician as soon as he or she returns

43. A terminally ill patient under the care of the physician for the last 3 days dies. The medical assistant should assist the physician in the preparation of a death certificate, which is signed
    A. after the remains have been sent to a mortician
    B. after autopsy
    C. after funeral arrangements have been made
    D. within 72 hours
    E. as quickly as possible as a courtesy to the family

44. When a notifiable disease is called in to the health department, each of the following is required information EXCEPT
    A. age of the patient
    B. occupation of the patient
    C. suspected disease
    D. date of disease onset
    E. name of the patient's employer

45. On immunization records, the National Childhood Vaccine Injury Act of 1986 mandates the inclusion of each of the following EXCEPT
    A. signed informed consent form
    B. manufacturer and lot number of the vaccine
    C. name and title of person administering the vaccine
    D. address of the person administering the vaccine
    E. any adverse events following administration of the vaccine

46. The National Childhood Vaccine Injury Act, passed by Congress in 1986, regulates each of the following childhood immunizations EXCEPT
    A. DTP
    B. TT
    C. MMR
    D. polio, inactivated
    E. polio, live

47. In all 50 states, laws require health care professionals to report each of the following EXCEPT
    A. rape
    B. drug abuse
    C. spousal abuse
    D. elder abuse
    E. child abuse

48. When rendering first aid, Good Samaritan laws apply to
    A. medical offices
    B. clinics
    C. both A and B
    D. public places
    E. both A and D

49. Which of the following is a circumstance that requires the patient to sign an informed consent form?
    A. when a patient makes an appointment for a throat culture
    B. when a patient rolls up her sleeve to have her blood drawn
    C. when a physician administers first aid to a patient who collapses to the floor
    D. when a patient agrees to release records to a consultant
    E. when a patient decides not to have radiation treatments

50. After signing an informed consent, a patient begins crying and states he isn't sure he is doing the right thing. The medical assistant should
    A. ask the physician to speak with the patient
    B. ask the patient to think about it some more and call back tomorrow with a final decision
    C. comfort the patient and assure him he is doing the right thing
    D. suggest the patient talk with family members or clergy
    E. suggest the patient cancel the procedure until a time when he feels more sure of what he wants

51. A minor child was living with his mother following a divorce but now is in the care of foster parents. In this situation, who signs for the release of the child's medical records?
    A. natural father
    B. natural mother
    C. foster parents
    D. the courts
    E. social services

52. Which of the following secondary containers may be used without a hazard warning label?
    A. 70% isopropyl alcohol dispenser
    B. soap dispenser
    C. Betadine dispenser
    D. Gram's stain dispensers
    E. bleach dispenser

53. Under the OSHA hazardous and toxic substance law, the employer is required to
    A. list all hazardous and toxic substances in the workplace
    B. give employees a list of all toxic substances within 24 hours after hiring
    C. both A and B
    D. give employees Material Safety Data Sheets within 1 day of employment
    E. both A and D

54. During a patient interview, the patient gives a brief summary of his symptoms over a 2-month period, then begins talking about the weather. The medical assistant listens and then replies, "Let's get back to what you were saying about your leg pains." This is an interview technique called
    A. mirroring
    B. restating
    C. pinpointing
    D. feedback
    E. probing

55. A patient will not make eye contact with the medical assistant. Poor eye contact is an example of
    A. verbal communication
    B. nonverbal communication
    C. indirect communication
    D. therapeutic communication
    E. nontherapeutic communication

56. A patient mentions an upsetting incident, and the medical assistant replies, "Tell me more about that." This communication is an example of
    A. reflection
    B. feedback
    C. clarification
    D. closed statement
    E. open-ended statement

57. A 54-year-old patient tells the medical assistant she has been having vaginal bleeding for several days. After making note of the patient's problem, the medical assistant's most appropriate response is to
    A. reassure the patient that occasional vaginal bleeding is normal for her age
    B. reassure her that the bleeding will stop
    C. explain to her that she needs to tell the physician when he examines her
    D. ask her to keep the office informed if her symptoms persist or get any worse
    E. explain that vaginal bleeding can be a symptom of serious disease

58. As a medical assistant attempts to administer an IM medication, the patient strikes the medical assistant's hand. The syringe falls to the floor, and the patient breaks into tears. The medical assistant's FIRST response should be to
    A. comfort the patient
    B. ask the patient to be quiet
    C. clean up the spill
    D. prepare a second injection
    E. call for assistance

59. Obsessive-compulsive disorder is characterized by
    A. delusions
    B. hallucinations
    C. hyperactivity
    D. ritualistic actions
    E. depression

60. Deficits in hyperactive children are characterized as
    A. intellectual
    B. physical
    C. mental retardation
    D. temperamental
    E. behavioral

61. In mental health terminology, a bipolar disorder is a disorder of
    A. mood and thought
    B. personality
    C. interpersonal deficits
    D. intelligence
    E. self-image

62. Measurements that are termed "anthropometric" include
    A. weight
    B. blood pressure
    C. both A and B
    D. head circumference
    E. both A and D

63. The correct term for the instrument used to test reflexes is
    A. tines
    B. tuning fork
    C. caliper
    D. percussion hammer
    E. knee-knocker

64. Each of the following is spelled correctly EXCEPT
    A. *Nocardia asteroides*
    B. *Escherischia coli*
    C. *Klebsiella pneumoniae*
    D. *Staphylococcus aureus*
    E. *Entamoeba histolytica*

65. A sudden occurrence of symptoms such as pain is described as
    A. parenchymal
    B. adnexal
    C. paroxysmal
    D. eccentric
    E. transient

66. Material obtained from the posterior cul-de-sac by aspiration is used to determine a ruptured ectopic pregnancy. The procedure is called a
    A. biopsy
    B. culdocentesis
    C. laparoscopy
    D. laparotomy
    E. dilatation and curettage

67. The term meaning the destruction of red blood cells is
    A. hemolysis
    B. hematopoiesis
    C. hemoptysis
    D. hemostasis
    E. hemophilia

68. Basal is an adjective to denote
    A. fundamental or primary importance
    B. toward the base of a structure
    C. a known value for comparison
    D. all-purpose
    E. alkalinity

69. Choose the word that is spelled correctly.
    A. hemmorhagic
    B. nephrotosis
    C. gastrorhaphy
    D. sphygnomanometer
    E. polycythemia

70. Choose the word that is spelled correctly.
    A. exopthalmic
    B. gonorrhia
    C. pharnyx
    D. ankylodactylia
    E. antiflexion

71. Choose the word that is spelled correctly.
    A. colangiogastrectomy
    B. iliojejunostomy
    C. interstitial
    D. spleenectomy
    E. dispepsia

72. Hemiplegia is defined as
    A. weakness on one side of the body
    B. paralysis on one side of the body
    C. bleeding into a body cavity
    D. weakness of the lower extremities
    E. paralysis of the lower extremities

73. An unsteady gait is defined as
    A. ataxia
    B. agnosia
    C. hemiparesis
    D. dysphagia
    E. aphagia

74. One medical word element that relates to the English term "two" is
    A. poly
    B. semi
    C. hemi
    D. diplo
    E. bi

75. In the laboratory, cytology is used to differentiate
    A. normal from neoplastic cells
    B. the structure of tissues
    C. anatomical size, position, and extent of tumors
    D. the extent of invasion of malignant cells
    E. the developmental stages of blood cells

76. One medical word element that relates to the English term "within" is
    A. intra
    B. inter
    C. infra
    D. antero
    E. meso

77. The abbreviation "CA" is used to mean
    A. chronic-acute
    B. cancer
    C. caudal-anterior
    D. calcium
    E. coronary arteries

78. Cerumen is an example of
    A. excrement
    B. secretion
    C. excretion
    D. discharge
    E. exudation

79. Choose the word that is spelled correctly.
    A. alopecia
    B. diaphram
    C. emphisema
    D. supperative
    E. inflamation

80. The term for the Korotkoff sound that disappears during phase II of a blood pressure reading is termed
    A. ausculatory gap
    B. diastole
    C. systole
    D. fading sound
    E. asystole

81. Surgery that uses the transference of light into a visible beam of radiation focused at close range is known as
    A. electrosurgery
    B. hyfrecation
    C. stereotactic surgery
    D. laser surgery
    E. cryosurgery

82. A woman who has never produced a viable offspring after several pregnancies is
    A. primigravida
    B. multigravida
    C. multipara
    D. nulligravida
    E. nullipara

83. During a health history, a woman reports one abortion and one viable birth. This patient is recorded as
    A. gravida 1, para 0
    B. gravida 1, para 1
    C. gravida 1, para 2
    D. gravida 2, para 1
    E. gravida 2, para 2

84. Painless intermittent uterine contractions, usually occurring in the last trimester, are called
    A. Chadwick's sign
    B. Goodell's sign
    C. Hegar's sign
    D. Nagele's rule
    E. Braxton Hicks' sign

85. The abbreviation "c/o" stands for
    A. coronary obstruction
    B. cancel out
    C. carbon dioxide
    D. complains of
    E. chronic obstructive disease

86. On a patient history is found the following notation: Hx HBP; DM +, neurologic WNL. "WNL" indicates
    A. normal
    B. not present
    C. negative
    D. not done
    E. absent

87. In the previous question, the "+" symbol means
    A. increased
    B. positive
    C. primary
    D. present
    E. equal

88. The potential of a substance to exert a harmful effect on humans is termed
    A. toxicity
    B. reactivity
    C. lethal concentration
    D. threshold
    E. hazardous

89. The term applied to an agent or substance that may cause physical defects in the developing embryo or fetus, when a pregnant woman is exposed to that substance, is
    A. carcinogen
    B. irritant
    C. mutagen ✓
    D. sensitizer
    E. teratogen

90. The local death of cells is termed
    A. necrosis ✓
    B. infarction
    C. anoxia
    D. somatic death
    E. ischemia

91. Hypoplasia is defined as
    A. absence of tissue
    B. wasting of tissue
    C. underdevelopment of tissues
    D. diminished strength
    E. diminished sense of smell

92. In women, the most common cystic lesion affecting the vulva is the
    A. Bartholin's gland cyst
    B. Nabothian cyst
    C. Gartner's cyst
    D. functional cyst
    E. Stein-Leventhal cyst

93. The medical term most closely associated with health is
    A. compliance
    B. morbidity
    C. homeostasis ✓
    D. prevention
    E. treatment

94. A small hemorrhage the size of a pinhead is termed
    A. hematoma
    B. ecchymosis
    C. petechia ✓
    D. extravasation
    E. thrombosis

95. Diseases caused by the medical profession may be termed
    A. iatrogenic
    B. idiopathic
    C. both A and B
    D. nosocomial
    E. both A and D

96. A chronic disease characterized by scaling of the scalp is known as
    A. seborrheic dermatitis
    B. eczema
    C. psoriasis ✓
    D. dermatophytoses
    E. urticaria

97. Psychoneurologic causes of acute or chronic headache include
    A. nitrites in food ✓
    B. rapid temperature change
    C. rapid altitude change
    D. fatigue
    E. motion sickness

98. A therapeutic procedure in which the patient self-induces an electrical impulse into large nerve fibers to block painful impulses is called
    A. biofeedback
    B. trigger point therapy
    C. stereotaxis
    D. electrodialysis
    E. transcutaneous electrical nerve stimulation (TENS)

99. A disease that results from unexpressed negative emotions is described as
    A. psychoneurologic
    B. psychosomatic
    C. psychotropic
    D. a personality disorder
    E. psychoneurosis

100. It is thought that migraine headaches are caused by
    A. physical changes in brain circulation
    B. negative emotions
    C. stress and distress
    D. poor nutrition
    E. environmental factors

Part 2—Administrative Procedures

Directions: *Each of the following questions or incomplete statements precedes five suggested answers or completions. Select the ONE answer or completion that is BEST in each case, and fill in the circle containing the corresponding letter on the answer sheet.*

101. Diagnostic tests may present a risk of allergic reaction in some patients. The medical assistant should question the patient concerning any allergies when scheduling
    A. angiography
    B. cholangiography
    C. both A and B
    D. pneumoencephalography
    E. both A and D

102. During office hours, if a patient thinks an illness is urgent the medical assistant should
    A. cancel another patient's appointment to open a time for this patient
    B. calm the patient and set the appointment for the same day
    C. turn the call over to the physician
    D. schedule the patient immediately
    E. send the patient to an emergency room

103. When choosing a computerized appointment system, which of the following features might be excluded?
    A. programmed time frames
    B. sound tone signaling an appointment
    C. cancellation tracking
    D. no-show tracking
    E. printout schedules

104. In a lactating woman, an appointment should be scheduled for the same day if the patient reports
    A. breast engorgement
    B. nipple cracks and redness
    C. both A and B
    D. incomplete emptying during breast-feeding
    E. both A and D

105. Which of the following statements is true regarding the scheduling of office appointments?
    A. Determining time frames for different procedures is an accurate science.
    B. Hours of availability cannot be accurately calculated.
    C. People need to accept and work for the appointment book.
    D. As a practice changes, so should the appointment book.
    E. After study, unpredictable problems can be anticipated.

106. Which of the following is correct vitae format?
    A. abbreviated organizations and agencies
    B. abbreviated titles
    C. underlined journals and books in citations
    D. children's names included
    E. marital status included

107. Which of the following should be underscored for italics?
    A. punctuation marks following underscored material
    B. foreign expressions that are not considered part of the English language
    C. translations of foreign expressions
    D. plural ending added on to an underscored word
    E. possessive ending added to an underscored word

108. Once used in a manuscript, each of the following abbreviations is correct EXCEPT
    A. T4
    B. mm Hg
    C. Rh
    D. Val
    E. Jan.

109. Each of the following medical abbreviations is correct EXCEPT
    A. *E. coli*
    B. *Staphylococcus a.*
    C. *H. influenzae*
    D. kg
    E. lymphs

110. Each of the following medical abbreviations is correct EXCEPT
    A. pH
    B. HGB
    C. mEq
    D. mOsm
    E. PKU

111. In an article, each of the following abbreviations has correct punctuation EXCEPT
    A. et al.
    B. et. al.
    C. MS
    D. ms
    E. ibid.

112. Which of the following editing definitions is correct?
    A. The abbreviation "e.g." means "that is."
    B. The abbreviation "i.e." means "for example."
    C. The abbreviation "Ibid." refers to "in the work cited."
    D. The abbreviation "op cit." refers to "in the same place."
    E. "Sic" is used to indicate that a misspelled word is not the author's doing.

113. Each of the following requires diacritical (` ´ ^ ~) marks EXCEPT
    A. cul-de-sac
    B. Roentgen rays
    C. Turk's cell
    D. fiancee
    E. a la carte

114. Each of the following symbols with numbers is correct EXCEPT
    A. 36°C
    B. 2+
    C. grade IV/V
    D. 4×4
    E. 45 ½%

115. Each of the following is correct usage of a question mark EXCEPT
    A. Will you answer my question, "Who manufactures this brace"?
    B. The manufacturer answered my original question, "Who makes this brace?"
    C. "Can you dictate the report on Mr. Smith for me"? she asked.
    D. The CBC showed a 27,000 (?) WBC.
    E. Should I invite Dr. Smith? Dr. Jones? Dr. Terry?

116. Which of the following requires two spaces after punctuation?
    A. colon before a series
    B. colon used with the time of day
    C. colon used to express a dilute solution
    D. colon used to separate a journal issue and page number
    E. semicolon

117. Which of the following requires one space after punctuation?
    A. period at the end of a sentence
    B. exclamation point at the end of a sentence
    C. question mark at the end of a sentence
    D. quotation mark at the end of a sentence
    E. period following an initial

118. A proofreader's mark that indicates a question to the author is
    A. ?
    B. ⑦
    C. //
    D. stet
    E. @

119. The physician has prepared a presentation for a scientific meeting. The final copy consists of 20 double-spaced pages, with 200 to 250 words on each page. The estimated time for delivering this presentation is
    A. 5 minutes
    B. 10 minutes
    C. 20 minutes
    D. 40 minutes
    E. 60 minutes

120. Which of the following is organized in the *Index Medicus*?
    A. list of diseases
    B. list of procedures
    C. list of current journal articles
    D. online computer services
    E. medical e-mail services

121. When preparing a manuscript, a series of three periods with one space between each indicates
    A. the beginning of a long quotation
    B. the end of a long quotation
    C. omissions in quoted material
    D. the writer's insertions within quoted material
    E. paraphrased material

122. In the following bibliography, which element is usually excluded?
    Author, AA, Author, BB, Author, CC et al: The title of the chapter. In Editor, AA, Editor, BB (eds): The Title of the Book, ed 3. Publisher, New York, New York, Year, p #.
    A. et al.
    B. In
    C. (eds)
    D. ed 3
    E. State

123. Additional copies of articles published in journals are called
    A. abstracts
    B. reprints
    C. galley proofs
    D. page proofs
    E. editions

124. An online computer database accessed through the National Library of Medicine to locate a scientific article in a journal is
    A. Medline
    B. American Standard Code for Information Exchange
    C. ERIC
    D. *Index Medicus*
    E. Internet

125. One computer file extension (.xxx) designating a spreadsheet file is
    A. DBF
    B. DTF
    C. IDX
    D. WK1
    E. DAT

126. A report is to be prepared on 8.5 × 11-inch bond paper in the landscape format. Specifications require a 12 cpi font and right and left margins of 1 inch each. The number of spaces available to the typed line would be approximately
    A. 68 characters
    B. 88 characters
    C. 102 characters
    D. 108 characters
    E. 240 characters

127. In WordPerfect 5.1, special European accent characters can be typed by using
    A. macros
    B. control-V codes
    C. graphics
    D. text in/out commands
    E. reveal codes

128. Each of the following is a special feature of WordPerfect 5.1 EXCEPT
    A. numbers calculation
    B. automatic typing
    C. automatic outlining
    D. split screen viewing
    E. indexing

129. For which of the following is a spreadsheet application the best choice?
    A. employee records
    B. vendor files
    C. insurance claims
    D. patient files
    E. monthly inventory tracking

130. When purchasing a computer printer, a standard laser printer has a print resolution known as
    A. near–letter quality
    B. desktop publishing quality
    C. letter quality
    D. correspondence quality
    E. draft quality

131. A good collection rate is considered to be
    A. 10%
    B. 20%
    C. 50%
    D. 80%
    E. 90%

132. Capital equipment is a term that designates equipment
    A. purchases with a long life expectancy
    B. purchases that cost $100 or more
    C. both A and B
    D. that appreciates over time
    E. both A and D

133. During a comparison of ledger card totals to the accounts receivable total, the ledger cards totaled $6450 and the AR totaled $6540, creating a $90 discrepancy. If this discrepancy is the result of only one error, the possible error to look for first is
    A. whether an account balance was omitted on the day sheet
    B. whether a ledger card is missing
    C. whether digits were transposed on one of the records
    D. whether a decimal point is in the wrong place
    E. whether a debit was entered as a credit

134. Which of the following can be used to disburse money from petty cash to mail a package?
    A. petty cash voucher
    B. employee reimbursement voucher
    C. both A and B
    D. post office receipt
    E. both A and D

135. A report of all taxes owed by a business must be submitted at least
    A. every 2 weeks
    B. monthly
    C. quarterly
    D. semiannually
    E. annually

136. In the cash basis accounting system, which of the following "chart of account" categories is considered income?
    A. recovery of bad debts
    B. accounts receivable
    C. savings account
    D. checking account
    E. retained earning

137. On the balance sheet, the accounts receivable category represents a business
    A. fixed asset
    B. asset
    C. capital
    D. expense
    E. liability

138. A deposit of payroll taxes greater than $500 but less than $3000 must be submitted at least
    A. every 2 weeks
    B. monthly
    C. quarterly
    D. semiannually
    E. annually

139. At year end, which of the following forms must an employer prepare for mailing directly to the Social Security Administration?
    A. W-2
    B. W-3
    C. W-4
    D. 1096
    E. 1099

140. Which of the following is an example of a third-party payer?
    A. Medicare
    B. health maintenance organization
    C. preferred provider organization
    D. parent of a young child
    E. patient's spouse

141. Checks that are acceptable for patient payment include
    A. counter checks
    B. government tax refunds
    C. travelers' checks
    D. insurance checks made out to the patient
    E. endorsed money orders

142. An example of an accounts payable record is the
    A. day sheet
    B. patient ledger card
    C. petty cash voucher
    D. transaction slip
    E. cash receipt

143. Under which of the following accounts should income from a collection agency be entered?
    A. accounts receivable
    B. recovery of bad debts
    C. professional fees
    D. accounts payable
    E. checking

144. An established patient brings his 22-year-old son into the office. They work at the same plant, and the son has been injured on the job. Under which name should the account card be set up?
    A. father's name
    B. son's name
    C. workers' compensation
    D. company name
    E. local disability agency name

145. A fee of $128 was turned over to a collection agency, who in turn charges a 50% fee for collecting the debt. A check for $128 subsequently was submitted by the patient to the office. The correct handling of the check is to
    A. send the check back to the patient, requesting a new check made out to the agency
    B. endorse the check, then forward it to the agency
    C. post the check, then forward it to the agency
    D. post 50% of the check, deposit the $128, and write a $64 check to the agency
    E. post and deposit the full amount, then notify the agency of the deposit

146. A patient's $300 account is written off to a zero balance when is it turned over to a collection agency as "uncollectable." The agency recovers $100 and retains 50% as its fee. The reinstatement entry would be
    A. charge $50; payment $50
    B. charge $100; payment $50
    C. charge $100; payment $50; credit adjustment $50
    D. payment $50; credit adjustment $50
    E. payment $50; debit adjustment $50

147. If an account card does not have an adjustment column, a returned patient check is
    A. deducted from the checkbook
    B. entered in the account card charge column
    C. both A and B
    D. entered in the account card payment column in brackets
    E. both A and D

148. Which of the following statements is true concerning coordination of benefits?
    A. It is the sharing of insurance costs among multiple insurance plans.
    B. It is the sharing of insurance costs between the insurer and the patient.
    C. It is a small flat rate that may be payable when services are rendered.
    D. It is a percentage of the total benefits.
    E. The provider agrees to accept the insurance company's approved fee.

149. A Medicare patient being treated by a participating physician is financially responsible for
    A. the difference between the Medicare Fee Schedule and the 80% Medicare payment
    B. the difference between the physician's charge and the 80% Medicare payment
    C. the physician's charge and the Medicare Fee Schedule
    D. the deductible amount only
    E. the entire charge of a service

150. In which of the following instances will Medicare be the primary payer?
    A. automobile accident injury covered by auto insurance
    B. patient eligible for Medicaid benefits
    C. employed 65-year-old patient covered by employer group plan
    D. retired 65-year-old patient covered by working spouse's group plan
    E. 69-year-old patient injured on the job

151. In an HMO plan, services covered include
    A. emergency treatment, out-of-plan, with authorization obtained within 24 hours
    B. emergency treatment, in-plan, without authorization obtained
    C. gynecologic consultation obtained in-plan by the patient with no prior authorization obtained
    D. elective cosmetic surgery
    E. experimental treatments

152. When registering a new patient who has Blue Shield insurance, the medical assistant should ask for the
    A. name of the carrier
    B. case ID number
    C. both A and B
    D. address of the carrier
    E. both A and D

153. A subscriber to a Preferred Provider Organization goes outside of the network to receive special services. The patient's primary care physician provides a referral and notifies the carrier. This patient will pay
    A. no out-of-pocket expenses
    B. the deductible amount
    C. the copayment
    D. the deductible amount and the copayment
    E. the total cost of the services

154. A patient calls for an initial appointment and states he has a Medical Assistance card. Telephone verification designates the patient a member of a federal HMO. The medical assistant should
    A. register the patient as a managed care patient
    B. call the patient's HMO and request a referral
    C. tell the patient to be prepared to pay in full for the visit
    D. tell the patient that the office can provide services only in an emergency
    E. tell the patient that he will be responsible for the deductible amount and copayments

155. In which of the following plans do physicians provide health care services on a discounted fee-for-service basis?
    A. PPO
    B. HMO
    C. Medical Assistance
    D. Blue Cross/Blue Shield
    E. workers' compensation

156. In a preferred provider network, patients who go outside of the network to receive service without a referral
    A. do not have any additional out-of-pocket expenses
    B. will have to pay deductible amounts
    C. will have to pay copayments
    D. will have to pay deductible amounts and copayments
    E. will have to pay the total expense

157. For payment purposes, Medicare insurance is primary to
    A. Blue Cross/Blue Shield
    B. Workers' Compensation
    C. Medigap
    D. disability insurance
    E. all other insurance plans

158. Services for Medical Assistance patients that require preapproval by a primary care provider include
    A. annual physical examinations
    B. family planning services
    C. sexually transmitted disease services
    D. obstetric care
    E. outpatient alcohol/drug abuse services

159. A Blue Shield card with a picture of the United States in the upper-right corner, indicating a "Government-Wide Service Benefit Plan," designates the
    A. BS National Account
    B. BS Federal Employee Program
    C. BS Medicare Plan
    D. BS Out-of-Sate Reciprocity Plan
    E. BS Preferred Provider Network

160. Which of the following types of managed care permits enrollees to retain coverage when the patient seeks services from noncontracted providers?
    A. open-ended or point-of-service providers
    B. preferred provider organization (PPO)
    C. both A and B
    D. staff model HMO
    E. both A and D

161. Under which of the following circumstances should an operative note accompany a claim form?
    A. adult patient undergoing bilateral inguinal hernia repair
    B. adult patient undergoing multiple-level cervical laminectomy
    C. patient returning 1 month postoperatively to the OR for complications
    D. team of specialty-skilled surgeons performing a multidisciplined procedure
    E. physician performing a modified radical mastectomy as a second procedure planned at the time of a biopsy procedure 1 week earlier

162. Which of the following charges could result from releasing medical information without the authorization of the patient?
    A. battery
    B. assault
    C. invasion of privacy
    D. defamation of character
    E. libel

163. That the patient has the right to refuse treatment to the extent permitted by law and to be informed of the medical consequences of this action is a part of which universal document?
    A. Medical Assisting Code of Ethics
    B. Declaration of Geneva
    C. Hippocratic Oath
    D. AMA Code of Ethics
    E. Patient's Bill of Rights

164. To which of the following patient questions regarding organ donation is the answer "Yes"?
    A. "Will my hospital care suffer if I am an organ donor?"
    B. "Will the recipient be told my name?"
    C. "Will my family have to pay for having my organs donated?"
    D. "Can my organs be sold?"
    E. "Can I change my mind later on?"

165. A 13-year-old girl is to have an elective abdominal CT scan within the next 30 days. Her LMP was January 1 to January 7. One acceptable date for the examination is
    A. January 17
    B. January 24
    C. January 31
    D. February 1
    E. February 7

166. The physician requests the capability to retrieve messages on a computer by dialing a special code number or calling an operator. The medical assistant would purchase
    A. an electronic message service
    B. a computer network service
    C. a radio pager
    D. a mobile telephone
    E. a voice mail service from the telephone company

167. During clinic hours, calls immediately put through to the physician include
    A. prescription refills
    B. other physicians
    C. laboratory reports
    D. status reports
    E. patient family members

168. When alphabetically filing the following, which is the last indexing unit? Ms. Carol Rogers Miller (Mrs. James C.)
    A. Rogers
    B. Miller
    C. Mrs. James C.
    D. James C.
    E. Carol

169. In the problem-oriented medical records system, the initial database includes information regarding the patient's
    A. progress
    B. numbered list of past medical problems
    C. numbered list of present problems
    D. numbered list of social problems
    E. physical examination

170. A notation on the patient's chart contains an error. The method for making a correction is to
    A. re-enter the entire notation correctly
    B. draw a single line through the error and correct with a carat
    C. strike out the error and write the correction in the right margin
    D. strike out the error and write the correction at the end of the entry
    E. erase the error and write in the correction

171. A procedure was charted but then not done. The medical assistant should
    A. erase the entry
    B. ink-out the entry
    C. draw a single line through the entry, and write "err"
    D. draw a single line through the entry, and write the words "not done"
    E. discard the section containing the entry

172. The Office of Subpoenas calls to request patient records. The medical assistant should
    A. require receipt of the subpoena first
    B. give the information to the caller
    C. request a release of records from the patient
    D. take the phone number and return the call
    E. refer the caller to the physician's attorney

173. For which of the following coding would colored medical history folders be useful?
    A. cases assigned to a particular physician
    B. allergies
    C. ICD-9 codes
    D. inactive patients
    E. past-due accounts

174. Records may be released without the patient's signature when
    A. communicable diseases are reported to the health department
    B. faxing information from one health care facility to another
    C. both A and B
    D. the patient is unable to sign in an emergency
    E. both A and D

175. A calendar of scientific meetings should include
    A. names of meeting participants
    B. the inclusive dates of each conference
    C. the dates the physician intends to travel
    D. the number of continued education credits
    E. detailed schedules of each day

176. For every on-hold patient telephone call, the minimum information collected should be
    A. the patient's name
    B. the patient's telephone number
    C. both A and B
    D. the reason for the call
    E. both A and D

177. While registering a patient by telephone, another telephone line rings. The medical assistant should say to the caller
    A. " I have to answer another line. Hold please."
    B. "Can you call me back? I have to answer another line."
    C. "I have to put you on hold."
    D. "Will you please hold?"
    E. "May I call you back at a more convenient time?"

178. A patient calls to obtain a first refill for methylphenidate (Ritalin), a schedule II drug. The medical assistant should
    A. route the call to the physician immediately
    B. schedule an appointment before approving a refill
    C. ask the patient to have the pharmacist call the office
    D. pull the patient's chart and check with the physician
    E. take the message for the physician to return the call

179. In the previous case, the physician approves the refill. The prescription should be
    A. called in to the pharmacist
    B. faxed to the pharmacist
    C. picked up by the patient
    D. faxed to the patient
    E. signed for at the pharmacy by the patient

180. At the patient's request, a cover letter is prepared for mailing with a laboratory report to his business address. The letter and two-page report contain information concerning test results of a highly sensitive nature. The envelope should include the on-arrival notation
    A. "Attention: patient's name"
    B. "Enclosure"
    C. "Certified"
    D. "Personal"
    E. "Confidential"

181. In the previous case, the on-arrival notation should be placed on the envelope
    A. below the return address
    B. in the lower-left corner
    C. in the lower-right corner
    D. two lines below the address
    E. centered above the address

182. The envelope size used for this mailing is
    A. no. 5 ½
    B. no. 7
    C. no. 10
    D. 8 ½ × 11 large
    E. 9 × 12 large

183. When addressing an envelope for the patient in the previous case, uppercase letters should be used for
    A. everything on the envelope
    B. the address only
    C. the patient's name only
    D. the on-arrival notation only
    E. the state abbreviation only

184. Continuing with the foregoing case, the cover letter explains that a copy of a two-page laboratory report is included in the mailing. Therefore,
    A. an enclosure notation at the bottom of the letter is unnecessary
    B. "Enclosures" should be typed two lines below the reference initials
    C. "Laboratory Report Enclosed" should be typed two lines below the reference initials
    D. "Enclosure 2" should be typed two lines below the reference initials
    E. "Enclosures" should be typed two lines below the complimentary close

185. Of the following items received in the day's mail, which item(s) should be placed on top for the physician's reading?
    A. notification of a meeting
    B. consultation letter
    C. patient letter of appreciation
    D. journals
    E. personal letter

186. Correspondence that can be signed by the medical assistant include
    A. letters to professional associations
    B. written advice to patients
    C. patient notifications
    D. hospital correspondence
    E. medical reports to insurance companies

187. Signature stamps may be used for
    A. Workers' Compensation claims
    B. disability reports
    C. "return to work" forms
    D. dictated operative notes
    E. dictated discharge summaries

188. When using the U.S. postal system, x-ray films should be mailed
    A. special delivery
    B. certified, return receipt requested
    C. special handling
    D. registered
    E. parcel post

189. A trauma patient undergoes anastomosis of extracranial and intracranial arteries (61711) and an elevation of a depressed compound skull fracture (62005-51). The modifier "-51" is used to indicate
    A. multiple sites
    B. additional team members
    C. an unrelated service the same day as surgery
    D. bilateral surgery
    E. multiple same-day procedures

190. In the previous case, the 90-day postoperative global fee applies to code
    A. 61711
    B. 62005
    C. both A and B
    D. 62005-51
    E. both A and D

191. In the same case, the patient has a second surgery 96 days after the first surgical service to repair a skull defect. The CPT code for reparative brain surgery is 62145. The claim should be coded
    A. 62145
    B. 62145-51 (multiple procedures)
    C. 52145-78 (return to OR for related procedure during postoperative period)
    D. 62145-79 (unrelated procedure by same physician during postoperative period)
    E. 61711, 62005-51, 62145

192. A patient has cataract surgery on the right eye. The ophthalmologist performs the surgery and turns the postoperative management over to an optometrist. The opthalmologist should code the claim as
    A. 66984 RT
    B. 66984 54
    C. 66984-54 RT
    D. 66984-55
    E. 66984-55 RT

193. In the same case, the optometrist should code the claim as
    A. 66984 RT
    B. 66984 54
    C. 66984-54 RT
    D. 66984-55
    E. 66984-55 RT

194. In the previous case, the patient returns to the ophthalmologist 60 days later to have the left cataract removed, with postoperative management by the same optometrist. CPT-4 code 66984 has a 90-day global fee period. The ophthalmologist's claim should be coded
    A. 66984-50
    B. 66984-54 79 LT
    C. 66984-55 50
    D. 66984-50 78
    E. 66984-54 78 LT

195. An established patient incurs a head injury with a laceration to the scalp. The physician sutures the head wound and also performs a neurologic evaluation to rule out any complications caused by the trauma. The claim should include the CPT code 99213 with
    A. the modifier "-00" (unspecified)
    B. the modifier "-21" (prolonged evaluation)
    C. the modifier "-25" (unrelated E & M service, same day as surgery)
    D. the modifier "-55" (postoperative care only)
    E. no modifier

196. A physician admits a new patient to the hospital because of an MI (410). Because of the patient's deteriorating condition, the physician spends a significant amount of time above the 70-minute, highest-level initial inpatient CPT-4 E & M code. This claim should be coded with the modifier "21" (prolonged evaluation), typed as follows:
    A. 99221
    B. 99223-21
    C. 410.00-21
    D. 410.21
    E. 412.21

197. The patient has four nerve block injections on the same day (64510, 64520, 64508, 64505), each at a different body site. The claim should be coded
    A. 64510
    B. 64510, 64520, 64508, 64505
    C. 64510, 64520-51, 64508-51, 64505-51
    D. 64510-51, 64520-51, 64508-51, 64505-51
    E. 64510, 64520-50, 64508-51, 64505-51

198. A CPT-4 modifier indicates that a service or procedure
  A. has been altered by a particular circumstance
  B. has changed the definition of the standard CPT code
  C. is part of a global procedure
  D. is not commonly performed for a particular ICD-9 code
  E. is performed for a diagnosis that has no ICD-9 code

199. Special codes indicating injuries caused by a motor vehicle traffic accident are
  A. V codes
  B. E codes
  C. ICD-O codes
  D. CPT modifiers
  E. 5th-digit codes

200. According to surgical global packaging policies, which of the following services can be reimbursed separately?
  A. 1-day preoperative services
  B. usual and necessary intraoperative services
  C. additional medical-surgical services resulting from complications during a surgical procedure
  D. an initial consultation
  E. 90-day postoperative visits

Part 3—Clinical Procedures

Directions: *Each of the following questions or incomplete statements precedes five suggested answers or completions. Select the ONE answer or completion that is BEST in each case, and fill in the circle containing the corresponding letter on the answer sheet.*

201. Which ECG part controls the height of the ECG standardization mark?
    A. sensitivity
    B. stylus
    C. both A and B
    D. SDT control
    E. both A and D

202. The ECG lead that is placed at the fourth intercostal space at the right of the sternum is lead
    A. V_1
    B. V_2
    C. V_4
    D. V_5
    E. V_6

203. The medical assistant is asked to rerun a rhythm strip. The rhythm is the same as
    A. lead I
    B. lead II
    C. lead III
    D. aVR
    E. lead V_1

204. Which of the following is used to measure atrial sinus rhythm?
    A. P-P rate
    B. R-R rate
    C. height of R waves
    D. depth of S waves
    E. ST segment elevation and depression

205. If the R wave is equal to or larger than the S wave in lead V_1, and is accompanied by a right-axis deviation where the QRS complex is predominantly negative in lead I, the most probable diagnosis is
    A. left atrial hypertrophy
    B. right atrial hypertrophy
    C. left ventricular hypertrophy
    D. right ventricular hypertrophy
    E. complete AV block

206. Rhythms that may occur in healthy hearts include
    A. atrial tachycardia
    B. atrial flutter
    C. junctional tachycardia
    D. ventricular tachycardia
    E. ventricular flutter

207. A beat that arrives early in the cardiac cycle, has no P wave of its own, and displays a wide and bizarre QRS complex is
    A. an atrial premature contraction
    B. a ventricular premature contraction
    C. a junctional premature contraction
    D. an atrial premature contraction with aberration
    E. a junctional premature contraction with aberration

208. For which patient group is potassium a particularly important daily requirement?
    A. osteoporosis in the elderly
    B. anemia during pregnancy
    C. both A and B
    D. persons taking diuretics
    E. both A and D

209. When teaching a patient about a high-iron diet, correct selections include
    A. skinless chicken
    B. fish
    C. whole-grain cereals
    D. shellfish
    E. egg whites

210. What is the expected delivery date for a pregnant woman whose first day of the last menstrual period was May 3, 1995?
    A. January 27, 1996
    B. January 28, 1996
    C. February 3, 1996
    D. February 10, 1996
    E. February 26, 1996

211. Over which of the following muscle areas is the diabetic patient taught by demonstration to self-administer insulin?
    A. deltoid
    B. biceps brachii
    C. external oblique
    D. rectus femoris
    E. vastus lateralis

212. Among the viral childhood diseases that produce a rash, the appearance of papules on the oral mucosa is a distinct characteristic of
    A. German measles (rubella)
    B. measles (rubeola)
    C. chickenpox (varicella)
    D. roseola infantum
    E. scarlet fever

213. A patient's chart reads as follows: "1/12/9–: F, age 71; T = 37(o); P = 72, +1, regular; R = 18; BP (10:30a sitting) R/A 110/70, AP 72; (10:35 lying) R/A 118/76, AP 74; (10:40 standing) R/A 96/68, AP 80, PD = 80/76; Ht 63"; Wt 85 kg." Which of the following readings is considered outside the normal range?
    A. T = 37(o)
    B. P = 72, +1, regular
    C. R = 18
    D. AP = 72
    E. PD = 80/76

214. For the same patient, convert the temperature to Fahrenheit degrees [F = (9/5 × C) + 32].
    A. 96.8
    B. 98.0
    C. 98.4
    D. 98.6
    E. 100.4

215. On standing, this patient's pulse pressure measures
    A. 96/98
    B. 94/92
    C. 80
    D. 28
    E. 4

216. In the previous case, the patient's blood pressure and pulse variations can be attributed to
    A. orthostatic hypotension
    B. orthostatic hypertension
    C. atherosclerotic hypertension
    D. an auscultatory gap
    E. anxiety about the examination

217. In the same patient, "PD = 80/86" represents the recording of
    A. the average pulse rate
    B. the average blood pressure reading
    C. premature heartbeats
    D. arrhythmia
    E. apical heartbeat and radial heartbeat

218. In the previous patient, which of the patient findings is most unusual in view of her blood pressure readings?
    A. postural changes
    B. pulse rates
    C. respiration rates
    D. weight
    E. age

219. The infrared tympanic thermometer is able to record body temperature in
    A. 3 seconds
    B. 10 seconds
    C. 30 seconds
    D. 1 minute
    E. 3 minutes

220. At a patient's first assessment, blood pressure readings are taken in both arms. When comparing right and left arms, blood pressure is usually
    A. the same in both arms
    B. 1–2 mm Hg different
    C. 5–10 mm Hg different
    D. 12–15 mm Hg different
    E. up to 20 mm Hg different

221. Transillumination can be used to examine the
    A. frontal sinuses
    B. ethmoid sinuses
    C. both A and B
    D. maxillary sinuses
    E. both A and D

222. Neurologic examination of the olfactory nerve includes:
    A. irritating the nasal mucosa with an ammonia fumes
    B. sugar, salt, vinegar, and quinine placed on the tongue
    C. asking the patient to whistle, blow, and wrinkle the forehead
    D. testing sensitivity to sounds with an audiometer
    E. flashlight inspection of the eyes

223. For which of the following is Gelfoam the trade name?
    A. contraceptive jelly
    B. colloid product used to keep wound edges together
    C. antacid suspension of aluminum hydroxide
    D. gelatinous base used to support bacterial growth
    E. absorbable sponge to control oozing of blood in wounds

224. Regions that contain major nerves and are, therefore, contraindicated for injections include the
    A. anterior part of the gluteal region
    B. triangular area bounded by the anterior superior iliac spine, the tubercle of the iliac crest, and the greater trochanter
    C. both A and B
    D. gluteus maximus, between the greater trochanter and the ischial tuberosity
    E. both A and D

225. While preparing a patient for a minor surgical procedure, the patient responds "Yes" when questioned about having an iodine allergy. Which of the following must be eliminated from the procedure?
    A. Gamophen
    B. Prepodyne
    C. normal saline solution
    D. Gelfoam
    E. Zephiran Chloride

226. During a postoperative visit, the medical assistant prepares a patient by cleansing an incision site containing a Penrose drain. When cleansing the wound, the medical assistant should
    A. remove the drain and replace it with a new, sterile drain
    B. flush the drain with sterile saline
    C. cleanse from the drain site outward, leaving the drain untouched
    D. cleanse the wound edge several times with a cotton swab and sterile saline
    E. cleanse the wound edges with antiseptic, then rise with normal saline

227. Sutures in the lower extremities should be left in place
    A. 24–48 hours
    B. 3 days
    C. 4–5 days
    D. 7–10 days
    E. 14 days

228. Which of the following may NOT rest on a sterile tray field?
    A. transfer forceps
    B. syringe and needle packet
    C. vial of anesthesia
    D. used operating instruments
    E. specimen container

229. The instrument used to directly visualize a joint, such as the knee, by inserting a cannula and fine telescope is called
    A. an arthrometer
    B. an arthrotome
    C. an arthroscope
    D. an orthoscope
    E. a pneumoarthrograph

230. A middle-aged man with benign prostatic hypertrophy is to have a transurethral resection of the prostate. Where would this patient have a surgical incision?
    A. anterior to the anus
    B. on the anterior surface of the penis
    C. on the lower abdominal wall
    D. in the left or right groin area
    E. internally in the urinary tract

231. The culdoscopic examination is performed in which position?
    A. knee-chest
    B. lithotomy
    C. dorsal recumbent
    D. Trendelenburg's
    E. jackknife

232. When excess fluid occurs in the peritoneal cavity, the surgical procedure used to withdraw the fluid is
    A. gastric lavage
    B. paracentesis
    C. cisternal puncture
    D. sternal puncture
    E. peritoneal dialysis

233. A skeletal structure that may be used for bone marrow aspiration is the
    A. fifth lumbar vertebra
    B. sacrum
    C. sternum
    D. pubic symphysis
    E. clavicle

234. To assess blood pressure properly, the medical assistant should
    A. position the patient's arm, slightly flexed, lower than heart level
    B. position the patient's arm, extended, at heart level
    C. position the patient's arm, slightly flexed, above heart level
    D. position the lower edge of the cuff just above the crease of the elbow
    E. center the arrow marker on the cuff over the stethoscope

235. When comparing the popliteal blood pressure to the brachial blood pressure, which finding is within normal limits?
    A. systole 10–40 mm Hg higher; diastole the same
    B. systole the same; diastole 10–40 mm Hg higher
    C. systole and diastole both 10–40 mm Hg higher
    D. systole and diastole both 10–40 mm Hg lower
    E. systole and diastole the same

236. After a biopsy, specimens should be transported to the laboratory in formalin or normal saline in a ratio of liquid medium to specimen of
    A. 1:1
    B. 2:1
    C. 5:1
    D. 10:1
    E. 20:1

237. During a surgical procedure, the area that is considered sterile on a draped towel on a Mayo stand is
    A. the entire surface
    B. within a 1-inch circle from the center of the tray
    C. within a 2-inch circle from the center of the tray
    D. within a 1-inch border around the sterile field
    E. within a 2-inch border around the sterile field

238. A CO_2 laser unit is used to cauterize tissue during a surgical procedure. Items that may not be used during the procedure include
    A. vinyl gloves
    B. cotton swabs
    C. 4 × 4 gauze
    D. a cloth fenestrated drape
    E. an absorbent-backed disposable aperture drape

239. A dressing adheres to a draining wound. The dressing should be released by
    A. peeling the edges toward the wound
    B. peeling the skin away from the dressing
    C. soaking the dressing first with hydrogen peroxide
    D. soaking the dressing first with sterile saline
    E. soaking the dressing in warm sudsy water

240. The proper technique for removing adhesive tape from the skin is to
A. pull tape toward the wound
B. pull tape away from the wound
C. pull the tape from the skin held taut
D. remove the tape quickly
E. remove the tape in one single motion

241. When applying an elastic bandage, one should
A. begin at the proximal part
B. hold the roll away from the body part
C. unroll the entire bandage and then wrap
D. hold the roll downward as it is rolled
E. overlap each layer by one half the width of the strip

242. For which of the following purposes may heat, as a form of therapy, be applied to the extremities?
A. to decrease blood supply to a part
B. to reduce swelling
C. to decrease suppuration
D. to relieve muscle spasm
E. to stop bleeding

243. Early signs of spontaneous septic abortion include
A. chills and fever
B. bleeding
C. rupture of membranes
D. products of conception passing through the cervical canal
E. nausea and vomiting

244. A patient returns to have a TB tine test read in 48 hours. There is induration of doubtful interpretation. The usual next step would be for the patient
A. to return in another 24 hours
B. to receive a Mantoux test
C. to receive a chest x-ray examination
D. to receive a repeated tine test
E. to undergo allergy testing

245. A positive tuberculin test result is characterized by
A. erythema
B. macules
C. pustules
D. a weal
E. induration

246. When treating a patient's right eye with drops, the medical assistant should have the patient
A. seated, looking up
B. lying, with the head turned right
C. either A or B
D. lying, with the head turned left
E. either A or D

247. Equipment necessary for a posterior rhinoscopic visualization includes
A. nasal speculum
B. otoscope
C. Krause nasal snare
D. laryngeal mirror
E. pharyngoscope

248. Which is a true characteristic of a simple knee jerk (reflex arc) during examination?
A. It requires thought.
B. It is initiated by painful stimuli.
C. It involves two nerves and one synapse.
D. Impulses go from sensory nerves to spinal nerves to motor nerves.
E. It involves spinal nerves and motor nerves only.

249. Which of the following may occur if an adhesive dressing is applied for too long?
A. swollen extremities
B. swollen joints
C. decreased circulation
D. softening of scar tissue
E. tissue damage

250. A patient calls and reports a blister that has become infected. The patient should be instructed to
A. cleanse the area with mild soap
B. puncture the blister with a sterile needle and apply antibiotic cream
C. both A and B
D. come into the office for treatment and tetanus prophylaxis as required
E. both A and D

251. For surgery on the sole of the foot or palm of the hand, it is advisable to prepare the skin first using
    A. warm scrubbing or soaking with liberal amounts of tincture of green soap
    B. warm scrubbing or soaking with liberal amounts of Betadyne
    C. soaking with liberal amounts of 70% alcohol
    D. soaking with liberal amounts of hydrogen peroxide
    E. scrubbing with plain soap and water

252. A child with a live insect in one ear is brought into the office. There is pain and noise in the ear. The treatment is
    A. to lure the insect from the ear canal with a bright light
    B. to instill a drop of oil and float the insect out
    C. to dislodge the insect with a sudden tap on the same side of the head above the ear
    D. to instill a few drops of 70% alcohol to kill the insect, then remove it with bayonet forceps
    E. to lavage the ear with an ear syringe and warm water

253. Each of the following statements about impetigo is true, EXCEPT
    A. it is noncommunicable and treated with hydrocortisone
    B. it is characterized by pustules that rupture and form yellow crusts
    C. it occurs in children who have been swimming in ponds and streams
    D. its lesions must be removed and cleaned two to three times a day
    E. patients should be advised to come into the office for treatment

254. A furuncle is usually treated nonsurgically with
    A. hydrocortisone cream
    B. hot wet compresses
    C. both A and B
    D. dry icepacks
    E. both A and D

255. A nulliparous, postmenopausal woman is taking estrogen for relief of menopausal symptoms. She is obese and has diabetes mellitus and hypertension. This patient is at particular risk for developing
    A. chronic endometritis
    B. endometrial polyps
    C. carcinoma of the endometrium
    D. cervical carcinoma in situ (CIS)
    E. osteomalacia

256. For the previous patient, an office procedure done annually or semiannually is
    A. pap smear
    B. aspiration biopsy of the endometrium
    C. laparoscopy
    D. colposcopy
    E. extended pelvic examination

257. Tincture of benzoin is used on the skin as
    A. a topical antibiotic ointment
    B. an anticoagulant
    C. a thin layer of liquid protectant
    D. a hemostatic
    E. a dye

258. When managing airway obstruction, it is important to know that irreversible brain damage can occur within
    A. 30 seconds
    B. 1 minute
    C. 2 minutes
    D. 3 minutes
    E. 4 minutes

259. A patient is bleeding profusely from a stab wound in the shoulder just above the armpit. The correct pressure point is the
    A. brachial
    B. subclavian
    C. temporal
    D. facial
    E. carotid

260. After an injury, a patient enters the office with blood slowly oozing from the left forearm. Immediate management includes
    A. firmly applying a pressure dressing and bandage to the area
    B. locating and compressing pressure points
    C. both A and B
    D. applying ice to the area
    E. both A and D

261. A patient calls from her home and reports she has spilled boiling water over her hands. Immediate management includes
    A. covering the area with sterile dressing to reduce contact with the air
    B. application of zinc oxide ointment
    C. application of aloe or other soothing topical cream
    D. application of household remedies, such as butter or tea bags
    E. application of ice water

262. The medical assistant should prepare the patient for intravenous access for each of the following office emergencies, EXCEPT
    A. cerebrovascular accident
    B. diabetic coma
    C. hypertensive crisis
    D. bone fracture
    E. myocardial infarction

263. Which of the following is contraindicated for inducing vomiting?
    A. ipecac syrup
    B. stimulating the uvula or posterior pharynx
    C. both A and B
    D. salt solutions
    E. both A and D

264. For each of the following emergencies, transfer to a hospital is necessary EXCEPT
    A. diabetic coma
    B. diabetic insulin shock that does not improve
    C. epilepsy
    D. status epilepticus
    E. hypertensive crisis

265. The chin-lift airway technique is contraindicated in patients
    A. who are unconscious
    B. with neck and spinal injuries
    C. whose tongue is blocking the airway
    D. with a hyperactive gag reflex
    E. who wear dentures

266. To remove fresh blood stains from fabric
    A. allow hot water to run through the fabric, then wash in hot soap solution
    B. soak fabric in acetone followed by warm chlorine bleach rinse
    C. soak fabric in cold water, then wash in lukewarm soap solution
    D. soak fabric in alcohol, then wash with baking soda and hot water
    E. soaked fabric in skimmed milk, lemon juice, or salt water; then wash in lukewarm soap solution

267. When a specimen is being prepared for transport, specimen labels should be placed on the
    A. requisition
    B. lid
    C. both A and B
    D. container
    E. both A and D

268. When fixing cervical smears, spraying the cytology fixative close to the slide can cause the cells to
    A. aggregate
    B. be washed from the slide
    C. lyse
    D. dilute
    E. coagulate

269. During a wet prep examination, nonmotile forms of *Trichomonas vaginalis* can be easily confused with
    A. epithelial cells
    B. yeast cells
    C. clue cells
    D. white blood cells
    E. mucous threads

270. A pregnancy test that provides information about fetal size, age, and sex is
    A. amniocentesis
    B. ultrasound examination
    C. fetal heart rate (FHR) tracing
    D. oxytocin challenge test
    E. alpha-fetoprotein (AFP) test

271. Blood tests necessary at the first postpartum visit include
    A. hematocrit
    B. hemoglobin
    C. both A and B
    D. rubella titer
    E. both A and D

272. After collection in transport media, throat swabs should be processed within
   A. 10 minutes
   B. 20–30 minutes
   C. 2–3 hours
   D. 24 hours
   E. 48 hours

273. Which of the following is interpreted as a positive Hemoccult II slide test result?
   A. pink symbol in the test area
   B. trace of blue on or near the edge of the test area
   C. pale blue ring on the test paper
   D. pale pink ring on the test paper
   E. no color in the test area

274. False-negative Hemoccult II test results may be due to ingestion of
   A. ascorbic acid
   B. iron preparations
   C. aspirin
   D. corticosteroids
   E. alcohol in excess

275. If an ssA culture plate incubates for 24 hours and no beta-hemolytic colonies are seen,
   A. the test result is interpreted as positive
   B. the test result is interpreted as negative
   C. the plate is reincubated for an additional 24 hours
   D. a new specimen is obtained
   E. the specimen is replated onto a fresh plate

276. For which of the following tests is a first morning urine specimen preferred?
   A. slide test for C-reactive protein
   B. Color Slide II Mononucleosis Test
   C. Rheumaton Slide Test for rheumatoid factor
   D. Rapid Plasma Reagin Card Test
   E. Tandem ICON II pregnancy test

277. Eating or drinking in the laboratory is prohibited under OSHA standards because hazardous or toxic substances may be unknowingly
   A. inhaled
   B. absorbed
   C. spilled
   D. contaminated
   E. ingested

278. Which of the following microscopic morphology would be reported as "seen"?
A. white blood cells
B. casts
C. epithelial cells
D. red blood cells
E. yeast

279. After charging a hemacytometer with a Unopette, how much time should elapse before counting the cells?
A. None
B. 1–2 minutes
C. 10 minutes
D. 15 minutes
E. 20–30 minutes

Using the following types of specimens, answer the next three questions:
A. throat culture swab
B. wound swab
C. urine culture
D. genital culture
E. serum specimens

280. Which type of specimen needs to be held at room temperature until the test(s) can be performed? D Genital Culture

281. Which type of specimen usually needs to be frozen until the test(s) can be performed? E Serum Specimens

282. Which type of specimen is collected by placing a swab directly into suppurative material? B Wound Swab

283. An 8-year-old child needs a tetanus and diphtheria booster. Acceptable toxoids include
A. DT
B. Td
C. both A and B
D. DPT
E. both A and D

284. Of the following routes, medications are most rapidly absorbed when applied
A. orally
B. subcutaneously
C. intramuscularly
D. intravenously
E. by Z-track

285. For which of the following immunizations is the subcutaneous route used?
A. diphtheria-tetanus
B. measles-mumps-rubella (MMR)
C. inactivated poliovirus vaccine (IPV)
D. typhoid
E. rabies

286. In which childhood diseases must antipyretics be limited to Tylenol?
A. chickenpox (varicella)
B. influenza
C. both A and B
D. acute tonsillitis
E. both A and D

287. Fever is now thought to be of benefit to the patient, and the automatic use of antipyretic therapy invalid in most cases EXCEPT
A. dehydration
B. heat exhaustion or stroke
C. both A and B
D. febrile convulsions
E. both A and D

288. The treatment for scalp lice and other skin infestations is an insecticide known as
A. chlorophothane (DDT)
B. antivenin
C. methoxalen (Oxsoralen)
D. gamma benzene hexachloride (Kwell)
E. streptokinase

289. In the pregnant woman, daily dietary recommendations include an increase in each of the following supplements EXCEPT
A. protein
B. folic acid
C. calcium
D. sodium
E. iron

290. In the first trimester, pregnant women are expected to gain how much weight per month?
A. None
B. 0.8 lb
C. 1 lb
D. 2 lb
E. 4 lb

291. Breast-feeding mothers should alter their nutritional requirements by
    A. subtracting 500 calories per day
    B. adding 500 calories per day
    C. increasing whole milk to 1 qt per day
    D. avoiding consumption of meats, poultry, fish, eggs, and dairy products
    E. avoiding foods high in fiber

292. According to OSHA standards, surfaces used for laboratory analyses of patient specimens must be decontaminated
    A. before each patient analysis
    B. after each patient analysis
    C. both A and B
    D. before leaving an area for lunch or a break
    E. both A and D

293. The diamond system hazard label uses the numbers 0 to 4 to rate the
    A. severity of a chemical reaction
    B. degree of flammability of a substance
    C. exposure limits with no adverse affects
    D. hazard of a material during a fire
    E. the type of fire extinguisher to use

294. Which of the following reprocessing methods is required for equipment that comes into contact with the mucous membranes?
    A. environmental disinfection
    B. low-level disinfection
    C. intermediate disinfection
    D. high-level disinfection
    E. sterilization

295. An OSHA-rated hazard associated with the reagents used with the Color Slide II Mononucleosis Test Kit and other serology test kits is categorized as
    A. explosion hazard
    B. fire hazard
    C. respiratory hazard
    D. skin hazard
    E. ingestion hazard

296. The lowest temperature at which a liquid gives off enough vapor to form an ignitable mixture and burn when exposed to open flames, such as when using a Bunsen or alcohol burner, is the
    A. threshold
    B. melting point
    C. flash point
    D. boiling point
    E. ignition point

297. Which of the following information is important to read on a Material Safety Data Sheet before mixing two chemicals?
    A. Section III—Physical Data
    B. Section IV—Fire and Explosion Hazard Data
    C. Section V—Reactivity Data
    D. Section VI—Health Hazard Data
    E. Section VII—Special Protection Information

298. A patient asks how long an MRI will take. The correct response is
    A. 1 min
    B. 10–15 min
    C. 30 min
    D. 45–60 min
    E. 60–90 min

299. The purpose of a transcatheter embolization is to
    A. increase vessel lumen diameter
    B. stop localized bleeding
    C. remove calculi
    D. remove atherosclerotic plaque from arteries
    E. restore blood flow

300. Radiographic views to show the vertebrae include
    A. anterior
    B. posterior
    C. both A and B
    D. lateral
    E. both A and D

ANSWER KEY FOR SIMULATION TEST 1

1. **A.** Pyrexia is one term for fever. Shivering and chills occur when the body manufactures heat and continue until the fever falls. *Frew, Lane, and Frew, p. 345.*

2. **E.** The Monospot detects the presence of a nonspecific antibody called the heterophile antibody. It is present in the serum of patients with infectious mononucleosis. It occurs shortly after the appearance of symptoms and provides only presumptive evidence of the disease. *Gylys and Wedding, p. 192.*

3. **C.** The final stage of urine production occurs when specialized cells of the collecting tubules secrete ammonia, uric acid, and other substances directly into the lumen of the collecting tubules. The formation of urine is now complete and it is passed from the collecting tubules to the renal pelvis, or the basin of the kidney. *Gylys and Wedding, p. 242.*

4. **D.** A vasectomy is the removal of all or a segment of the vas deferens. A bilateral vasectomy results in sterility. *Gylys, p. 204.*

5. **C.** An electrolyte is a solution that conducts electricity and then is decomposed by the passage of an electrical current. *Sheldon, p. 104.*

6. **B.** Herpes simplex is transmitted orally. Transmission of HBV or HIV infections during mouth-to-mouth resuscitation has not been documented; however, possible transmission of herpes simplex through saliva has been documented. Because of this and the theoretical transmission of HIV and HBV via wounds or bleeding, disposable airway equipment and air bags should be used. Universal precautions do not apply to saliva. The use of gloves when examining the mucous membranes of the mouth, as well as hand washing after exposure to saliva, further minimizes the risk. *Sheldon, p. 216; Lane, Medications, p. 786.*

7. **E.** From infancy through childhood, children have a greater distribution of interstitial and intracellular fluid and a lesser distribution of dry weight (e.g., bone). Compared with adults, children have a greater body surface area and, therefore, greater rates of metabolism, including temperature, pulse, and respiration. *Sheldon, p. 24; Frew, Lane, and Frew, p. 351.*

8. **C.** As the follicles grow in the ovary, estrogen is produced by the surrounding cells. The endometrium responds to estrogen by growth of epithelium and connective tissue, and by forming other tissues necessary to receive a fertilized egg. *Sheldon, p. 433.*

9. **E.** *Haemophilus vaginalis* produces a grayish discharge with a disagreeable odor. It gives little inflammation of the underlying tissue, in contrast to candida (fungal infection) and trichomonas (protozoan). The diagnosis may be made by finding "clue cells" in the vaginal secretions (epithelial cells filled with bacteria). Herpes simplex and condyloma acuminatum are both viral infections. *Sheldon, p. 447.*

10. **E.** Epidemiologists have documented that there is a correlation between the risk of developing cervical cancer and the number of male sexual partners, the sexual promiscuity of these partners, and the age of the woman at the time of first intercourse. This indicates that cancer of the cervix behaves like a sexually transmitted disease. To support this concept, it has been established that close to 100% of patients with cervical cancer have evidence of prior HPV infection. *Sheldon, p. 449; Tamparo and Lewis, p. 110.*

11. **A.** Gonorrhea is the most frequently reported communicable disease in the United States. Pelvic inflammatory disease is the most common serious complication of gonorrhea and is considered a major public health problem. *Sheldon, p. 455.*

12. **D.** Tuberculosis is considered a disease not now eradicable. Currently, there are 8 to 10 million new cases and 2 to 3 million deaths per year worldwide. There is a great need for improved diagnostic testing, improved chemotherapy, vaccine, and better access to those affected. ***Sheldon, p. 50.***

13. **D.** The coagulation sequence begins with fibrinogen and ends with the formation of fibrin. Thrombin and calcium are essential cofactors. ***Sheldon, p. 505.***

14. **E.** The most common ectopic site is within one of the fallopian tubes, but ectopic implantation can occur in the abdominal cavity or the ovary. ***Tamparo and Lewis, p. 129.***

15. **D.** Cholesterol concentrations are below normal in hyperthyroidism, during increased levels of estrogen, and during malnutrition. ***Scanlon, p. 538.***

16. **A.** The hematocrit measures how much of the patient's blood is made up of red blood cells, an indication of how well the blood can transport oxygen to body tissues. ***Tamparo and Lewis, p. 401.***

17. **B.** Symptoms related to hypercalcemia include weak, brittle bones, joint pain, and the presence of kidney stones. ***Tamparo and Lewis, p. 278.***

18. **D.** O-negative blood is the universal donor type because type O blood lacks both the A and B antigen and therefore will not be agglutinated by any other blood type. ***Scanlon, p. 250.***

19. **B.** Collagen is a fibrous, insoluble protein in the connective tissue of skin, bone, ligaments, and cartilage. ***Taber's, p. 414.***

20. **B.** The ureters are tubes 10 to 12 inches long that carry urine to the bladder. ***Scanlon, p. 427.***

21. **D.** Yellow-brown urine usually contains bilirubin resulting from excessive destruction of RBCs, obstruction of the bile duct, or diminished function of the liver cells. ***Tamparo and Lewis, p. 54.***

22. **E.** Bilirubin enters the gallbladder and is excreted through the intestines. In the intestines, it is converted to a colorless compound called urobilinogen. ***Taber's, p. 2089.***

23. **C.** Warts are caused by infection from one of five possible papilloma viruses, each tending to infect different parts of the body. ***Tamparo and Lewis, p. 321.***

24. **B.** Insulin promotes the movement of glucose through cell membranes, lowering the blood glucose levels. ***Tamparo and Lewis, p. 268.***

25. **C.** Pediculosis is a skin infestation with lice, a parasitic insect. ***Tamparo and Lewis, p. 318.***

26. **B.** The liquid portion of clotted blood is called serum; the liquid portion of uncoagulated blood after centrifuging is plasma. ***Wedding and Toenjes, p. 132.***

27. **D.** Unlike the Living Will, this document allows another person to make decisions even if the illness is not terminal. The document is not in effect as long as the patient is able to make medical decisions. ***Frew, Lane, and Frew, p. 59.***

28. **B.** In 1988, Congress passed the Clinical Laboratory Improvement Amendment (CLIA), which regulates all human testing and applies to anyone who performs testing of human specimens for the diagnosis, prevention, or treatment of disease or health problems. This includes physicians who perform the most basic tests. In some states, MAs cannot perform venipuncture. Some states also regulate who can practice radiography procedures and protocol. ***Frew, Lane, and Frew, p. 708.***

29. **B.** Overtime compensation is a rate of not less than 1.5 times the regular rate of pay for hours worked over 40 hours in a workweek. ***Lane, Keenon, Coleman (eds.), p. 235.***

30. **E.** Some states require unlicensed health care personnel to have a permit or be registered with the state if they perform venipuncture, injections, allergy testing, or in some other way pierce human tissue. The ESR is considered a "waiver" test under the Clinical Laboratory Improvement Amendment of 1988 and able to be performed by the medical assistant in all states. *Lane, Keenon, Coleman (eds.), p. 280.*

31. **A.** The general rule is that employers do not have the right to see an employee's medical records without the employee's consent, unless the physician provides a pre-employment physical examination requested and paid for by the employer. *Lane, Keenon, Coleman (eds.), p. 32.*

32. **D.** A DEA registration certificate is always specific to a single site. Separate DEA registration certificates must be obtained if the physician dispenses controlled substances at different sites. Each DEA certificate is valid for 3 years. A separate certificate must be obtained if the physician dispenses and/or administers controlled substances at another hospital or office. *Lane, Medications, p. 31–34.*

33. **E.** Sixty days before the expiration of the DEA certificate, the DEA will send a renewal application. If the renewal application is not received within 45 days of the expiration date, it is the physician's responsibility to notify the DEA that the renewal has not been received. *Lane, Medications, p. 34.*

34. **B.** Only the physician is responsible for the explanation of medical procedures to the patient. The medical assistant prepares the consent forms; the medical assistant's signature is witness that the signature is that of the patient and no one else. *Lewis and Tamparo, p. 104.*

35. **E.** By law, patients have a right to access their records. Patients may be expected to make an appointment to obtain record copies and pay reproduction fees. Access should be withheld only when the law prohibits such access or when, in the physician's opinion, great harm would be done to the patient. *Lewis and Tamparo, p. 113.*

36. **D.** A licensed NP can function alone or under the supervision of an MD in a medical facility. An LPN works under the direct supervision of an MD or RN, as does the MA, RMA or CMA. The MLT works under the direct supervision of an MT or MD. A registered nurse also works under the direction of an MD. *Lewis and Tamparo, p. 29–30.*

37. **E.** Most states' statutes of frauds include a section on third-party payments for medical services, but to be binding, this agreement must be in the form of a contract and in writing with the third party's signature affixed to the agreement. *Lewis and Tamparo, p. 63.*

38. **A.** Although each of the negligent practices mentioned is a potential malpractice suit, failing to return a telephone call within a reasonable time could result in charges of abandonment, if patient harm resulted from the lack of care while waiting for the physician or office staff to return the call. *Lewis and Tamparo, p. 63.*

39. **C.** Defamation is spoken or written words that tend to injure another person's reputation and for which damages can be recovered. *Lewis and Tamparo, pp. 64–65.*

40. **C.** The statute of limitations begins at the occurrence of a negligence but can be further extended until after the discovery of an alleged negligence, which could be years later. *Lewis and Tamparo, p. 66.*

41. **B.** Employment in a corporation, HMO, or hospital does not guarantee professional liability coverage. Many employers or institutions carry insurance only on themselves or the institution, and not on the employees. In some cases, patients sue both the physician and the employee. If employees are covered by an employer's policy, the employees should be specifically named. Medical assistants who are not otherwise covered should purchase their own professional liability insurance. *Lewis and Tamparo, p. 67.*

42. **D.** A schedule II drug cannot be refilled. Only a DEA-registered physician can make the decision to sign an order for a new prescription. A patient who expresses a need for a narcotic analgesic should not be put off until the physician returns to town. The patient's condition could be serious and in need of immediate medical attention. Referring this patient to the physician on call permits the patient access to medical care and protects the physician from possible charges of abandonment. *Lewis and Tamparo, pp. 70–72.*

43. **E.** The physician should not send the remains to a mortician or perform an autopsy without authorization from the next of kin or other person responsible for funeral expenses. Funeral and financial arrangements cannot begin until a Certificate of Death is signed. An autopsy cannot be performed without a Certificate of Death. Many states require completion of the certificate in 24 to 48 hours. Death certificates should be completed and signed as quickly as possible as a courtesy to the family members. *Lewis and Tamparo, pp. 80–86.*

44. **E.** Reports of communicable and notifiable diseases called into to local health departments must include the patient's name, address, age, occupation, disease or suspected disease, date of the onset of the disease, and the person reporting the disease. The name of the patient's employer is not necessary. *Lewis and Tamparo, p. 86.*

45. **A.** By law, the information recorded must include the date of administration; the vaccine manufacturer and lot number; the name, address, and title (MD) of the person administering the vaccine; and any adverse events following the administration of the vaccine. Although many offices are requiring a signed informed consent form prior to administration, it is not required by law. *Lewis and Tamparo, pp. 86–87.*

46. **B.** The law regulates vaccinations of childhood: diphtheria, tetanus, and pertussis vaccine (DTP); pertussis vaccine; measles, mumps, and rubella vaccine (MMR); poliovirus vaccine, live, oral; and poliovirus vaccine inactivated. Tetanus Toxoid (TT) is not given as a childhood immunization but is used as a booster injection every 10 years throughout adulthood or as needed after an injury. *Lewis and Tamparo, pp. 86–87.*

47. **B.** All 50 states have laws governing the reporting of rape (a criminal offense), spousal rape, and other injuries resulting from the violence of another person. The majority of states have enacted legislation addressing elder abuse, and every state has laws defining child abuse and neglect reporting. In some states, failure to report elder or spousal abuse may result in misdemeanor charges. Few statutes relate to drug abuse other than the Controlled Substances Act; however, health professionals have a public duty to be alert to and do everything possible to prevent the increase of drug abuse. *Lewis and Tamparo, pp. 87–91.*

48. **D.** Good Samaritan statutes apply to situations in which the patient-physician relationship does not exist. The statute is a legal doctrine meant to encourage doctors and health care professionals to render emergency first aid to accident victims. Most of the laws, however, are very vague or unclear. *Lewis and Tamparo, p. 92.*

49. **E.** Informed consent implies an intentional and deliberate decision. The Doctrine of Informed Consent occurs when the patient gives permission to treat or refuses treatment after being told what a procedure is, how it is performed, the possible risks involved, the expected outcome, any alternative procedures or treatments, and the results if no treatment is given. Ideally every consent is informed (which is assumed in answer choices *A* to *D*); however, *E* involves a procedure that is considered beyond the usual patient understanding, and therefore, detailed information is necessary for rational decision making on the part of the patient. In this case, the patient should sign a "Refusal to Consent to Treatment" form. *Lewis and Tamparo, p. 97.*

50. **A.** Informed consent implies an intentional and deliberate decision. If this patient has more questions concerning what he has just consented to, he should be referred back to the physician immediately. Although informed consent does not imply that the patient is necessarily pleased with a recommendation and decision, it does imply that the patient thoroughly agrees with what he has consented to. The physician must be sure that the patient's hesitation is not due to a misunderstanding or a lack of understanding that could later turn into a lawsuit. Informed consent is a process that must be seen through to the end by the patient with his or her physician. *Lewis and Tamparo, pp. 97–104*.

51. **C.** A minor's legal guardian authorizes release of the child's records. Foster parents qualify as care providers appointed by the courts. *Lewis and Tamparo, pp. 99–100*.

52. **B.** Under OSHA rules, portable or secondary containers must be labeled in the same way as the original container. Common household soap and other common consumer products may not be labeled to indicate hazards of their use. *OSHA "Hazard Communication" Rule (29 CFR 1910.1200)*.

53. **A.** Under OSHA's "Hazardous Communication" ruling, employers are required to list all hazardous and toxic substances in the work place. Employers are required to provide employees a personal list of all substances and/or Material Data Safety Sheets within 5 days of employment. *OSHA "Hazard Communication" Rule (29 CFR 1910.1200)*

54. **E.** Interrupting the patient to clarify important points or focus on critical events is probing. *Frew, Lane, and Frew, p. 331*.

55. **B.** In nonverbal communication, messages can be sent without words. Nonverbal communication can be intentional or unintentional, such as in not making good eye contact. *Frew, Lane, and Frew, p. 56*.

56. **E.** Open-ended statements or questions encourage the patient to elaborate freely and unpredictably. *Frew, Lane, and Frew, p. 58*.

57. **C.** One should never assume the physician's role or go beyond the physician's guidelines or what he or she has revealed to the patient. The patient should be referred to the physician when it would be more appropriate for the physician to answer the question. *Frew, Lane, and Frew, p. 70*.

58. **E.** The medical assistant should call for assistance. If the medical assistant cannot gain the patient's cooperation, other personnel or family should assist immediately. With both the spill to clean and the patient to calm, more than one person is needed. *Lane, Medications, p. 187*.

59. **D.** Obsessions manifest as persistent thoughts. Compulsions are repetitive, ritualistic behavior in response to an obsession. *St. Anthony's Color-Coded ICD-9-CM Code Book for Physician Payment, p. 295*.

60. **E.** Hyperactivity or hyperkinetic syndrome in childhood commonly refers to manifestations of disturbed behavior in children, characterized by constant overactivity, inability to concentrate, and aggressiveness. Hyperkinetic activity usually disappears during adolescence. *Taber's, p. 930; St. Anthony's Color-Coded ICD-9-CM Code Book for Physician Payment, p. 291*.

61. **A.** Bipolar affective disorder is a disorder in which the patient exhibits both manic and depressive episodes. These alterations in mood are usually episodic and recurrent. *Taber's, pp. 229, 1165; St. Anthony's Color-Coded ICD-9-CM Code Book for Physician Payment, p. 287*.

62. **E.** An anthropometric measurement is a measure of body dimensions such as weight, height, and circumference. *Frew, Lane, and Frew, p. 359*.

63. **D.** The reflex or percussion hammer has a rubber, triangular-shaped head for testing neurologic reflexes such as in the tendons of the knee. *Frew, Lane, and Frew, p. 404*.

64. **B.** *Escherichia coli. Frew, Lane, and Frew, p. 773*.

65. **C.** Paroxysmal. *Gylys and Wedding, p. 126*.

66. **B.** Culdocentesis means a puncture in the posterior vaginal cul-de-sac to obtain material from the uterus or uterine tubes for examination. *Gylys and Wedding, p. 11.*

67. **A.** Hemolysis. *Gylys and Wedding, pp. 12, 189.*

68. **A.** "Basal" means basic, fundamental, or primary. *Taber's, p. 206.*

69. **E.** Polycythemia. *Taber's, p. 1552.*

70. **D.** Ankylodactylia. *Gylys and Wedding, pp. 213, 215.*

71. **C.** Interstitial. *Gylys and Wedding, p. 296.*

72. **B.** Hemiplegia is paralysis on one side of the body. *Gylys and Wedding, p. 326.*

73. **A.** Ataxia. *Gylys and Wedding, p. 326.*

74. **E.** The prefix "bi" refers to two; "diplo" means double; "semi" or "hemi" means half or partial; and "poly" means many. *Gylys and Wedding, p. 35.*

75. **A.** Cytology is the study of cells—their origin, structure, and function. *Gylys and Wedding, p. 44.*

76. **A.** The prefix "intra" refers to in or within, as does the prefix "endo." "Inter" refers to between. *Gylys and Wedding, pp. 34, 36.*

77. **B.** The abbreviation CA stands for cancer. *Gylys and Wedding, p. 382.*

78. **B.** Cerumen is the waxlike, soft brown secretion found in the ear canal. It is produced by modified sweat glands lining the external auditory canal. "Secretion" is used to describe substances produced by the glandular organs. "Excretion" is the elimination of waste products from the body. "Excrement" is a term usually limited to describing the elimination of feces. "Discharge" is the flowing away of pus, feces, urine, and so on. "Exudation" is the oozing of pathologic fluids, usually the result of inflammatory conditions. *Gylys and Wedding, p. 347.*

79. **A.** Alopecia. *Gylys and Wedding, pp. 65, 66.*

80. **A.** The loss of sound during phase II is called an auscultatory gap. *Lane, Keenon, Coleman (eds.), pp. 316–317.*

81. **D.** Laser, the acronym for *l*ight *a*mplification by *s*timulated *e*mission of *r*adiation, is a device that emits intense heat and power at close range. *Lane, Keenon, Coleman (eds.), p. 388.*

82. **E.** "Nullipara" is used to describe a woman who has not produced a viable offspring, regardless of the number of pregnancies. *Lane, Keenon, Coleman (eds.), p. 467.*

83. **D.** "Gravida" means pregnancy and "para" a pregnancy that results in a viable birth. *Lane, Keenon, Coleman (eds.), p. 467.*

84. **E.** Braxton Hicks' sign refers to painless, intermittent uterine contractions in the last trimester. *Lane, Keenon, Coleman (eds.), p. 473.*

85. **D.** The abbreviation "c/o" stands for "complains of." *Lane, Keenon, Coleman (eds.), p. 696.*

86. **A.** WNL is the abbreviation for within normal limits. *Lane, Keenon, Coleman (eds.), p. 698.*

87. **B.** The "+" means positive, slight trace, plus, excess, acid reaction, or slight reaction. *Lane, Keenon, Coleman (eds.), p. 731.*

88. **A.** Toxicity. *OSHA "Hazard Communication" Rule (29 CFR 1910. 1200).*

89. **E.** Teratogen. *OSHA "Hazard Communication" Rule (29 CFR 1910.1200).*

90. **A.** Necrosis is the local death of cells. It is derived from the Greek "nekros," meaning corpse. *Sheldon, p. 22.*

91. **C.** Hypoplasia is the incomplete development or underdevelopment of tissues or organs. *Taber's, p. 555.*

92. **A.** The most common cystic lesion affecting the vulva is the Bartholin's gland cyst or abscess. *Sheldon, p. 446.*

93. **C.** Homeostasis is the preservation of the balance of electrolytes and water that serves to maintain the constancy of the normal, internal environment. *Sheldon, p. 71.*

94. **C.** Hemorrhages as small as a pinhead are called petechiae. *Sheldon, p. 87.*

95. **E.** Any adverse mental or physical condition induced in a patient by effects of treatment by a physician is termed iatrogenic ("iatric" referring to physicians). A nosocomial infection is one that is acquired in a hospital. Idiopathic, on the other hand, refers to a condition without recognizable cause. *Tamparo and Lewis, pp. 22, 384.*

96. **A.** Seborrheic dermatitis is characterized by skin eruptions on areas of the scalp, face, or trunk that produce dry, moist, or greasy scales. *Tamparo and Lewis, p. 323.*

97. **D.** Psychoneurologic causes include fatigue, nervous tension, exhaustion, worry, excitement, and psychoneuroses. *Tamparo and Lewis, p. 245.*

98. **E.** Transcutaneous electrical nerve stimulation (TENS). *Tamparo and Lewis, p. 360.*

99. **B.** A disease resulting from unexpressed negative emotion is psychosomatic. The symptoms of the disease are very real, but the cause cannot be traced to any real underlying pathology other than negative emotions. *Tamparo and Lewis, p. 369.*

100. **A.** Migraine headaches are accompanied by changes in cerebral blood flow, presumably caused by vasoconstriction and subsequent vasodilation of cerebral-cranial arteries. What initiates the process, however, is not known. Susceptibility to migraine headaches may be hereditary. *Tamparo and Lewis, p. 245.*

101. **C.** Both angiography and cholangiography require the use of a contrast media. Many patients are allergic to one or more components of contrast media (e.g., iodine). A pneumoencephalogram involves the injection of air into the brain ventricles. *Frew, Lane, and Frew, pp. 417, 855–856.*

102. **D.** The appointment schedule should never come between physician access and an ill patient. If the patient thinks an illness is urgent, office personnel must assume the same urgency. *Lane, Keenon, Coleman (eds.), p. 13.*

103. **B.** Sound tone signaling is not a necessary feature; however, an automated appointment system must be able to track activity, dates, and times and to print out schedules. *Lane, Keenon, Coleman (eds.), p. 13.*

104. **B.** If nipples are cracked or there are signs of infection, the patient should be seen. *Lane, Keenon, Coleman (eds.), p. 473.*

105. **D.** The best system is the one that works right for the practice. As a practice evolves or changes, so should the appointment book. *Lane, Keenon, Coleman (eds.), p. 9.*

106. **E.** Personal information beyond office address and telephone number, birth date, birth place, and marital status should not be included. Names of organizations, agencies, and titles should be spelled out. Publication citations should not be underlined, but the genus and species of microorganisms and Latin words should. *Fordney and Diehl, p. 471.*

107. **B.** Foreign expressions that are not considered a part of the English language should be underscored or word processed in italics. *Fordney and Diehl, p. 39.*

108. **E.** The days of the week and months of the year should not be abbreviated. Known chemical and mathematical abbreviations should be written in a combination of both uppercase and lowercase letters without periods. *Fordney and Diehl, pp. 6, 8.*

109. **B.** The genus but not the species should be abbreviated after the genus has been used once in the text. *Fordney and Diehl, p. 173.*

110. **B.** Hemoglobin is abbreviated in upper and lowercase as Hgb. *Fordney and Diehl, p. 177.*

111. **B.** "et al." is the abbreviation for "and elsewhere" or "and others." *Fordney and Diehl, p. 216.*

112. E. "Sic," meaning "thus," is used to emphasize that an unlikely looking expression or spelling is not a typographic error but is written as meant. "E.g." means "for example" and "i.e.," "that is." "Ibid." means in the same place, and "op.cit." means in the work cited. ***Fordney and Diehl, p. 216.***

113. A. Cul-de-sac requires no diacritical marks. ***Fordney and Diehl, p. 438.***

114. E. Simple fractions should not be used with the percent symbol. It is acceptable to describe temperature without the degree symbol if it is not dictated or is not represented on the keyboard. ***Fordney and Diehl, pp. 448–449.***

115. C. When a quoted sentence stands alone or is at the beginning of a sentence, quotation marks are used outside the closing quotation mark. A question mark is placed outside a closing quotation mark if the entire sentence is in the form of a question. A question mark goes inside a closing quotation mark if only the quoted material is a question. It is proper to use question marks to indicate a series of questions or to show doubt. ***Fordney and Diehl, p. 412.***

116. A. Two spaces are required after a colon, except when used with the time of day, when expressing a dilute solution, or to separate volumes and pages in bibliographies. ***Fordney and Diehl, p. 412.***

117. E. One space is required after an initial or single letter, except when used to end a sentence. ***Fordney and Diehl., p. 412.***

118. B. All queries to the author are enclosed in a circle to distinguish them from manuscript material. The "?" or "Qu" are two symbols used to question the author. ***Frew, Lane, and Frew, p. 135.***

119. D. Each page of 200 to 250 words can be read in 2 minutes. A 20-page presentation would take approximately 40 minutes to deliver. ***Frew, Lane, and Frew, p. 149.***

120. C. The *Index Medicus* is an index to current medical articles in journals catalogued by author and subject. ***Lane, Keenon, Coleman (eds.), p. 42.***

121. C. Omissions in quoted material are indicated by three periods with one space between each. The writer's insertions within quoted material are added in brackets. ***Lane, Keenon, Coleman (eds.), p. 43.***

122. E. The bibliography should include the author or editor, title of the book, name of the publisher, the city of the publisher, and the year of publication. The state is usually not required, unless the city name would be unknown to most readers. ***Lane, Keenon, Coleman (eds.), p. 43.***

123. B. Additional copies are called reprints. ***Lane, Keenon, Coleman (eds.), p. 43.***

124. A. Medline is the biomedical referencing program online with the National Library of Medicine. ***Frew, Lane, and Frew, pp. 220–221.***

125. D. " .WK1" is the extension for a worksheet created by the Lotus 1-2-3 spreadsheet program. The other extensions are created by database software programs. ***Walter, p. 80.***

126. D. At 12 characters per inch (cpi) × 11 inches wide in the landscape format, the total cpi would be 132 characters. After subtracting 12 cpi for the right margin and 12 for the left margin (total 24), the approximate number of spaces available in a uniform font would be 108 cpi. ***Walter, p. 128.***

127. B. WordPerfect V-Codes are used to compose special language accent symbols as well as symbols for scientific writing and foreign languages. They are created by typing Control-V and then selecting the proper numbers or keys from the list of V-Codes. ***Walter, p. 132.***

128. A. WordPerfect is a word processing program and does not feature a calculator pad for numbers calculation. ***Walter, p. 148.***

129. E. Spreadsheets are tables of numbers. A spreadsheet can show how many dollars are earned or spent, how much inventory is on hand, and how people scored on a certification examination. ***Walter, p. 172.***

130. **B.** The standard laser printer prints 300 dots per inch and is called desktop quality because it is capable of printing quality newsletters. *Walter, p. 34.*

131. **E.** Collection rates of 95% to 98% are considered excellent. Collection rates vary according to the type of practice, and a 90% collection rate would be considered a good rate. *Frew, Lane, and Frew, p. 256.*

132. **C.** Capital equipment usually refers to purchases of equipment costing more than a set amount ($100, $300, $500) and lasting a long time (items that are not expendable). *Frew, Lane, and Frew, p. 266.*

133. **C.** If an error involves only two digits, in this case $90, and the discrepancy is divisible by 9, the first thing to do is look for a transposition of digits. *Frew, Lane, and Frew, pp. 269–270.*

134. **E.** A payment from the petty cash fund requires a written receipt. A special form, called a petty cash voucher, or an actual purchase receipt should be used to verify the expenditure. A reimbursement voucher would be used if the employee used his or her own money. *Frew, Lane, and Frew, pp. 272–273.*

135. **C.** Every 3 months, an employer must complete and submit a quarterly federal tax return. *Frew, Lane, and Frew, p. 278.*

136. **A.** Professional fees, laboratory fees, and recovery of bad debts are considered income on the chart of accounts. In cash accounting, the accounts receivable account is not active on a day-to-day basis. The category is kept separate to represent an asset to bankers or investors and to indicate that additional monies have been earned but not yet received. *Lane, Keenon, Coleman (eds.), pp. 124–125.*

137. **B.** On the balance sheet, the accounts receivable is considered a business asset, as it represents income (money earned but not yet realized). *Lane, Keenon, Coleman (eds.), p. 141.*

138. **B.** If at the end of any month the total undeposited taxes are $500 or more but less than $3000, the taxes must be deposited within 15 days after the end of the month. There are no exceptions to this rule. *Lane, Keenon, Coleman (eds.), p. 147.*

139. **B.** At year end, employers must disburse W-2 forms to employees. The physician keeps one copy and the remaining copies (W-3 forms) are forwarded to the Social Security Administration. At the same time, 1099 forms are disbursed to independent contractors and a 1096, summary of 1099s, is mailed to the IRS. *Lane, Keenon, Coleman (eds.), pp. 152–155.*

140. **A.** A third-party payer is any person, insurance company, or government agent other than the patient or the patient's family who pays the patient's account. *Frew, Lane, and Frew, p. 248.*

141. **C.** Travelers' checks are the same as cash and better than out-of-town personal checks, unless the medical assistant is acquainted with the patient. Preprinted personal checks are safer than blank or counter checks. Accepting an endorsed insurance check, money order, or tax refund check is accepting a third-party check and often requires change be paid back to the patient. *Lane, Keenon, Coleman (eds.), p. 101.*

142. **C.** Accounts payable records include disbursements, payroll, and petty cash. *Lane, Keenon, Coleman (eds.), p. 79.*

143. **B.** The recommended way is to post collection receipts into a separate income account to reflect the collection of a bad debt and not to run collection recoveries through the normal accounts receivable account. *Lane, Keenon, Coleman (eds.), pp. 129–130.*

144. **D.** Some accounts are best kept by a company name. In the case of a workers' compensation case, where a patient's record should be kept separate from non–case-related medical services rendered in the past or future, the charges can be entered on the company ledger card, including the name of the patient treated. *Lane, Keenon, Coleman (eds.), p. 84.*

145. **B.** Once an account has been turned over to a collection agency, no further payment arrangements with the patient are made. If payments are mistakenly mailed to the practice, the collection company should be notified and the check endorsed and sent on to the collection agency. *Lane, Keenon, Coleman (eds.), p. 85.*

146. **E.** Only the percentage amount paid to the practice is reinstated and not the percentage retained by the agency *Lane, Keenon, Coleman (eds.), pp. 87–88.*

147. **E.** Both the deposit entry and the account card payment must be reversed. A patient check returned by the bank must be subtracted from the checkbook and reentered onto the patient's account card. *Lane, Keenon, Coleman (eds.), p. 90.*

148. **A.** The coordination of benefits is the sharing of insurance costs when a patient has more than one insurance plan. One plan will be designated as the primary provider and the other plan as the secondary provider. *Frew, Lane, and Frew, p. 286.*

149. **A.** The patient is responsible for the difference between the Medicare Fee Schedule and the 80% Medicare payment. *Frew, Lane, and Frew, pp. 289–290.*

150. **B.** For crossover, dual Medicare-Medicaid recipients, Medicare is billed first, then the balance is transferred to the Medicaid office for further processing. *Frew, Lane, and Frew, p. 290.*

151. **A.** Emergency services will be covered provided authorization is obtained within 48 hours of the emergency. Noncovered services include those that are cosmetic, experimental, or not medically necessary. All authorized services within a plan must be approved in advance by the primary care physician or the plan managers. *Frew, Lane, and Frew, p. 301.*

152. **E.** The medical assistant should ask for the carrier address and telephone number on the card. *Frew, Lane, and Frew, p. 302.*

153. **D.** Unlike HMOs in the traditional sense, PPO enrollees retain coverage when services are secured from noncontracted providers. The patient may go to a nonparticipating doctor if he or she chooses but will still be responsible for a deductible and copayment, which may be at a higher rate to the patient. *Gylys, 203.*

154. **D.** If the patient is a managed-care Medicaid recipient and the verification system states he or she is a member of an HMO, then, except in an emergency, prior authorization is minimally necessary, if the patient can be treated outside of the HMO at all. This patient should be referred back to his or her HMO. *Gylys, pp. 202–203.*

155. **A.** A Preferred Provider Organization is a formal agreement among health care providers to treat a specific patient population at a discount. *Gylys, p. 203.*

156. **D.** The patient may go to a nonparticipating doctor, but the fee will not be covered at the same rate. The patient is responsible for deductibles and copayments. *Gylys, p. 203.*

157. **C.** Medicare is the payer of last resort. The exception is Medicare is billed as the primary payer when the patient's only other coverage is a Medigap plan or Medicaid. *Gylys, p. 211.*

158. **A.** Medicaid services include inpatient and outpatient medical and surgical care, laboratory services, x-ray, dental, and family planning services, care in a skilled nursing facility, and early diagnostic screening and treatment for children under the age of 21. Medicaid will not pay for not medically necessary services, such as an annual physical examination. *Gylys, p. 193.*

159. **B.** Enrollees in the Federal Employee plan have been issued new cards containing a picture of the United States in the upper-right corner. The older cards contained the words "Government-Wide Service Benefit Plan." Enrollees are federal government employees. *Lane, Keenon, Coleman (eds.), p. 160.*

160. C. The staff model is a type of closed HMO. HMOs usually require their enrollees to receive care only from physicians who belong to the HMO. If a referral to a specialist is needed, the HMO doctors decide which specialist is to be seen and under what circumstances. ***Lane, Keenon, Coleman (eds.), p. 186.***

161. D. Team surgeries are highly complex procedures, often of different specialties. Such circumstances may be identified by each participating physician with the modifier "-66" or the modifier code 09966. A report must accompany the claim for payment. ***Lane, Keenon, Coleman (eds.), p. 717.***

162. C. Invasion of privacy is the unauthorized disclosure of information regarding the patient to a third party. ***Frew, Lane, and Frew, p. 36.***

163. E. The right to refuse treatment is encorporated in the Patient's Bill of Rights as declared by the Joint Commission on Accreditation of Health Care Organizations. ***Frew, Lane, and Frew, pp. 44–45.***

164. E. After signing a donor card, all a person has to do is tear up the organ donor card and notify the family that he or she has had a change of mind. ***Frew, Lane, and Frew, p. 48.***

165. A. Always follow the "10-day rule," which consists of scheduling elective abdominal x-ray examinations on girls and women of childbearing age (10 to 50 years old) during the 10 days after their last menstrual period. This eliminates the possibility of performing an abdominal x-ray examination on a patient who is unaware of her pregnancy. ***Frew, Lane, and Frew, p. 869.***

166. A. An electronic message service is a system that records messages on a computer system. Messages can then be retrieved by using a special code number, calling the operator, or obtaining a printout at a terminal point. ***Frew, Lane, and Frew, p. 181.***

167. B. Calls to be put through immediately to the physician include emergencies and other physicians. ***Lane, Keenon, Coleman (eds.), p. 15.***

168. D. Married women are indexed by surname, followed by given name, then middle name or initial. The husband's given and middle names are noted parenthetically. ***Frew, Lane, and Frew, pp. 108–109.***

169. E. The initial database includes the patient's complete health and family and social history, the physical examination, the physician's assessment, available patient profiles, and available laboratory data. A separate problem list is a numbered list of past and present medical, social, environmental, and psychologic problems that is derived from the initial database. Progress notes are listed separately during subsequent visits. ***Frew, Lane, and Frew, p. 323.***

170. B. Specific additions and corrections are made by drawing a single line through the error and writing the correction above it, indicated by a carat. ***Frew, Lane, and Frew, p. 335.***

171. D. Inclusions of procedures that were not done are potentially damaging. If an entry is made in the wrong record or entered in the record incorrectly, the error is identified by a single line through the entry with an explanation of the error placed immediately above it. ***Frew, Lane, and Frew, p. 88.***

172. A. The Office of Subpeonas should be asked to forward the subpeona before any information is given out. ***Frew, Lane, and Frew, p. 89.***

173. A. Color coding is useful for quick identification without cross reference, such as in a practice with multiple physicians. ICD-9 codes are too numerous and varied to remember without cross reference. Allergies are too critical and specific to be generalized by color. Color coding past due accounts is recommended, but this should be done on the patient's ledger card rather than the medical history. ***Lane, Keenon, Coleman (eds.), p. 19.***

174. **E.** Certain information must be reported, with or without the authorization of the patient. These include reporting communicable diseases required by law to the health department and information about the commission of a crime. In addition, medical information on a "need to know" basis about a patient can be released in an emergency without the patient's permission. *Lane, Keenon, Coleman (eds.), p. 32.*

175. **C.** Calendar notations of scientific meeting should include the inclusive dates the physician intends to be away from the office, title and purpose of the meeting, and the place of the meeting. *Frew, Lane, and Frew, pp. 150–151.*

176. **C.** The patient's name and telephone number should be obtained as early as possible because the patient may be cut off. In an emergency, the patient's location is also very important. *Frew, Lane, and Frew, p. 165.*

177. **D.** The medical assistant should ask the patient if it is all right to place him or her on hold. Waiting for a response gives the caller the option to hold or call back. *Frew, Lane, and Frew, p. 180.*

178. **D.** Schedule II drugs may not be refilled unless they are written and presented to the pharmacist, except in an emergency. *Lane, Medications, p. 41.*

179. **C.** Schedule II drugs must be presented to the pharmacist in written form, except in a bona fide emergency. Prescription facsimile (fax) copies are not an acceptable written form, again except in a bona fide emergency. Even in an emergency, the amount dispensed must be limited to the emergency period and the written order received by the pharmacy within 72 hours. *Lane, Medications, p. 41.*

180. **E.** In cases of sensitive material, "Confidential" is typed on the front and on the envelope. *Frew, Lane, and Frew, p. 139.*

181. **D.** On-arrival notations are typed two to four lines below the last entry on the envelope. *Lane, Keenon, Coleman (eds.), p. 38.*

182. **C.** The standard business envelope is the No. 10 envelope. *Frew, Lane, and Frew, p. 138.*

183. **A.** Everything in the address is capitalized and all punctuation is eliminated. *Frew, Lane, and Frew, pp. 138, 139.*

184. **D.** The word "enclosure" is typed two lines below the reference initials, and the number of enclosures specified. *Frew, Lane, and Frew, pp. 129–130.*

185. **B.** When establishing priorities for incoming mail, letters take precedence. Professional letters take precedence over letters not directly involved in patient care. *Frew, Lane, and Frew, p. 140.*

186. **C.** The medical assistant may sign patient notifications. The physician must sign his or her own patient correspondence, advice to patients, referral and consultations reports to colleagues, letters to professional associations, and medical reports to insurance companies. *Frew, Lane, and Frew, p. 133.*

187. **C.** Signature stamps may be used to endorse checks and for completing office-generated forms. *Frew, Lane, and Frew, pp. 133, 299.*

188. **B.** Certified mail, return receipt requested, provides proof that mail was delivered and received. The return receipt should be kept in the x-ray film log for tracking any missing films. *Lane, Keenon, Coleman (eds.), p. 36.*

189. **E.** When multiple procedures are performed on the same day or at the same session, the major procedure or service is reported first. Any secondary procedures are identified with the modifier "-51." *CPT-94, p. 91; Lane, Keenon, Coleman (eds.), p. 717.*

190. **E.** Each procedure code involves a 90-day postoperative global fee period. *Lane, Keenon, Coleman (eds.), p. 716.*

191. **A.** No modifiers are required because the second surgery occurred after the 90-day global fee period of the prior surgery. *Lane, Keenon, Coleman (eds.), p. 716.*

192. **C.** The ophthalmologist uses the modifier "-54" to bill for the surgical care only. *CPT-94, p. 92.*

193. **D.** The optometrist uses the modifier "-55" to report that the service rendered is postoperative care only. *CPT-94, p. 92.*

194. **B.** The modifier "-54" designates surgical care only and is required first because the claim is priced according to the surgical and postoperative percentage for the CPT-4 code 66984. Modifier "-79" designates a procedure unrelated to the original procedure and is ranked second in importance to modifier "-54." LT further differentiates the surgery from the original surgery. If the "-79" and "LT" were missing, the claims could be denied. *CPT-94, pp. 92, 94.*

195. **C.** This circumstance is reported by adding modifier "-25" to the appropriate level of service since the examination was not one that resulted in a decision to perform surgery, but was a separate same-day procedure. *CPT-94, p. 8.*

196. **B.** Usually in problems of high severity requiring admission, the physician typically spends 70 minutes at the bedside and on the unit. When this service is prolonged, it is identified by adding the modifier "-21" to the E/M code. *CPT-94, pp. 8, 28.*

197. **C.** When multiple procedures are performed on the same day or at the same session, the major procedure or service may be reported as listed without a modifier. The secondary additional procedures may be identified by adding the modifier "-51" or by the use of the separate five-digit modifier code 09951. Code "-50" is incorrect because it designates a bilateral procedure. *CPT-94, p. 91.*

198. **A.** Modifiers indicate that a standard procedure has been altered by a particular circumstance but has not changed the definition of the code. Modifiers have a direct impact on how claims are processed and paid by third-party payers. *Frew, Lane, and Frew, p. 306; Lane, Keenon, Coleman, p. 717.*

199. **B.** E codes provide a supplementary classification of external causes of injury or poisoning. *Lane, Keenon, Coleman (eds.), p. 194.*

200. **D.** Under the major surgical global package, an initial consultation can be submitted as a separate payment. *Lane, Keenon, Coleman (eds.), p. 716.*

201. **A.** The sensitivity control adjusts the voltage (height) of the standardization mark. *Frew, Lane, and Frew, p. 841.*

202. **A.** Lead V_1 is the first lead placed at the fourth intercostal space at the right of the sternum (right sternal border). *Frew, Lane, and Frew, p. 842.*

203. **B.** The rhythm strip is the same as lead II. *Frew, Lane, and Frew, p. 842.*

204. **A.** Sinus rhythm is measured on the horizontal axis. The P-P measures atrial rate and the R-R ventricular rate. In normal sinus rhythm, the P-P and R-R rates are exactly the same and the PR interval remains constant. *Lane, Keenon, Coleman (eds.), p. 502.*

205. **D.** Right ventricular hypertrophy is diagnosed when the R wave is equal to or larger than the S wave in lead V_1 accompanied by a right-axis deviation. A right axis can be recognized either by a QRS complex that is predominantly negative in lead I or by one in which the R wave and S wave have approximately equal voltages. *Lane, Keenon, Coleman (eds.), p. 509.*

206. **A.** Atrial arrhythmias may occur in healthy hearts although atrial flutter and fibrillation are usually associated with heart disease. Junctional tachycardia occurs in the presence of heart disease or digitalis toxicity. All rapid ventricular rhythms create emergency situations and are usually associated with heart disease. *Lane, Keenon, Coleman (eds.), p. 512.*

207. **B.** A ventricular premature contraction (VPC) is a beat that arrives early in the cardiac cycle, has no P wave of its own, and displays a wide and bizarre QRS complex. In an atrial premature contraction (APC), the P wave records different from the sinus P wave and the QRS complex resembles that of a normal cardiac rhythm. The junctional premature contraction records an inverted P wave that precedes a normal QRS complex. Although aberrations can produce a bizarre QRS complex in both APCs and JPCs, P waves are still present. *Lane, Keenon, Coleman (eds.), p. 512.*

208. **D.** Potassium helps regulate water retention and acid-base balance and is of significant importance to persons taking diuretics ("fluid pills"). *Frew, Lane, and Frew, p. 515.*

209. **C.** High iron sources include liver, egg yolks, beans, and whole grain cereals. *Frew, Lane, and Frew, p. 534.*

210. **D.** Nagele's rule: estimated date of confinement (EDC) = first day of last menstrual period + 7 days − 3 months + 1 year. *Lane, Keenon, Coleman (eds.), p. 467.*

211. **E.** The vastus lateralis is the largest and most accessible muscle area for subcutaneous self-injection of insulin and is the area of choice for patient instruction. At home, the patient will rotate injection sites according to a personalized injection log. *Lane, Medications, p. 252.*

212. **B.** In measles, papules appear on the oral mucosa by the second or third day of clinical symptoms. These are small red spots with bluish-white centers on the oral mucosa, particularly in the region opposite the molars. *Tamparo and Lewis, p. 41.*

213. **B.** A +1 pulse is difficult to palpate; is weak and thready; and is easy to obliterate with slight pressure. A normal pulse is easy to palpate and not easily obliterated. As the pulse deficit was measured only one time, it could be due to the difficulty palpating the radial pulse. *Frew, Lane, and Frew, p. 352.*

214. **D.** (9/5 × 37) + 32 = 98.6. *Frew, Lane, and Frew, p. 350.*

215. **D.** The pulse pressure is the difference between the systolic and diastolic pressures. *Frew, Lane, and Frew, p. 357.*

216. **A.** Orthostatic hypotension occurs when a person quickly changes from a supine to an upright position or stands for a prolonged period of time. *Frew, Lane, and Frew, p. 357.*

217. **E.** The pulse deficit is the difference between the apical and radial pulses. When arrhythmias are suspected, the pulse deficit should be determined. *Lane, Keenon, Coleman (eds.), p. 312.*

218. **D.** 1 kg = 2.2 lb; 85 × 2.2 = 187 lb. The patient's weight for her age and height should be approximately 143 lb. *Frew, Lane, and Frew, p. 360.*

219. **A.** The newest technique for measuring body temperature is the infrared tympanic thermometer, which can record body temperature in 3 seconds. *Frew, Lane, and Frew, p. 348.*

220. **C.** A difference of 5 to 10 mm Hg is normal. *Frew, Lane, and Frew, p. 378.*

221. **D.** Information regarding the clarity of the maxillary sinuses can be obtained in a dark room by means of a strong light placed inside the mouth with the sinuses being observed through the face. The other sinuses must be examined radiographically with or without the injection of a radiopaque medium. *Frew, Lane, and Frew, pp. 405, 860.*

222. **A.** All tests are used to examine the various cranial nerves. The patient is asked to identify common odors with the eyes closed, to test the olfactory (smell) nerve. *Frew, Lane, and Frew, p. 416.*

223. **E.** Gelfoam is absorbable gelatin sponge, U.S.P. It is a local hemostatic agent that gives a good surface for and aids in clot formation. *Frew, Lane, and Frew, p. 558.*

224. **D.** The sciatic nerve descends, under cover of the gluteus maximus, between the greater trochanter and the ischial tuberosity, and should never be a site for injections. The upper and lateral quadrant of the buttock and the anterior part of the gluteal region are relatively avascular and free of major nerves. An alternative site for injections is the triangular area bounded by the anterior superior iliac crest, and the greater trochanter. *Frew, Lane, and Frew, p. 570.*

225. **B.** Patients who are allergic to iodine should not come in contact with iodine-based antiseptics such as Betadine, Isodine, and Prepodyne. *Frew, Lane, and Frew, p. 600.*

226. **C.** The skin is cleansed in a circular motion, working from the site outward and passing over an area only once. The drain is not touched or cleansed unless the physician gives the order to do so. Wound edges should be left untouched and may be covered with a 4 × 4 sterile gauze for extra protection during cleansing. *Frew, Lane, and Frew, pp. 618, 646.*

227. **D.** Sutures in the lower extremities and over large joints should be removed between the 7th and 10th days. *Frew, Lane, and Frew, p. 634.*

228. **D.** Once the surgical site is made ready by skin prepping and applying a fenestrated drape, sterile instruments and materials can be exchanged between the operative field and the sterile field on the tray stand. *Frew, Lane, and Frew, p. 636.*

229. **C.** Arthroscopy is the examination of a joint using an arthroscope. Arthrometry is the measuring of joints; arthroplasty, the surgical repair of joints; pneumoarthrography, radiographic examination with air; and orthoscopy, the examination of corneal refraction used in ocular examinations. *Gylys and Wedding, p. 223.*

230. **E.** In this procedure, pieces of the prostate gland are removed through a cystoscope, which is inserted into the prostate gland via the urethra. A suprapubic or retropubic prostatectomy incision is made on the lower abdominal wall. The perineal site is the site of entry for a radical prostatectomy. *Gylys and Wedding, p. 246.*

231. **A.** A patient is placed in the knee-chest position for a culdoscopic examination. The culdoscope is inserted into the vagina and then into the pelvis through a small incision in the posterior fornix. *Taber's, p. 475.*

232. **B.** Paracentesis is the surgical puncture of a cavity for the aspiration of fluid. In peritoneal dialysis, fluid is introduced into the abdominal cavity by means of a catheter and then, after a period of time, is drained. Gastric lavage is the washing of the contents of the intestine. Cisternal puncture is used to remove cerebrospinal fluid and sternal puncture is used to remove bone marrow. *Gylys and Wedding, p. 351.*

233. **C.** Because of its accessibility and the thinness of its compacta, the sternum can be easily punctured and marrow aspirated for study. *Gylys and Wedding, p. 388.*

234. **B.** One should assist the patient into a comfortable position with the arm at heart level. Having the arm above heart level may produce a falsely low reading. The cuff should be positioned 1 to 2 inches above the antecubital space. The stethoscope should not be placed under the cuff. *Lane, Keenon, Coleman (eds.), p. 318.*

235. **A.** Systolic pressure in the popliteal artery is usually 10 to 40 mm Hg higher than in the brachial artery; the diastolic pressure is usually the same as in the brachial artery. *Lane, Keenon, Coleman (eds.), p. 319.*

236. **E.** The ratio of liquid (10% formalyn or normal saline) to specimen is ideally 20:1. *Lane, Keenon, Coleman (eds.), p. 381.*

237. **D.** A 1-inch border around a sterile field on a sterile tray is considered unsterile, because this area may have become contaminated during the setup of the tray. *Lane, Keenon, Coleman (eds.), p. 383.*

238. **E.** Paper products should not be used for a barrier on the patient. Laser-beam flash fire on the paper could burn the patient's skin. *Lane, Keenon, Coleman (eds.), p. 388.*

239. **D.** Antiseptic technique includes the use of sterile products such as sterile saline. *Lane, Keenon, Coleman (eds.), p. 392.*

240. **A.** Tape is removed by pulling it toward the wound, peeling the edges by holding the skin taut and pushing it away from the tape. Pushing the skin away from the tape is less traumatic than pulling the tape from the skin. *Lane, Keenon, Coleman (eds.), p. 392.*

241. **E.** Bandaging is begun at the distal end while holding the roll upward and close to the part being bandaged. The bandage is unrolled as the body part is wrapped and each turn is overlapped by one-half to one-third the width of the bandage. *Lane, Keenon, Coleman (eds.), p. 395.*

242. **D.** Heat is applied to relieve pain, congestion, muscle spasms, and inflammation in an area by increasing the blood supply. *Lane, Keenon, Coleman (eds.), p. 398.*

243. **A.** Septic abortion refers to an abortion that results in maternal infection characterized by fever, chills, and abdominal pain. If treatment is delayed, the condition progresses to septicemia and septic shock. *Lane, Keenon, Coleman (eds.), p. 470.*

244. **B.** Any doubtful reaction to the tine test should be rechecked by a Mantoux test before ordering a follow-up chest x-ray examination. *Lane, Medications, p. 198.*

245. **E.** The result is considered positive if there is induration (raised area) at the test site. *Lane, Medications, p. 199.*

246. **C.** The patient is positioned lying down with the head turned right so that the medication flows away from the nose, or is seated with the head tilted backward. *Lane, Medications, p. 215.*

247. **D.** In posterior rhinoscopy, the back part of the nasal cavity is inspected by inserting a mirror into the mouth and pharynx. *Taber's, 1722; Frew, Lane, and Frew, p. 405.*

248. **C.** A simple reflex arc involves two nerves and one synapse. The stimulus sends an impulse along a sensory nerve that is relayed to a motor nerve by synapse. The stimulus is a tap or stretch and is not painful. This reflex occurs while the brain is just becoming aware of the tape and needs no thought for the motor response. *Taber's, p. 1686.*

249. **E.** If a bandage is applied too tightly or for a prolonged period, tissue damage may occur. *Taber's, p. 201.*

250. **D.** If infection develops, one should treat as for any other wound, including tetanus prophylaxis or booster as required. *Taber's, p. 239.*

251. **A.** In operations on the palm of the hand or sole of the foot, it is advisable to scrub with warm water and tincture of green soap and then rinse. *Taber's, p. 559.*

252. **B.** One should not attempt to lure an insect from the ear canal with a bright light, as this could stimulate the insect to crawl deeper. Bland oil should be dropped in and the insect floated out. In the case of a solid foreign body, however, oil or water should not be used. *Taber's, p. 597.*

253. **A.** Impetigo is highly contagious and antibiotics are essential. Patients must be seen. A thorough cleansing of the lesions is necessary two to three times a day. *Tamparo and Lewis, p. 318.*

254. **B.** Furuncles are cleansed with soap and water, and hot, wet compresses are applied. *Tamparo and Lewis, p. 318.*

255. **C.** Adenocarcinoma of the endometrium commonly occurs in postmenopausal women. The typical patient is an obese, diabetic, hypertensive women who has never had children. Estrogens for the relief of menopausal symptoms may increase the risk. *Sheldon, p. 452.*

256. **B.** Because the Pap smear is not a reliable detector of endometrial carcinoma, aspiration biopsies of the endometrium are performed as an office procedure on an annual or semiannual basis. *Sheldon, p. 452.*

257. **C.** Tincture of benzoin or Mastisol is applied to the skin a thin layer of liquid protectant to enhance sticking of the tape and help protect the skin. *Lane, Keenon, Coleman (eds.), p. 392.*

258. **E.** Timing is critical. Irreversible brain damage can occur within 4 to 5 minutes if oxygen is not restored to the cerebral circulation. *Lane, Keenon, Coleman (eds.), p. 668.*

259. **B.** The correct pressure point to compress for control of bleeding of the upper arm, shoulder, and lateral chest is the subclavian vein. *Lane, Keenon, Coleman (eds.), p. 670.*

260. **E.** Blood oozing from the site indicates either capillary bleeding or that the bleeding is stopping on its own. Firm direct pressure or application of a pressure dressing and bandage should control the bleeding. If the bleeding is not severe, ice is applied to the area and the affected limb elevated to decrease blood flow to the injury. *Lane, Keenon, Coleman (eds.), p. 671.*

261. **E.** Immediate management is immerse in ice water or wrap in ice-cold towels. *Lane, Keenon, Coleman (eds.), p. 671.*

262. **D.** Immediate management for bone fractures is immobilization, control of bleeding, and stabilization while waiting for transport to the hospital. *Lane, Keenon, Coleman (eds.), pp. 671–674.*

263. **D.** Removal of stomach contents is best performed either by stimulating the gag reflex or by giving the patient syrup of ipecac. Oral salt solutions can be absorbed by the body and be lethal in some cases. *Lane, Keenon, Coleman (eds.), p. 672.*

264. **C.** Immediate management includes protecting the patient, maintaining an open airway, and interfering as little as possible. Transfer to a hospital is usually not necessary unless the patient has another seizure. Status epilepticus are rapid, successive seizures that constitute a medical emergency requiring rapid intervention. *Lane, Keenon, Coleman (eds.), p. 673.*

265. **B.** The chin-lift airway technique, head tilt, is not to be used in patients with neck or spinal injuries. *Taber's, p. 368.*

266. **C.** Blood stains are removed by first soaking in cold water, then washing in a lukewarm soap solution. *Taber's, p. 125.*

267. **E.** Each slide, cup, or tube must be individually labeled with the patient's name. The laboratory requisition must also include the patient's name. *Frew, Lane, and Frew, p. 718.*

268. **C.** Spraying the cytology fixative too close to the slide may permanently damage the cells. *Lane, Keenon, Coleman (eds.), p. 443.*

269. **D.** Nonmotile forms of *T. vaginalis* are easily confused with white blood cells. *Lane, Keenon, Coleman (eds.), p. 448.*

270. **B.** Ultrasound is used to assess the size, age, and sex of the fetus, to diagnose multiple fetuses, and to diagnose some abnormal conditions. *Lane, Keenon, Coleman (eds.), p. 472.*

271. **C.** Blood levels obtained at the first postpartum visit include hematocrit and hemoglobin levels. *Lane, Keenon, Coleman (eds.), p. 473.*

272. **D.** Throat swabs placed in transport media should be processed within 24 hours. Throat swabs not collected in a swab-transport media should be processed within 2 to 3 hours. *Lane, Keenon, Coleman (eds.), p. 543.*

273. **B.** Any trace of blue on or at the edge of the smear indicates the test result is positive for occult blood. Hemoccult developer may produce a pale blue ring on the test paper and is not interpreted as a positive reaction. No blue on or at the edge of the smear indicates the test result is negative for occult blood. *Lane, Keenon, Coleman (eds.), p. 630.*

274. **A.** False-negative results may be due to ascorbic acid intake of more than 250 mg/day. *Lane, Keenon, Coleman (eds.), p. 631.*

275. **C.** If no beta-hemolytic colonies are seen, reincubate for an additional 24 hours. If no beta-hemolytic colonies are seen after 48 hours, the culture is reported as negative. *Lane, Keenon, Coleman (eds.), p. 633.*

276. **E.** The Tandem ICON II pregnancy test is performed on 5 drops of urine and requires a more concentrated sample. *Lane, Keenon, Coleman (eds.), p. 640.*

277. **E.** Under OSHA requirements, employees are required to refrain from smoking, eating, or drinking around hazardous substances. Eating or drinking in the laboratory may result in the ingestion of contaminated foods or liquids. *OSHA "Hazard Communication" Rule (29 CFR 1910.1200).*

278. **E.** Yeasts are frequently found as a contaminant in the urine of women with *Candida albican* infection of the vagina. When observed, they should be noted on the request slip. *Wedding and Toenjes, p. 117.*

279. **B.** After dispensing a small amount of fluid directly under the cover glass, one should allow 2 minutes for the cells to settle. Waiting too long will allow the sample to evaporate. *Wedding and Toenjes, p. 257.*

280. **D.** Genital cultures and viral cultures should be kept at room temperature or incubated, if possible, until tests can be performed. *Lane, Keenon, Coleman (eds.), p. 545.*

281. **E.** Serum specimens are routinely frozen if it is impractical to perform tests immediately. It is best to check with the laboratory first, as a few tests deteriorate if frozen. *Lane, Keenon, Coleman (eds.), p. 545.*

282. **B.** A wound culture is collected by placing a swab directly into the pus present in a wound. *Frew, Lane, and Frew, p. 772.*

283. **B.** DT toxoid is used in children under age 7. Td toxoid is used in persons over 7 years old. Td contains the same amount of tetanus as DPT and DT but a reduced dose of diphtheria toxoid. *Lane, Keenon, Coleman (eds.), p. 424.*

284. **D.** Drugs administered intravenously or by inhalation are absorbed within seconds; injectable drugs, within a few minutes to 20 minutes; and oral drugs, on average, 30 minutes to 1 hour. *Lane, Medications, p. 189.*

285. **B.** MMR is a live vaccine that is administered subcutaneously. Vaccines with adjuvants (aluminum hydroxide or aluminum phosphate) should be given intramuscularly because adsorbed toxoids remain in the human tissues longer. *Lane, Medications, p. 237.*

286. **C.** Patients should be told not to use aspirin when treating children with chickenpox or flulike illness owing to the risk of Reye's syndrome. *Lane, Medications, p. 243.*

287. **C.** Except in cases of dehydration, heat stroke, or heat exhaustion, fever may be of benefit to the patient. *Taber's, p. 723.*

288. **D.** For scalp lice, a special shampoo, Kwell, is used. *Tamparo and Lewis, p. 319; Taber's, p. 775.*

289. **D.** Sodium should not be restricted because of blood volume maintenance and fetal requirements. However, sodium intake must be watched with caution and not increased, to prevent excessive weight gain and possible hypertension or toxemia in pregnancy (eclampsia or preeclampsia). *Frew, Lane, and Frew, p. 526.*

290. **C.** Although physicians differ on the desired amount of weight gain, most usually recommend a 2- to 4.5-lb gain in the first trimester. *Frew, Lane, and Frew, p. 526.*

291. **B.** Caloric demands for the breast-feeding, or lactating, woman are greater than those for pregnancy. The recommended dietary allowances include an additional 500 calories per day. *Frew, Lane, and Frew, pp. 526–527.*

292. **D.** Surfaces used for laboratory analysis must be cleaned when they become obviously contaminated; after any spill of blood or other potentially infectious materials; and at the end of a work shift or before leaving an area for lunch or a break. Employees need not decontaminate the work area after each patient procedure, but only after those that actually result in contamination. *Frew, Lane, and Frew, p. 383.*

293. **D.** The National Fire Protection Association has developed a diamond rating system. Inside each diamond is a number from zero to four, with four being extremely hazardous in a fire. *Frew, Lane, and Frew, p. 737.*

294. **D.** High-level disinfection is used for reusable instruments or devices that come into contact with mucous membranes (e.g., laryngoscope blades, endotracheal tubes). Methods include a 6- to 10-hour exposure to an EPA-approved sterilant or shorter exposure times of 10 to 45 minutes as directed by the manufacturer. High-level disinfection kills all forms of microbial life except high numbers of bacterial spores. *Frew, Lane, and Frew, p. 899.*

295. **A.** Reagents and controls contain sodium azide, which may react with lead and copper plumbing to form highly explosive metal azides. If discarded into a sink, they should be flushed with a large volume of water to prevent azide buildup. *Lane, Keenon, Coleman (eds.), p. 644.*

296. **C.** The flash point is the temperature at which a substance will burst into flames spontaneously. *OSHA "Hazard Communication" Rule (29 CFR 1910.1200).*

297. **C.** On the MSDS, the reactivity section covers a substance's compatability with other materials and substance stability. *OSHA "Hazard Communication" Rule (29 CFR 1910.1200).*

298. **E.** General patient instructions should include informing patients that the usual MRI examination will take, on average, 60 to 90 minutes, although the time varies from 45 minutes to 2 hours, depending on the examination. *Frew, Lane, and Frew, p. 865.*

299. **B.** A transcatheter embolization is the process by which a substance is injected via a catheter to occlude a blood vessel and stop a hemorrhage or the possibility of one. *Frew, Lane, and Frew, p. 867.*

300. **E.** Radiographs are usually taken in the anterior and lateral views. Oblique views may be necessary to show foramina and joints only in more detailed studies. *Lane, Keenon, Coleman (eds.), p. 480.*

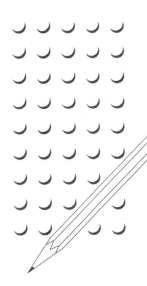

Sample Examination Simulation 2

- The following pages contain 300 test items.

- The examination is divided into:

  Part 1—General Medical Knowledge
  Part 2—Administrative Procedures
  Part 3—Clinical Procedures

- Answer sheets are provided for your use.

- The answer key immediately follows the test items and includes references with page numbers.

- References and suggested readings are at the end of the book.

Name _____ Date _____
Last   First   Middle

Directions for Marking Answers

- Use a black lead pencil (No. 2 or softer). Do NOT use pen or a pencil with hard lead.
- Make each mark heavy and black enough to completely obliterate the letter within the circle. Marks should fill the circles.
- Erase clearly any answer you wish to change.
- Make no stray marks on this answer sheet.
- Mark one and only one answer for each question. Multiple answers will be counted as wrong.

Example

WRONG   Ⓐ Ⓑ̸ Ⓒ Ⓓ Ⓔ
WRONG   Ⓐ Ⓑ̷ Ⓒ Ⓓ Ⓔ
WRONG   Ⓐ Ⓑ Ⓒ Ⓓ Ⓔ
RIGHT   Ⓐ Ⓑ Ⓒ ● Ⓔ

1 Ⓐ Ⓑ Ⓒ Ⓓ Ⓔ	26 Ⓐ Ⓑ Ⓒ Ⓓ Ⓔ	51 Ⓐ Ⓑ Ⓒ Ⓓ Ⓔ	76 Ⓐ Ⓑ Ⓒ Ⓓ Ⓔ
2 Ⓐ Ⓑ Ⓒ Ⓓ Ⓔ	27 Ⓐ Ⓑ Ⓒ Ⓓ Ⓔ	52 Ⓐ Ⓑ Ⓒ Ⓓ Ⓔ	77 Ⓐ Ⓑ Ⓒ Ⓓ Ⓔ
3 Ⓐ Ⓑ Ⓒ Ⓓ Ⓔ	28 Ⓐ Ⓑ Ⓒ Ⓓ Ⓔ	53 Ⓐ Ⓑ Ⓒ Ⓓ Ⓔ	78 Ⓐ Ⓑ Ⓒ Ⓓ Ⓔ
4 Ⓐ Ⓑ Ⓒ Ⓓ Ⓔ	29 Ⓐ Ⓑ Ⓒ Ⓓ Ⓔ	54 Ⓐ Ⓑ Ⓒ Ⓓ Ⓔ	79 Ⓐ Ⓑ Ⓒ Ⓓ Ⓔ
5 Ⓐ Ⓑ Ⓒ Ⓓ Ⓔ	30 Ⓐ Ⓑ Ⓒ Ⓓ Ⓔ	55 Ⓐ Ⓑ Ⓒ Ⓓ Ⓔ	80 Ⓐ Ⓑ Ⓒ Ⓓ Ⓔ
6 Ⓐ Ⓑ Ⓒ Ⓓ Ⓔ	31 Ⓐ Ⓑ Ⓒ Ⓓ Ⓔ	56 Ⓐ Ⓑ Ⓒ Ⓓ Ⓔ	81 Ⓐ Ⓑ Ⓒ Ⓓ Ⓔ
7 Ⓐ Ⓑ Ⓒ Ⓓ Ⓔ	32 Ⓐ Ⓑ Ⓒ Ⓓ Ⓔ	57 Ⓐ Ⓑ Ⓒ Ⓓ Ⓔ	82 Ⓐ Ⓑ Ⓒ Ⓓ Ⓔ
8 Ⓐ Ⓑ Ⓒ Ⓓ Ⓔ	33 Ⓐ Ⓑ Ⓒ Ⓓ Ⓔ	58 Ⓐ Ⓑ Ⓒ Ⓓ Ⓔ	83 Ⓐ Ⓑ Ⓒ Ⓓ Ⓔ
9 Ⓐ Ⓑ Ⓒ Ⓓ Ⓔ	34 Ⓐ Ⓑ Ⓒ Ⓓ Ⓔ	59 Ⓐ Ⓑ Ⓒ Ⓓ Ⓔ	84 Ⓐ Ⓑ Ⓒ Ⓓ Ⓔ
10 Ⓐ Ⓑ Ⓒ Ⓓ Ⓔ	35 Ⓐ Ⓑ Ⓒ Ⓓ Ⓔ	60 Ⓐ Ⓑ Ⓒ Ⓓ Ⓔ	85 Ⓐ Ⓑ Ⓒ Ⓓ Ⓔ
11 Ⓐ Ⓑ Ⓒ Ⓓ Ⓔ	36 Ⓐ Ⓑ Ⓒ Ⓓ Ⓔ	61 Ⓐ Ⓑ Ⓒ Ⓓ Ⓔ	86 Ⓐ Ⓑ Ⓒ Ⓓ Ⓔ
12 Ⓐ Ⓑ Ⓒ Ⓓ Ⓔ	37 Ⓐ Ⓑ Ⓒ Ⓓ Ⓔ	62 Ⓐ Ⓑ Ⓒ Ⓓ Ⓔ	87 Ⓐ Ⓑ Ⓒ Ⓓ Ⓔ
13 Ⓐ Ⓑ Ⓒ Ⓓ Ⓔ	38 Ⓐ Ⓑ Ⓒ Ⓓ Ⓔ	63 Ⓐ Ⓑ Ⓒ Ⓓ Ⓔ	88 Ⓐ Ⓑ Ⓒ Ⓓ Ⓔ
14 Ⓐ Ⓑ Ⓒ Ⓓ Ⓔ	39 Ⓐ Ⓑ Ⓒ Ⓓ Ⓔ	64 Ⓐ Ⓑ Ⓒ Ⓓ Ⓔ	89 Ⓐ Ⓑ Ⓒ Ⓓ Ⓔ
15 Ⓐ Ⓑ Ⓒ Ⓓ Ⓔ	40 Ⓐ Ⓑ Ⓒ Ⓓ Ⓔ	65 Ⓐ Ⓑ Ⓒ Ⓓ Ⓔ	90 Ⓐ Ⓑ Ⓒ Ⓓ Ⓔ
16 Ⓐ Ⓑ Ⓒ Ⓓ Ⓔ	41 Ⓐ Ⓑ Ⓒ Ⓓ Ⓔ	66 Ⓐ Ⓑ Ⓒ Ⓓ Ⓔ	91 Ⓐ Ⓑ Ⓒ Ⓓ Ⓔ
17 Ⓐ Ⓑ Ⓒ Ⓓ Ⓔ	42 Ⓐ Ⓑ Ⓒ Ⓓ Ⓔ	67 Ⓐ Ⓑ Ⓒ Ⓓ Ⓔ	92 Ⓐ Ⓑ Ⓒ Ⓓ Ⓔ
18 Ⓐ Ⓑ Ⓒ Ⓓ Ⓔ	43 Ⓐ Ⓑ Ⓒ Ⓓ Ⓔ	68 Ⓐ Ⓑ Ⓒ Ⓓ Ⓔ	93 Ⓐ Ⓑ Ⓒ Ⓓ Ⓔ
19 Ⓐ Ⓑ Ⓒ Ⓓ Ⓔ	44 Ⓐ Ⓑ Ⓒ Ⓓ Ⓔ	69 Ⓐ Ⓑ Ⓒ Ⓓ Ⓔ	94 Ⓐ Ⓑ Ⓒ Ⓓ Ⓔ
20 Ⓐ Ⓑ Ⓒ Ⓓ Ⓔ	45 Ⓐ Ⓑ Ⓒ Ⓓ Ⓔ	70 Ⓐ Ⓑ Ⓒ Ⓓ Ⓔ	95 Ⓐ Ⓑ Ⓒ Ⓓ Ⓔ
21 Ⓐ Ⓑ Ⓒ Ⓓ Ⓔ	46 Ⓐ Ⓑ Ⓒ Ⓓ Ⓔ	71 Ⓐ Ⓑ Ⓒ Ⓓ Ⓔ	96 Ⓐ Ⓑ Ⓒ Ⓓ Ⓔ
22 Ⓐ Ⓑ Ⓒ Ⓓ Ⓔ	47 Ⓐ Ⓑ Ⓒ Ⓓ Ⓔ	72 Ⓐ Ⓑ Ⓒ Ⓓ Ⓔ	97 Ⓐ Ⓑ Ⓒ Ⓓ Ⓔ
23 Ⓐ Ⓑ Ⓒ Ⓓ Ⓔ	48 Ⓐ Ⓑ Ⓒ Ⓓ Ⓔ	73 Ⓐ Ⓑ Ⓒ Ⓓ Ⓔ	98 Ⓐ Ⓑ Ⓒ Ⓓ Ⓔ
24 Ⓐ Ⓑ Ⓒ Ⓓ Ⓔ	49 Ⓐ Ⓑ Ⓒ Ⓓ Ⓔ	74 Ⓐ Ⓑ Ⓒ Ⓓ Ⓔ	99 Ⓐ Ⓑ Ⓒ Ⓓ Ⓔ
25 Ⓐ Ⓑ Ⓒ Ⓓ Ⓔ	50 Ⓐ Ⓑ Ⓒ Ⓓ Ⓔ	75 Ⓐ Ⓑ Ⓒ Ⓓ Ⓔ	100 Ⓐ Ⓑ Ⓒ Ⓓ Ⓔ

Name _____ **Date** _____

Last   First   Middle

Directions for Marking Answers

- Use a black lead pencil (No. 2 or softer). Do NOT use pen or a pencil with hard lead.
- Make each mark heavy and black enough to completely obliterate the letter within the circle. Marks should fill the circles.
- Erase clearly any answer you wish to change.
- Make no stray marks on this answer sheet.
- Mark one and only one answer for each question. Multiple answers will be counted as wrong.

Example

WRONG   (A) (B̸) (C) (D) (E)

WRONG   (A) (X̸) (C) (D) (E)

WRONG   (A) (B) (©) (D) (E)

RIGHT   (A) (B) (C) (●) (E)

---

101 (A) (B) (C) (D) (E)   126 (A) (B) (C) (D) (E)   151 (A) (B) (C) (D) (E)   176 (A) (B) (C) (D) (E)
102 (A) (B) (C) (D) (E)   127 (A) (B) (C) (D) (E)   152 (A) (B) (C) (D) (E)   177 (A) (B) (C) (D) (E)
103 (A) (B) (C) (D) (E)   128 (A) (B) (C) (D) (E)   153 (A) (B) (C) (D) (E)   178 (A) (B) (C) (D) (E)
104 (A) (B) (C) (D) (E)   129 (A) (B) (C) (D) (E)   154 (A) (B) (C) (D) (E)   179 (A) (B) (C) (D) (E)
105 (A) (B) (C) (D) (E)   130 (A) (B) (C) (D) (E)   155 (A) (B) (C) (D) (E)   180 (A) (B) (C) (D) (E)
106 (A) (B) (C) (D) (E)   131 (A) (B) (C) (D) (E)   156 (A) (B) (C) (D) (E)   181 (A) (B) (C) (D) (E)
107 (A) (B) (C) (D) (E)   132 (A) (B) (C) (D) (E)   157 (A) (B) (C) (D) (E)   182 (A) (B) (C) (D) (E)
108 (A) (B) (C) (D) (E)   133 (A) (B) (C) (D) (E)   158 (A) (B) (C) (D) (E)   183 (A) (B) (C) (D) (E)
109 (A) (B) (C) (D) (E)   134 (A) (B) (C) (D) (E)   159 (A) (B) (C) (D) (E)   184 (A) (B) (C) (D) (E)
110 (A) (B) (C) (D) (E)   135 (A) (B) (C) (D) (E)   160 (A) (B) (C) (D) (E)   185 (A) (B) (C) (D) (E)
111 (A) (B) (C) (D) (E)   136 (A) (B) (C) (D) (E)   161 (A) (B) (C) (D) (E)   186 (A) (B) (C) (D) (E)
112 (A) (B) (C) (D) (E)   137 (A) (B) (C) (D) (E)   162 (A) (B) (C) (D) (E)   187 (A) (B) (C) (D) (E)
113 (A) (B) (C) (D) (E)   138 (A) (B) (C) (D) (E)   163 (A) (B) (C) (D) (E)   188 (A) (B) (C) (D) (E)
114 (A) (B) (C) (D) (E)   139 (A) (B) (C) (D) (E)   164 (A) (B) (C) (D) (E)   189 (A) (B) (C) (D) (E)
115 (A) (B) (C) (D) (E)   140 (A) (B) (C) (D) (E)   165 (A) (B) (C) (D) (E)   190 (A) (B) (C) (D) (E)
116 (A) (B) (C) (D) (E)   141 (A) (B) (C) (D) (E)   166 (A) (B) (C) (D) (E)   191 (A) (B) (C) (D) (E)
117 (A) (B) (C) (D) (E)   142 (A) (B) (C) (D) (E)   167 (A) (B) (C) (D) (E)   192 (A) (B) (C) (D) (E)
118 (A) (B) (C) (D) (E)   143 (A) (B) (C) (D) (E)   168 (A) (B) (C) (D) (E)   193 (A) (B) (C) (D) (E)
119 (A) (B) (C) (D) (E)   144 (A) (B) (C) (D) (E)   169 (A) (B) (C) (D) (E)   194 (A) (B) (C) (D) (E)
120 (A) (B) (C) (D) (E)   145 (A) (B) (C) (D) (E)   170 (A) (B) (C) (D) (E)   195 (A) (B) (C) (D) (E)
121 (A) (B) (C) (D) (E)   146 (A) (B) (C) (D) (E)   171 (A) (B) (C) (D) (E)   196 (A) (B) (C) (D) (E)
122 (A) (B) (C) (D) (E)   147 (A) (B) (C) (D) (E)   172 (A) (B) (C) (D) (E)   197 (A) (B) (C) (D) (E)
123 (A) (B) (C) (D) (E)   148 (A) (B) (C) (D) (E)   173 (A) (B) (C) (D) (E)   198 (A) (B) (C) (D) (E)
124 (A) (B) (C) (D) (E)   149 (A) (B) (C) (D) (E)   174 (A) (B) (C) (D) (E)   199 (A) (B) (C) (D) (E)
125 (A) (B) (C) (D) (E)   150 (A) (B) (C) (D) (E)   175 (A) (B) (C) (D) (E)   200 (A) (B) (C) (D) (E)

Name _____ **Date** _____
　　　　　Last　　　　　　　First　　　　　　Middle

201 Ⓐ Ⓑ Ⓒ Ⓓ Ⓔ　　226 Ⓐ Ⓑ Ⓒ Ⓓ Ⓔ　　251 Ⓐ Ⓑ Ⓒ Ⓓ Ⓔ　　276 Ⓐ Ⓑ Ⓒ Ⓓ Ⓔ
202 Ⓐ Ⓑ Ⓒ Ⓓ Ⓔ　　227 Ⓐ Ⓑ Ⓒ Ⓓ Ⓔ　　252 Ⓐ Ⓑ Ⓒ Ⓓ Ⓔ　　277 Ⓐ Ⓑ Ⓒ Ⓓ Ⓔ
203 Ⓐ Ⓑ Ⓒ Ⓓ Ⓔ　　228 Ⓐ Ⓑ Ⓒ Ⓓ Ⓔ　　253 Ⓐ Ⓑ Ⓒ Ⓓ Ⓔ　　278 Ⓐ Ⓑ Ⓒ Ⓓ Ⓔ
204 Ⓐ Ⓑ Ⓒ Ⓓ Ⓔ　　229 Ⓐ Ⓑ Ⓒ Ⓓ Ⓔ　　254 Ⓐ Ⓑ Ⓒ Ⓓ Ⓔ　　279 Ⓐ Ⓑ Ⓒ Ⓓ Ⓔ
205 Ⓐ Ⓑ Ⓒ Ⓓ Ⓔ　　230 Ⓐ Ⓑ Ⓒ Ⓓ Ⓔ　　255 Ⓐ Ⓑ Ⓒ Ⓓ Ⓔ　　280 Ⓐ Ⓑ Ⓒ Ⓓ Ⓔ
206 Ⓐ Ⓑ Ⓒ Ⓓ Ⓔ　　231 Ⓐ Ⓑ Ⓒ Ⓓ Ⓔ　　256 Ⓐ Ⓑ Ⓒ Ⓓ Ⓔ　　281 Ⓐ Ⓑ Ⓒ Ⓓ Ⓔ
207 Ⓐ Ⓑ Ⓒ Ⓓ Ⓔ　　232 Ⓐ Ⓑ Ⓒ Ⓓ Ⓔ　　257 Ⓐ Ⓑ Ⓒ Ⓓ Ⓔ　　282 Ⓐ Ⓑ Ⓒ Ⓓ Ⓔ
208 Ⓐ Ⓑ Ⓒ Ⓓ Ⓔ　　233 Ⓐ Ⓑ Ⓒ Ⓓ Ⓔ　　258 Ⓐ Ⓑ Ⓒ Ⓓ Ⓔ　　283 Ⓐ Ⓑ Ⓒ Ⓓ Ⓔ
209 Ⓐ Ⓑ Ⓒ Ⓓ Ⓔ　　234 Ⓐ Ⓑ Ⓒ Ⓓ Ⓔ　　259 Ⓐ Ⓑ Ⓒ Ⓓ Ⓔ　　284 Ⓐ Ⓑ Ⓒ Ⓓ Ⓔ
210 Ⓐ Ⓑ Ⓒ Ⓓ Ⓔ　　235 Ⓐ Ⓑ Ⓒ Ⓓ Ⓔ　　260 Ⓐ Ⓑ Ⓒ Ⓓ Ⓔ　　285 Ⓐ Ⓑ Ⓒ Ⓓ Ⓔ
211 Ⓐ Ⓑ Ⓒ Ⓓ Ⓔ　　236 Ⓐ Ⓑ Ⓒ Ⓓ Ⓔ　　261 Ⓐ Ⓑ Ⓒ Ⓓ Ⓔ　　286 Ⓐ Ⓑ Ⓒ Ⓓ Ⓔ
212 Ⓐ Ⓑ Ⓒ Ⓓ Ⓔ　　237 Ⓐ Ⓑ Ⓒ Ⓓ Ⓔ　　262 Ⓐ Ⓑ Ⓒ Ⓓ Ⓔ　　287 Ⓐ Ⓑ Ⓒ Ⓓ Ⓔ
213 Ⓐ Ⓑ Ⓒ Ⓓ Ⓔ　　238 Ⓐ Ⓑ Ⓒ Ⓓ Ⓔ　　263 Ⓐ Ⓑ Ⓒ Ⓓ Ⓔ　　288 Ⓐ Ⓑ Ⓒ Ⓓ Ⓔ
214 Ⓐ Ⓑ Ⓒ Ⓓ Ⓔ　　239 Ⓐ Ⓑ Ⓒ Ⓓ Ⓔ　　264 Ⓐ Ⓑ Ⓒ Ⓓ Ⓔ　　289 Ⓐ Ⓑ Ⓒ Ⓓ Ⓔ
215 Ⓐ Ⓑ Ⓒ Ⓓ Ⓔ　　240 Ⓐ Ⓑ Ⓒ Ⓓ Ⓔ　　265 Ⓐ Ⓑ Ⓒ Ⓓ Ⓔ　　290 Ⓐ Ⓑ Ⓒ Ⓓ Ⓔ
216 Ⓐ Ⓑ Ⓒ Ⓓ Ⓔ　　241 Ⓐ Ⓑ Ⓒ Ⓓ Ⓔ　　266 Ⓐ Ⓑ Ⓒ Ⓓ Ⓔ　　291 Ⓐ Ⓑ Ⓒ Ⓓ Ⓔ
217 Ⓐ Ⓑ Ⓒ Ⓓ Ⓔ　　242 Ⓐ Ⓑ Ⓒ Ⓓ Ⓔ　　267 Ⓐ Ⓑ Ⓒ Ⓓ Ⓔ　　292 Ⓐ Ⓑ Ⓒ Ⓓ Ⓔ
218 Ⓐ Ⓑ Ⓒ Ⓓ Ⓔ　　243 Ⓐ Ⓑ Ⓒ Ⓓ Ⓔ　　268 Ⓐ Ⓑ Ⓒ Ⓓ Ⓔ　　293 Ⓐ Ⓑ Ⓒ Ⓓ Ⓔ
219 Ⓐ Ⓑ Ⓒ Ⓓ Ⓔ　　244 Ⓐ Ⓑ Ⓒ Ⓓ Ⓔ　　269 Ⓐ Ⓑ Ⓒ Ⓓ Ⓔ　　294 Ⓐ Ⓑ Ⓒ Ⓓ Ⓔ
220 Ⓐ Ⓑ Ⓒ Ⓓ Ⓔ　　245 Ⓐ Ⓑ Ⓒ Ⓓ Ⓔ　　270 Ⓐ Ⓑ Ⓒ Ⓓ Ⓔ　　295 Ⓐ Ⓑ Ⓒ Ⓓ Ⓔ
221 Ⓐ Ⓑ Ⓒ Ⓓ Ⓔ　　246 Ⓐ Ⓑ Ⓒ Ⓓ Ⓔ　　271 Ⓐ Ⓑ Ⓒ Ⓓ Ⓔ　　296 Ⓐ Ⓑ Ⓒ Ⓓ Ⓔ
222 Ⓐ Ⓑ Ⓒ Ⓓ Ⓔ　　247 Ⓐ Ⓑ Ⓒ Ⓓ Ⓔ　　272 Ⓐ Ⓑ Ⓒ Ⓓ Ⓔ　　297 Ⓐ Ⓑ Ⓒ Ⓓ Ⓔ
223 Ⓐ Ⓑ Ⓒ Ⓓ Ⓔ　　248 Ⓐ Ⓑ Ⓒ Ⓓ Ⓔ　　273 Ⓐ Ⓑ Ⓒ Ⓓ Ⓔ　　298 Ⓐ Ⓑ Ⓒ Ⓓ Ⓔ
224 Ⓐ Ⓑ Ⓒ Ⓓ Ⓔ　　249 Ⓐ Ⓑ Ⓒ Ⓓ Ⓔ　　274 Ⓐ Ⓑ Ⓒ Ⓓ Ⓔ　　299 Ⓐ Ⓑ Ⓒ Ⓓ Ⓔ
225 Ⓐ Ⓑ Ⓒ Ⓓ Ⓔ　　250 Ⓐ Ⓑ Ⓒ Ⓓ Ⓔ　　275 Ⓐ Ⓑ Ⓒ Ⓓ Ⓔ　　300 Ⓐ Ⓑ Ⓒ Ⓓ Ⓔ

Name _____ **Date** _____

Last   First   Middle

Directions for Marking Answers

- Use a black lead pencil (No. 2 or softer). Do NOT use pen or a pencil with hard lead.
- Make each mark heavy and black enough to completely obliterate the letter within the circle. Marks should fill the circles.
- Erase clearly any answer you wish to change.
- Make no stray marks on this answer sheet.
- Mark one and only one answer for each question. Multiple answers will be counted as wrong.

Example

WRONG   Ⓐ Ⓑ̶ Ⓒ Ⓓ Ⓔ
WRONG   Ⓐ Ⓑ̶ Ⓒ Ⓓ Ⓔ
WRONG   Ⓐ Ⓑ Ⓒ Ⓓ Ⓔ
RIGHT   Ⓐ Ⓑ Ⓒ ● Ⓔ

1 Ⓐ Ⓑ Ⓒ Ⓓ Ⓔ   26 Ⓐ Ⓑ Ⓒ Ⓓ Ⓔ   51 Ⓐ Ⓑ Ⓒ Ⓓ Ⓔ   76 Ⓐ Ⓑ Ⓒ Ⓓ Ⓔ
2 Ⓐ Ⓑ Ⓒ Ⓓ Ⓔ   27 Ⓐ Ⓑ Ⓒ Ⓓ Ⓔ   52 Ⓐ Ⓑ Ⓒ Ⓓ Ⓔ   77 Ⓐ Ⓑ Ⓒ Ⓓ Ⓔ
3 Ⓐ Ⓑ Ⓒ Ⓓ Ⓔ   28 Ⓐ Ⓑ Ⓒ Ⓓ Ⓔ   53 Ⓐ Ⓑ Ⓒ Ⓓ Ⓔ   78 Ⓐ Ⓑ Ⓒ Ⓓ Ⓔ
4 Ⓐ Ⓑ Ⓒ Ⓓ Ⓔ   29 Ⓐ Ⓑ Ⓒ Ⓓ Ⓔ   54 Ⓐ Ⓑ Ⓒ Ⓓ Ⓔ   79 Ⓐ Ⓑ Ⓒ Ⓓ Ⓔ
5 Ⓐ Ⓑ Ⓒ Ⓓ Ⓔ   30 Ⓐ Ⓑ Ⓒ Ⓓ Ⓔ   55 Ⓐ Ⓑ Ⓒ Ⓓ Ⓔ   80 Ⓐ Ⓑ Ⓒ Ⓓ Ⓔ
6 Ⓐ Ⓑ Ⓒ Ⓓ Ⓔ   31 Ⓐ Ⓑ Ⓒ Ⓓ Ⓔ   56 Ⓐ Ⓑ Ⓒ Ⓓ Ⓔ   81 Ⓐ Ⓑ Ⓒ Ⓓ Ⓔ
7 Ⓐ Ⓑ Ⓒ Ⓓ Ⓔ   32 Ⓐ Ⓑ Ⓒ Ⓓ Ⓔ   57 Ⓐ Ⓑ Ⓒ Ⓓ Ⓔ   82 Ⓐ Ⓑ Ⓒ Ⓓ Ⓔ
8 Ⓐ Ⓑ Ⓒ Ⓓ Ⓔ   33 Ⓐ Ⓑ Ⓒ Ⓓ Ⓔ   58 Ⓐ Ⓑ Ⓒ Ⓓ Ⓔ   83 Ⓐ Ⓑ Ⓒ Ⓓ Ⓔ
9 Ⓐ Ⓑ Ⓒ Ⓓ Ⓔ   34 Ⓐ Ⓑ Ⓒ Ⓓ Ⓔ   59 Ⓐ Ⓑ Ⓒ Ⓓ Ⓔ   84 Ⓐ Ⓑ Ⓒ Ⓓ Ⓔ
10 Ⓐ Ⓑ Ⓒ Ⓓ Ⓔ   35 Ⓐ Ⓑ Ⓒ Ⓓ Ⓔ   60 Ⓐ Ⓑ Ⓒ Ⓓ Ⓔ   85 Ⓐ Ⓑ Ⓒ Ⓓ Ⓔ
11 Ⓐ Ⓑ Ⓒ Ⓓ Ⓔ   36 Ⓐ Ⓑ Ⓒ Ⓓ Ⓔ   61 Ⓐ Ⓑ Ⓒ Ⓓ Ⓔ   86 Ⓐ Ⓑ Ⓒ Ⓓ Ⓔ
12 Ⓐ Ⓑ Ⓒ Ⓓ Ⓔ   37 Ⓐ Ⓑ Ⓒ Ⓓ Ⓔ   62 Ⓐ Ⓑ Ⓒ Ⓓ Ⓔ   87 Ⓐ Ⓑ Ⓒ Ⓓ Ⓔ
13 Ⓐ Ⓑ Ⓒ Ⓓ Ⓔ   38 Ⓐ Ⓑ Ⓒ Ⓓ Ⓔ   63 Ⓐ Ⓑ Ⓒ Ⓓ Ⓔ   88 Ⓐ Ⓑ Ⓒ Ⓓ Ⓔ
14 Ⓐ Ⓑ Ⓒ Ⓓ Ⓔ   39 Ⓐ Ⓑ Ⓒ Ⓓ Ⓔ   64 Ⓐ Ⓑ Ⓒ Ⓓ Ⓔ   89 Ⓐ Ⓑ Ⓒ Ⓓ Ⓔ
15 Ⓐ Ⓑ Ⓒ Ⓓ Ⓔ   40 Ⓐ Ⓑ Ⓒ Ⓓ Ⓔ   65 Ⓐ Ⓑ Ⓒ Ⓓ Ⓔ   90 Ⓐ Ⓑ Ⓒ Ⓓ Ⓔ
16 Ⓐ Ⓑ Ⓒ Ⓓ Ⓔ   41 Ⓐ Ⓑ Ⓒ Ⓓ Ⓔ   66 Ⓐ Ⓑ Ⓒ Ⓓ Ⓔ   91 Ⓐ Ⓑ Ⓒ Ⓓ Ⓔ
17 Ⓐ Ⓑ Ⓒ Ⓓ Ⓔ   42 Ⓐ Ⓑ Ⓒ Ⓓ Ⓔ   67 Ⓐ Ⓑ Ⓒ Ⓓ Ⓔ   92 Ⓐ Ⓑ Ⓒ Ⓓ Ⓔ
18 Ⓐ Ⓑ Ⓒ Ⓓ Ⓔ   43 Ⓐ Ⓑ Ⓒ Ⓓ Ⓔ   68 Ⓐ Ⓑ Ⓒ Ⓓ Ⓔ   93 Ⓐ Ⓑ Ⓒ Ⓓ Ⓔ
19 Ⓐ Ⓑ Ⓒ Ⓓ Ⓔ   44 Ⓐ Ⓑ Ⓒ Ⓓ Ⓔ   69 Ⓐ Ⓑ Ⓒ Ⓓ Ⓔ   94 Ⓐ Ⓑ Ⓒ Ⓓ Ⓔ
20 Ⓐ Ⓑ Ⓒ Ⓓ Ⓔ   45 Ⓐ Ⓑ Ⓒ Ⓓ Ⓔ   70 Ⓐ Ⓑ Ⓒ Ⓓ Ⓔ   95 Ⓐ Ⓑ Ⓒ Ⓓ Ⓔ
21 Ⓐ Ⓑ Ⓒ Ⓓ Ⓔ   46 Ⓐ Ⓑ Ⓒ Ⓓ Ⓔ   71 Ⓐ Ⓑ Ⓒ Ⓓ Ⓔ   96 Ⓐ Ⓑ Ⓒ Ⓓ Ⓔ
22 Ⓐ Ⓑ Ⓒ Ⓓ Ⓔ   47 Ⓐ Ⓑ Ⓒ Ⓓ Ⓔ   72 Ⓐ Ⓑ Ⓒ Ⓓ Ⓔ   97 Ⓐ Ⓑ Ⓒ Ⓓ Ⓔ
23 Ⓐ Ⓑ Ⓒ Ⓓ Ⓔ   48 Ⓐ Ⓑ Ⓒ Ⓓ Ⓔ   73 Ⓐ Ⓑ Ⓒ Ⓓ Ⓔ   98 Ⓐ Ⓑ Ⓒ Ⓓ Ⓔ
24 Ⓐ Ⓑ Ⓒ Ⓓ Ⓔ   49 Ⓐ Ⓑ Ⓒ Ⓓ Ⓔ   74 Ⓐ Ⓑ Ⓒ Ⓓ Ⓔ   99 Ⓐ Ⓑ Ⓒ Ⓓ Ⓔ
25 Ⓐ Ⓑ Ⓒ Ⓓ Ⓔ   50 Ⓐ Ⓑ Ⓒ Ⓓ Ⓔ   75 Ⓐ Ⓑ Ⓒ Ⓓ Ⓔ   100 Ⓐ Ⓑ Ⓒ Ⓓ Ⓔ

Name _____ **Date** _____

Last   First   Middle

Directions for Marking Answers

- Use a black lead pencil (No. 2 or softer). Do NOT use pen or a pencil with hard lead.
- Make each mark heavy and black enough to completely obliterate the letter within the circle. Marks should fill the circles.
- Erase clearly any answer you wish to change.
- Make no stray marks on this answer sheet.
- Mark one and only one answer for each question. Multiple answers will be counted as wrong.

Example

WRONG Ⓐ Ⓑ Ⓒ Ⓓ Ⓔ
WRONG Ⓐ Ⓧ Ⓒ Ⓓ Ⓔ
WRONG Ⓐ Ⓑ Ⓒ Ⓓ Ⓔ
RIGHT Ⓐ Ⓑ Ⓒ ● Ⓔ

101 Ⓐ Ⓑ Ⓒ Ⓓ Ⓔ   126 Ⓐ Ⓑ Ⓒ Ⓓ Ⓔ   151 Ⓐ Ⓑ Ⓒ Ⓓ Ⓔ   176 Ⓐ Ⓑ Ⓒ Ⓓ Ⓔ
102 Ⓐ Ⓑ Ⓒ Ⓓ Ⓔ   127 Ⓐ Ⓑ Ⓒ Ⓓ Ⓔ   152 Ⓐ Ⓑ Ⓒ Ⓓ Ⓔ   177 Ⓐ Ⓑ Ⓒ Ⓓ Ⓔ
103 Ⓐ Ⓑ Ⓒ Ⓓ Ⓔ   128 Ⓐ Ⓑ Ⓒ Ⓓ Ⓔ   153 Ⓐ Ⓑ Ⓒ Ⓓ Ⓔ   178 Ⓐ Ⓑ Ⓒ Ⓓ Ⓔ
104 Ⓐ Ⓑ Ⓒ Ⓓ Ⓔ   129 Ⓐ Ⓑ Ⓒ Ⓓ Ⓔ   154 Ⓐ Ⓑ Ⓒ Ⓓ Ⓔ   179 Ⓐ Ⓑ Ⓒ Ⓓ Ⓔ
105 Ⓐ Ⓑ Ⓒ Ⓓ Ⓔ   130 Ⓐ Ⓑ Ⓒ Ⓓ Ⓔ   155 Ⓐ Ⓑ Ⓒ Ⓓ Ⓔ   180 Ⓐ Ⓑ Ⓒ Ⓓ Ⓔ
106 Ⓐ Ⓑ Ⓒ Ⓓ Ⓔ   131 Ⓐ Ⓑ Ⓒ Ⓓ Ⓔ   156 Ⓐ Ⓑ Ⓒ Ⓓ Ⓔ   181 Ⓐ Ⓑ Ⓒ Ⓓ Ⓔ
107 Ⓐ Ⓑ Ⓒ Ⓓ Ⓔ   132 Ⓐ Ⓑ Ⓒ Ⓓ Ⓔ   157 Ⓐ Ⓑ Ⓒ Ⓓ Ⓔ   182 Ⓐ Ⓑ Ⓒ Ⓓ Ⓔ
108 Ⓐ Ⓑ Ⓒ Ⓓ Ⓔ   133 Ⓐ Ⓑ Ⓒ Ⓓ Ⓔ   158 Ⓐ Ⓑ Ⓒ Ⓓ Ⓔ   183 Ⓐ Ⓑ Ⓒ Ⓓ Ⓔ
109 Ⓐ Ⓑ Ⓒ Ⓓ Ⓔ   134 Ⓐ Ⓑ Ⓒ Ⓓ Ⓔ   159 Ⓐ Ⓑ Ⓒ Ⓓ Ⓔ   184 Ⓐ Ⓑ Ⓒ Ⓓ Ⓔ
110 Ⓐ Ⓑ Ⓒ Ⓓ Ⓔ   135 Ⓐ Ⓑ Ⓒ Ⓓ Ⓔ   160 Ⓐ Ⓑ Ⓒ Ⓓ Ⓔ   185 Ⓐ Ⓑ Ⓒ Ⓓ Ⓔ
111 Ⓐ Ⓑ Ⓒ Ⓓ Ⓔ   136 Ⓐ Ⓑ Ⓒ Ⓓ Ⓔ   161 Ⓐ Ⓑ Ⓒ Ⓓ Ⓔ   186 Ⓐ Ⓑ Ⓒ Ⓓ Ⓔ
112 Ⓐ Ⓑ Ⓒ Ⓓ Ⓔ   137 Ⓐ Ⓑ Ⓒ Ⓓ Ⓔ   162 Ⓐ Ⓑ Ⓒ Ⓓ Ⓔ   187 Ⓐ Ⓑ Ⓒ Ⓓ Ⓔ
113 Ⓐ Ⓑ Ⓒ Ⓓ Ⓔ   138 Ⓐ Ⓑ Ⓒ Ⓓ Ⓔ   163 Ⓐ Ⓑ Ⓒ Ⓓ Ⓔ   188 Ⓐ Ⓑ Ⓒ Ⓓ Ⓔ
114 Ⓐ Ⓑ Ⓒ Ⓓ Ⓔ   139 Ⓐ Ⓑ Ⓒ Ⓓ Ⓔ   164 Ⓐ Ⓑ Ⓒ Ⓓ Ⓔ   189 Ⓐ Ⓑ Ⓒ Ⓓ Ⓔ
115 Ⓐ Ⓑ Ⓒ Ⓓ Ⓔ   140 Ⓐ Ⓑ Ⓒ Ⓓ Ⓔ   165 Ⓐ Ⓑ Ⓒ Ⓓ Ⓔ   190 Ⓐ Ⓑ Ⓒ Ⓓ Ⓔ
116 Ⓐ Ⓑ Ⓒ Ⓓ Ⓔ   141 Ⓐ Ⓑ Ⓒ Ⓓ Ⓔ   166 Ⓐ Ⓑ Ⓒ Ⓓ Ⓔ   191 Ⓐ Ⓑ Ⓒ Ⓓ Ⓔ
117 Ⓐ Ⓑ Ⓒ Ⓓ Ⓔ   142 Ⓐ Ⓑ Ⓒ Ⓓ Ⓔ   167 Ⓐ Ⓑ Ⓒ Ⓓ Ⓔ   192 Ⓐ Ⓑ Ⓒ Ⓓ Ⓔ
118 Ⓐ Ⓑ Ⓒ Ⓓ Ⓔ   143 Ⓐ Ⓑ Ⓒ Ⓓ Ⓔ   168 Ⓐ Ⓑ Ⓒ Ⓓ Ⓔ   193 Ⓐ Ⓑ Ⓒ Ⓓ Ⓔ
119 Ⓐ Ⓑ Ⓒ Ⓓ Ⓔ   144 Ⓐ Ⓑ Ⓒ Ⓓ Ⓔ   169 Ⓐ Ⓑ Ⓒ Ⓓ Ⓔ   194 Ⓐ Ⓑ Ⓒ Ⓓ Ⓔ
120 Ⓐ Ⓑ Ⓒ Ⓓ Ⓔ   145 Ⓐ Ⓑ Ⓒ Ⓓ Ⓔ   170 Ⓐ Ⓑ Ⓒ Ⓓ Ⓔ   195 Ⓐ Ⓑ Ⓒ Ⓓ Ⓔ
121 Ⓐ Ⓑ Ⓒ Ⓓ Ⓔ   146 Ⓐ Ⓑ Ⓒ Ⓓ Ⓔ   171 Ⓐ Ⓑ Ⓒ Ⓓ Ⓔ   196 Ⓐ Ⓑ Ⓒ Ⓓ Ⓔ
122 Ⓐ Ⓑ Ⓒ Ⓓ Ⓔ   147 Ⓐ Ⓑ Ⓒ Ⓓ Ⓔ   172 Ⓐ Ⓑ Ⓒ Ⓓ Ⓔ   197 Ⓐ Ⓑ Ⓒ Ⓓ Ⓔ
123 Ⓐ Ⓑ Ⓒ Ⓓ Ⓔ   148 Ⓐ Ⓑ Ⓒ Ⓓ Ⓔ   173 Ⓐ Ⓑ Ⓒ Ⓓ Ⓔ   198 Ⓐ Ⓑ Ⓒ Ⓓ Ⓔ
124 Ⓐ Ⓑ Ⓒ Ⓓ Ⓔ   149 Ⓐ Ⓑ Ⓒ Ⓓ Ⓔ   174 Ⓐ Ⓑ Ⓒ Ⓓ Ⓔ   199 Ⓐ Ⓑ Ⓒ Ⓓ Ⓔ
125 Ⓐ Ⓑ Ⓒ Ⓓ Ⓔ   150 Ⓐ Ⓑ Ⓒ Ⓓ Ⓔ   175 Ⓐ Ⓑ Ⓒ Ⓓ Ⓔ   200 Ⓐ Ⓑ Ⓒ Ⓓ Ⓔ

201 Ⓐ Ⓑ Ⓒ Ⓓ Ⓔ	226 Ⓐ Ⓑ Ⓒ Ⓓ Ⓔ	251 Ⓐ Ⓑ Ⓒ Ⓓ Ⓔ	276 Ⓐ Ⓑ Ⓒ Ⓓ Ⓔ
202 Ⓐ Ⓑ Ⓒ Ⓓ Ⓔ	227 Ⓐ Ⓑ Ⓒ Ⓓ Ⓔ	252 Ⓐ Ⓑ Ⓒ Ⓓ Ⓔ	277 Ⓐ Ⓑ Ⓒ Ⓓ Ⓔ
203 Ⓐ Ⓑ Ⓒ Ⓓ Ⓔ	228 Ⓐ Ⓑ Ⓒ Ⓓ Ⓔ	253 Ⓐ Ⓑ Ⓒ Ⓓ Ⓔ	278 Ⓐ Ⓑ Ⓒ Ⓓ Ⓔ
204 Ⓐ Ⓑ Ⓒ Ⓓ Ⓔ	229 Ⓐ Ⓑ Ⓒ Ⓓ Ⓔ	254 Ⓐ Ⓑ Ⓒ Ⓓ Ⓔ	279 Ⓐ Ⓑ Ⓒ Ⓓ Ⓔ
205 Ⓐ Ⓑ Ⓒ Ⓓ Ⓔ	230 Ⓐ Ⓑ Ⓒ Ⓓ Ⓔ	255 Ⓐ Ⓑ Ⓒ Ⓓ Ⓔ	280 Ⓐ Ⓑ Ⓒ Ⓓ Ⓔ
206 Ⓐ Ⓑ Ⓒ Ⓓ Ⓔ	231 Ⓐ Ⓑ Ⓒ Ⓓ Ⓔ	256 Ⓐ Ⓑ Ⓒ Ⓓ Ⓔ	281 Ⓐ Ⓑ Ⓒ Ⓓ Ⓔ
207 Ⓐ Ⓑ Ⓒ Ⓓ Ⓔ	232 Ⓐ Ⓑ Ⓒ Ⓓ Ⓔ	257 Ⓐ Ⓑ Ⓒ Ⓓ Ⓔ	282 Ⓐ Ⓑ Ⓒ Ⓓ Ⓔ
208 Ⓐ Ⓑ Ⓒ Ⓓ Ⓔ	233 Ⓐ Ⓑ Ⓒ Ⓓ Ⓔ	258 Ⓐ Ⓑ Ⓒ Ⓓ Ⓔ	283 Ⓐ Ⓑ Ⓒ Ⓓ Ⓔ
209 Ⓐ Ⓑ Ⓒ Ⓓ Ⓔ	234 Ⓐ Ⓑ Ⓒ Ⓓ Ⓔ	259 Ⓐ Ⓑ Ⓒ Ⓓ Ⓔ	284 Ⓐ Ⓑ Ⓒ Ⓓ Ⓔ
210 Ⓐ Ⓑ Ⓒ Ⓓ Ⓔ	235 Ⓐ Ⓑ Ⓒ Ⓓ Ⓔ	260 Ⓐ Ⓑ Ⓒ Ⓓ Ⓔ	285 Ⓐ Ⓑ Ⓒ Ⓓ Ⓔ
211 Ⓐ Ⓑ Ⓒ Ⓓ Ⓔ	236 Ⓐ Ⓑ Ⓒ Ⓓ Ⓔ	261 Ⓐ Ⓑ Ⓒ Ⓓ Ⓔ	286 Ⓐ Ⓑ Ⓒ Ⓓ Ⓔ
212 Ⓐ Ⓑ Ⓒ Ⓓ Ⓔ	237 Ⓐ Ⓑ Ⓒ Ⓓ Ⓔ	262 Ⓐ Ⓑ Ⓒ Ⓓ Ⓔ	287 Ⓐ Ⓑ Ⓒ Ⓓ Ⓔ
213 Ⓐ Ⓑ Ⓒ Ⓓ Ⓔ	238 Ⓐ Ⓑ Ⓒ Ⓓ Ⓔ	263 Ⓐ Ⓑ Ⓒ Ⓓ Ⓔ	288 Ⓐ Ⓑ Ⓒ Ⓓ Ⓔ
214 Ⓐ Ⓑ Ⓒ Ⓓ Ⓔ	239 Ⓐ Ⓑ Ⓒ Ⓓ Ⓔ	264 Ⓐ Ⓑ Ⓒ Ⓓ Ⓔ	289 Ⓐ Ⓑ Ⓒ Ⓓ Ⓔ
215 Ⓐ Ⓑ Ⓒ Ⓓ Ⓔ	240 Ⓐ Ⓑ Ⓒ Ⓓ Ⓔ	265 Ⓐ Ⓑ Ⓒ Ⓓ Ⓔ	290 Ⓐ Ⓑ Ⓒ Ⓓ Ⓔ
216 Ⓐ Ⓑ Ⓒ Ⓓ Ⓔ	241 Ⓐ Ⓑ Ⓒ Ⓓ Ⓔ	266 Ⓐ Ⓑ Ⓒ Ⓓ Ⓔ	291 Ⓐ Ⓑ Ⓒ Ⓓ Ⓔ
217 Ⓐ Ⓑ Ⓒ Ⓓ Ⓔ	242 Ⓐ Ⓑ Ⓒ Ⓓ Ⓔ	267 Ⓐ Ⓑ Ⓒ Ⓓ Ⓔ	292 Ⓐ Ⓑ Ⓒ Ⓓ Ⓔ
218 Ⓐ Ⓑ Ⓒ Ⓓ Ⓔ	243 Ⓐ Ⓑ Ⓒ Ⓓ Ⓔ	268 Ⓐ Ⓑ Ⓒ Ⓓ Ⓔ	293 Ⓐ Ⓑ Ⓒ Ⓓ Ⓔ
219 Ⓐ Ⓑ Ⓒ Ⓓ Ⓔ	244 Ⓐ Ⓑ Ⓒ Ⓓ Ⓔ	269 Ⓐ Ⓑ Ⓒ Ⓓ Ⓔ	294 Ⓐ Ⓑ Ⓒ Ⓓ Ⓔ
220 Ⓐ Ⓑ Ⓒ Ⓓ Ⓔ	245 Ⓐ Ⓑ Ⓒ Ⓓ Ⓔ	270 Ⓐ Ⓑ Ⓒ Ⓓ Ⓔ	295 Ⓐ Ⓑ Ⓒ Ⓓ Ⓔ
221 Ⓐ Ⓑ Ⓒ Ⓓ Ⓔ	246 Ⓐ Ⓑ Ⓒ Ⓓ Ⓔ	271 Ⓐ Ⓑ Ⓒ Ⓓ Ⓔ	296 Ⓐ Ⓑ Ⓒ Ⓓ Ⓔ
222 Ⓐ Ⓑ Ⓒ Ⓓ Ⓔ	247 Ⓐ Ⓑ Ⓒ Ⓓ Ⓔ	272 Ⓐ Ⓑ Ⓒ Ⓓ Ⓔ	297 Ⓐ Ⓑ Ⓒ Ⓓ Ⓔ
223 Ⓐ Ⓑ Ⓒ Ⓓ Ⓔ	248 Ⓐ Ⓑ Ⓒ Ⓓ Ⓔ	273 Ⓐ Ⓑ Ⓒ Ⓓ Ⓔ	298 Ⓐ Ⓑ Ⓒ Ⓓ Ⓔ
224 Ⓐ Ⓑ Ⓒ Ⓓ Ⓔ	249 Ⓐ Ⓑ Ⓒ Ⓓ Ⓔ	274 Ⓐ Ⓑ Ⓒ Ⓓ Ⓔ	299 Ⓐ Ⓑ Ⓒ Ⓓ Ⓔ
225 Ⓐ Ⓑ Ⓒ Ⓓ Ⓔ	250 Ⓐ Ⓑ Ⓒ Ⓓ Ⓔ	275 Ⓐ Ⓑ Ⓒ Ⓓ Ⓔ	300 Ⓐ Ⓑ Ⓒ Ⓓ Ⓔ

SIMULATION TEST 2

Part 1—General Medical Knowledge

Directions: *Each of the following questions or incomplete statements precedes five suggested answers or completions. Select the ONE answer or completion that is BEST in each case, and fill in the circle containing the corresponding letter on the answer sheet.*

1. True statements concerning febrile convulsions include
   A. they are set off after the body temperature reaches 105°F
   B. they occur very early in an illness
   C. both A and B
   D. they occur very late in an illness
   E. both A and D

2. The artery behind the knees used to measure pulse rate is the
   A. brachial
   B. popliteal
   C. femoral
   D. dorsalis pedis
   E. vastus lateralis

3. The hormone mainly responsible for secondary sex characteristics in men is secreted by the
   A. adrenal cortex
   B. corpus luteum
   C. testes
   D. anterior pituitary gland
   E. posterior pituitary gland

4. A pregnant woman near term reports feeling lightheaded when she lies on her back. This is due to
   A. faulty implantation of the placenta
   B. preeclampsia
   C. the gravid uterus compressing the vena cava
   D. hormonal imbalance
   E. an increase of blood supply to the brain

5. The principal electrolyte associated with blood volume, blood pressure, and extracellular fluid retention/loss is
   A. sodium
   B. potassium
   C. calcium
   D. organic phosphate
   E. magnesium

6. Inflammation and pain are associated with an increase in
   A. prostaglandin
   B. endorphin
   C. both A and B
   D. histamine
   E. both A and D

7. The predominant symptom(s) of Lyme disease is (are)
   A. pruritus
   B. arthritis
   C. hyperactive reflexes and muscle spasm
   D. lethargy, vomiting, and hepatic dysfunction
   E. seizures

8. In the inflammatory process, pus is the result of
   A. destruction of cells by bacteria
   B. digestion of cells by leukocytic enzymes
   C. lack of blood supply
   D. increased body temperature
   E. release of fat enzymes

9. Functions of the endocrine glands include the
   A. control of metabolism
   B. regulation of waste products
   C. both A and B
   D. regulation of personality
   E. both A and D

10. In men, a walnut-sized organ found at the base of the bladder surrounding the urethra is the
    A. prostate gland
    B. epididymis
    C. scrotum
    D. testis
    E. bulbourethral gland

11. The menstrual cycle and the resulting structural changes in the endometrium depend on a system controlled by the ovary in combination with the
    A. hypothalamus
    B. anterior pituitary gland
    C. both A and B
    D. posterior pituitary gland
    E. both A and D

12. Ovulation is the release of the mature ovum brought about by the sudden surge of what hormone?
    A. follicle-stimulating hormone
    B. luteinizing hormone
    C. estrogen
    D. progesterone
    E. human chorionic gonadotropin

13. Which of the following is a function of the placenta?
    A. to filter out all chemicals to the fetus
    B. to mix maternal and fetal blood
    C. to bathe the fetus
    D. to connect the arteries and veins to the fetus
    E. to transfer nutrients and oxygen to the fetus

14. Advantages of breast-feeding include which of the following?
    A. uterine involution
    B. prevention of infant colic
    C. both A and B
    D. reliable method of birth control
    E. both A and D

15. When blood is shed, which of the following must be first neutralized to allow clotting to take place?
    A. fibrinogen
    B. fibrin
    C. thrombin
    D. heparin
    E. thromboplastin

16. A placenta implanted abnormally low in the uterus is called
    A. ectopic
    B. preeclampsia
    C. eclampsia
    D. placenta previa
    E. abruptio placenta

17. The release of stored glucose in the liver, which raises the blood glucose level, is stimulated by
    A. glycogen
    B. insulin
    C. both A and B
    D. glucagon
    E. both A and D

18. In men, a recent clinical history of mumps is associated with
    A. prostatitis
    B. orchitis
    C. cryptorchidism
    D. impotence
    E. infertility

19. A skin condition involving inflammation of the capillaries followed by the eruption of pale wheals, erythema, and itching is known as
    A. hives
    B. contact dermatitis
    C. both A and B
    D. urticaria
    E. both A and D

20. Psoriasis is a condition characterized by
    A. small skin vesicles and exudative eruptions
    B. greasy scaling and itching
    C. a painful macropapular rash
    D. thick, flaky scaling
    E. leathery vesicular eruptions

21. Premenstrual syndrome (PMS) is a cluster of symptoms particularly frequent in women
    A. who use oral contraceptives
    B. in their 30s and 40s
    C. with previous intrauterine diethylstilbestrol (DES) exposure
    D. also diagnosed with dysfunctional uterine bleeding (DUB)
    E. also diagnosed with dysfunction characterized by anxiety

22. A good cholesterol level ratio associated with protection against atherosclerosis is
    A. a low ratio of HDL to LDL
    B. a low ratio of HDL to VLDL
    C. a high ratio of HDL to LDL and VLDL
    D. a high ratio of LDL to VLDL
    E. a high ratio of HDL to LDL and a low ratio of LDL to VLDL

23. The universal recipient blood type is
    A. A
    B. B
    C. AB
    D. O
    E. Rh positive

24. During urine formation, glucose, water, and amino acids are reabsorbed back into the bloodstream in the
    A. glomerulus
    B. Bowman's capsule
    C. proximal tubule
    D. distal tubule
    E. collecting tubule

25. Following severe diarrhea and vomiting, dehydration is often accompanied by
    A. oliguria
    B. polyuria
    C. anuria
    D. nocturia
    E. diuresis

26. When blood or extracellular fluids change in pH, corrections must be made by the
    A. lungs
    B. parathyroid gland
    C. both A and B
    D. kidneys
    E. both A and D

27. Under which protection may the physician deny a patient access to medical records?
    A. Freedom of Information Act
    B. 1973 U.S. Privacy Protection Study Commission
    C. Commission on Medical Management
    D. Doctrine of Professional Discretion
    E. A physician may not deny patient access to records.

28. A log of occupational injuries and illness occurring as a result of employment in a medical facility must be kept
    A. until follow-up examinations and tests are negative for each incident
    B. for 1 year
    C. for 3 years
    D. for 5 years
    E. indefinitely

29. Each of the following is a recordable case of occupational injury or illness EXCEPT
    A. fall, sprained ankle, no lost work days
    B. cut finger bandaged, no lost work days
    C. broken glassware, seven sutures, temporarily assigned to front office, no lost days
    D. loss of consciousness during minor surgery, no injury, no lost days
    E. third-degree autoclave burn, right arm, one lost working day

30. Quality control under OSHA and CLIA regulations requires the medical assistant to
    A. pass an evaluation every year
    B. use only FDA-approved test kits and methods
    C. both A and B
    D. attend training classes two times per year
    E. both A and D

31. The OSHA Hazard Communication Program regulates
    A. hazardous chemicals
    B. fire extinguisher maintenance
    C. both A and B
    D. infection control for protection against hepatitis B virus and HIV
    E. both A and D

32. According to OSHA standards, which of the following items must be included on the labels of hazardous materials?
    A. name of chemical and hazard warning
    B. effects of overexposure
    C. both A and B
    D. name and address of the physician
    E. both A and D

33. Regardless of the specific length of time medical records must be maintained, the minimum length of time runs from the date of
    A. the first entry
    B. the last office visit
    C. the last treatment
    D. the last entry
    E. the last payment

34. Which of the following statements is true legally if a physician is asked to collect a patient specimen for drug screening purposes?
    A. Only licensed personnel may collect the specimen.
    B. The specimen must be tested on site.
    C. The specimen must be prepared for transport out of the sight of the patient.
    D. The patient's written consent is required.
    E. The physician is legally responsible for obtaining an informed consent from the patient.

35. After a Medicare audit of services rendered, it may be necessary to repay funds reimbursed by Medicare for services provided if a medical record lacks a
    A. copy of insurance claim
    B. patient registration form
    C. progress note signature
    D. release of records authorization
    E. informed consent signature

36. Language that exempts a medical assistant from licensing requirements and allows the MA to perform certain clinical tasks under the delegation and supervision of a licensed health care practitioner is found in which document?
    A. AMA Code of Ethics
    B. Allied Health Education Directory
    C. State Medical Practice Act
    D. Federal Omnibus Budget Reconciliation Act
    E. AHA Statement on the Patient's Bill of Rights

37. The legal document that expresses the patient's legal right to refuse treatment prolonging life is the
    A. Living Will Declaration
    B. Durable Power of Attorney
    C. Uniform Donor Card
    D. Withdrawal of Life Support Statement
    E. Verification of Informed Consent

38. In which of the following circumstances may a small fee be charged for patient record release?
    A. faxing records to a new physician
    B. mailing records to a new physician
    C. photocopying records to mail to a new physician
    D. photocopying records for release to the patient
    E. preparing a physician's summary for mailing to a consultant

39. In which of the following circumstances does Regulation Z stipulate that a Truth in Lending agreement must be completed by the physician and patient?
    A. when the office bills for a $500 copayment in full
    B. when the patient makes a partial payment on a $500 payment-in-full statement
    C. both A and B
    D. when the patient signs an agreement to pay $500 in five monthly payments and the physician waives finance charges
    E. both A and D

40. Collection practices to avoid include
    A. "Ms. Smith, your total charges today are $65."
    B. "Would you like to pay for today's charges in cash or by check?"
    C. both A and B
    D. "Shall we bill you?"
    E. both A and D

41. Which of the following are legal collection practices?
    A. blind postcards with "Call me" written on them
    B. calling the debtor's employer
    C. both A and B
    D. calling between 6 PM and 8 PM
    E. both A and D

42. If the physician denies a new patient credit on the basis of an adverse credit rating, the medical assistant is required by law to tell the patient
    A. the names of other physicians who are accepting new patients
    B. that the office policy is cash or check only
    C. that the office is not accepting any new patients
    D. that the office does not accept new patients without insurance coverage
    E. the name and address of the agency that gave the patient a poor credit rating

43. When hiring a medical assistant, possible discrimination problem areas include inquiries concerning an applicant's
    A. age
    B. birth date
    C. nationality
    D. citizenship
    E. child care arrangements

44. A male patient consistently makes lewd remarks and inappropriately touches the medical assistant when she takes his vital signs. The MA tells her coworkers of the problem, and they tell her to forget about it. The MA then tells the physician, who also tells her to ignore the patient's behavior. The MA resigns, giving 2 weeks' notice. According the sexual harassment law, who is liable in this situation?
    A. the patient
    B. the physician
    C. both A and B
    D. the coworkers
    E. both A and D

45. In the foregoing case, rather than quit her job, the medical assistant could seek help from the
    A. Office of Equal Employment Opportunities
    B. Department of Human Resources
    C. American Medical Association
    D. Occupational Safety and Health Review Committee
    E. local police department

46. The ideal solution to the previous harassment situation would be for the medical assistant to
    A. ask that another MA be assigned to the patient and ignore the offensive behavior
    B. ask the physician to finish taking the vital signs and ignore the behavior
    C. ask the physician to tell the harasser to stop his behavior
    D. threaten to tell the doctor if he does not stop
    E. tell the patient to stop his behavior

47. Which of the following is a legal requirement when preparing an informed consent form?
    A. The form blanks are typed in before meeting with the patient.
    B. A blanket form, covering all aspects of care, can be prepared for new patients.
    C. Forms should be signed the day of surgery, before the procedure begins.
    D. The form should contain an expiration date.
    E. A signed form is all that is necessary in the patient record.

48. When using active listening techniques, restatement (i.e., repeating back the words of the patient as you hear them) should be used
    A. one time
    B. in the initial phases of listening
    C. only when strong emotion is heard behind the patient's words
    D. throughout the interview
    E. to summarize the end of the interview

49. A patient is upset and the conversation begins with an emotion-laden statement from the patient about the poor bookkeeping methods in the office. The medical assistant's most helpful response would be
    A. "You're worried that your bill is wrong, and that you'll not be able to convince us?"
    B. "We have the best bookkeeper in town."
    C. "Please lower your voice. We have some very sick patients here."
    D. "I hand-picked our bookkeeper myself."
    E. "Why don't you just have a seat?"

50. During an employee evaluation, you feel frustrated over your employer's emphasis on what needs improving and the lack of emphasis on your accomplishments. You decide to express your frustration with "I" statements. In doing so, you know that sending "I" messages
A. involves taking a risk
B. minimizes your strong underlying feelings
C. places your employer on the defensive
D. immediately solves the problem
E. keeps the discussion one sided

51. When you have a problem with a coworker's behavior and need to get the problem resolved, "I" statements guarantee that the
A. coworker will actively listen
B. coworker will respond in a helpful way
C. responsibility is not owned by you or the coworker
D. responsibility is owned by the coworker
E. responsibility is owned by you

52. Therapeutic patient communication includes being able to
A. offer advice quickly
B. find a solution to a problem quickly
C. help the patient
D. help the patient help himself or herself
E. please the patient

53. Which of the following is an example of a nonassertive behavior?
A. saying no
B. saying nothing
C. being confrontive
D. expressing affection
E. expressing opinions

54. Erikson's theory on the stages of development of personality centers on the successful resolution of tension in a series of steps encountered by the growing person from birth onward. When care givers leave a crying baby to cry, which of the baby's tension resolutions are being jeopardized?
A. Trust vs. Mistrust
B. Autonomy vs. Shame and Doubt
C. Intimacy vs. Isolation
D. Identity vs. Identity Diffusion
E. Integrity vs. Despair

55. During which of Erikson's stages of development (see previous question) is adult suppression of a child's sexual curiosity the most harmful?
A. Trust vs. Mistrust
B. Autonomy vs. Shame and Doubt
C. Initiative vs. Guilt
D. Identity vs. Identity Diffusion
E. Intimacy vs. Isolation

56. Which of Erikson's conflicts (see previous questions) remain unresolved if "potty training" is attempted too early?
A. Mistrust
B. Shame and Doubt
C. Guilt
D. Inferiority
E. Isolation

57. The psychologist who first described young children as very "present-oriented" and concrete in their thinking, and who described abstract logic as developing much later is
A. Jean Piaget
B. Erik H. Erikson
C. Penelope Leach
D. Carl Jung
E. Abraham Maslow

58. According to Erikson's theories, an infant who is abused and neglected will carry over to adulthood the view that the world is
A. uncertain
B. chaotic
C. both A and B
D. hostile
E. both A and D

59. Adults who fail to mature with autonomy and individuality and are addicted to substances or the well-being of another person for happiness are
A. extroverted
B. introverted
C. codependent
D. neurotic
E. psychotic

60. The term most closely interchangeable with "empathy" is
A. sympathy
B. pity
C. identification
D. self transposal
E. oneness

61. When caring for patients, the therapeutic relationship is best created by
    A. remaining subjective
    B. offering advice
    C. displaying sympathy
    D. respectful interest
    E. remaining neutral

62. A patient says that whenever he gets upset he kicks his cat. This is an example of the defense mechanism known as
    A. compensation
    B. rationalization
    C. dissociation
    D. projection
    E. displacement

63. A patient states that he is worried about his upcoming outpatient surgery. The medical assistant should respond
    A. "Don't worry about the surgery."
    B. "I understand your concerns. Most people feel the same way you do."
    C. "I understand your concern. Do you have any specific questions about your surgery?"
    D. "I don't think you'll find your surgery difficult, and you'll be home the same day."
    E. "You don't need to worry, but why don't I see if you can have a sedative before you come in for your procedure?"

64. Schizophrenia is a disorder of
    A. thought
    B. personality
    C. adjustment
    D. coping
    E. mood

65. When evaluating a patient's elevated temperature reading, it does not make sense in relation to the patient's appearance. The medical assistant should
    A. take the patient's temperature with a different thermometer
    B. take the patient's temperature using another body area
    C. both A and B
    D. take the patient's temperature in the same area and stay with patient
    E. both A and D

66. While gathering a patient history, it can be anticipated that a patient with advanced Alzheimer's disease would describe
    A. overeating
    B. anxiety
    C. sensory deficit
    D. self-care problems
    E. pain

67. On a progress note is written the symbol "R." The symbol means
    A. respiration
    B. right
    C. range
    D. review of systems
    E. rectal

68. A term meaning a fever disappears is
    A. afebrile
    B. defervescence
    C. subsiding
    D. lysis
    E. crises

69. Inflammation of milk ducts in breasts 2 to 4 weeks postpartum is termed
    A. mastitis
    B. papillomatosis
    C. cystic mastitis
    D. gynecomastia
    E. fibroadenoma

70. Treatment for dysphagia includes
    A. injections of botulin to decrease facial paralysis
    B. special feeding instructions
    C. range-of-motion exercises
    D. speech therapy
    E. oxygen therapy

71. A colporrhaphy refers to a surgical procedure in which the vagina is
    A. stabilized
    B. suspended
    C. punctured
    D. fixed
    E. sutured

72. The medical term that means cancer-producing is
    A. carcinoma
    B. carcinogenic
    C. carcinoid
    D. tumorous
    E. neoplasm

73. The removal of a blood clot by means of a balloon catheter is called
    A. grafting
    B. angioplasty
    C. stenting
    D. embolectomy
    E. stripping and ligation

74. Which of the following words is spelled correctly?
    A. hematopioesis
    B. rachicentesis
    C. diarrhia
    D. perenchyma
    E. hemiplagia

75. One noninvasive technique used to evaluate the female genital tract and fetus in the obstetrical patient is
    A. ultrasonography
    B. hysterosalpingography
    C. uterotubography
    D. culdoscopy
    E. colposcopy

76. Which of the following plural forms is spelled correctly?
    A. maculi
    B. epiphyses
    C. appendixes
    D. bacilla
    E. vertebraes

77. The term "phacoemulsification" means
    A. ingestion and digestion of bacteria by white blood cells
    B. ingestion of poisonous plants
    C. cataract surgery
    D. paralysis of the pharynx
    E. removal of the larynx

78. The medical word element for "softening" is
    A. kerat
    B. malacia
    C. scirrh
    D. scler
    E. sclerosis

79. The loss of hair or baldness is known as
    A. alopecia
    B. seborrhea
    C. scleroderma
    D. trichiasis
    E. trichitis

80. A snoring sound caused by secretions in the trachea or large bronchi is termed
    A. stertor
    B. stridor
    C. wheeze
    D. Cheyne-Stokes respirations
    E. apneusis

81. A woman who has never been pregnant is recorded as
    A. nulligravida
    B. nullipara
    C. primigravida
    D. primipara
    E. gravida

82. Efforts to reduce liabilities resulting from untoward events is termed
    A. quality assurance
    B. total quality management
    C. risk management
    D. utilization review
    E. quality control

83. The abbreviation for "of each" is
    A. $\bar{a}\bar{a}$
    B. $\bar{a}$
    C. ea
    D. oe
    E. @

84. The abbreviation "Sx" stands for
    A. label
    B. signs
    C. immediately
    D. subcutaneous
    E. symptom

85. Medical informatics deals with the exchange of medical information
    A. through computer-based systems
    B. through fax transmissions
    C. between hospital medical records departments
    D. between any two medical facilities
    E. between patient and physician

86. Cancer confined to one place or a localized site is defined as
    A. de novo
    B. in situ
    C. dormant
    D. metastatic
    E. invasive

87. Hydrosalpinx is defined as
    A. a fluid-filled fallopian tube
    B. a pus-filled fallopian tube
    C. an ovary filled with fluid
    D. an ovarian abscess
    E. fluid absorbed into the uterine wall

88. A method used to measure cerebral blood flow and metabolism with radionuclides is
    A. nuclear medicine scan
    B. positron emission tomography (PET)
    C. magnetic resonance scan
    D. arteriogram
    E. ventriculography

89. Which of the following is the correct singular form?
    A. data
    B. media
    C. addenda
    D. larva
    E. ova

90. The term meaning the impairment of well-being or the decrease in the life expectancy of an individual compared to a specific population is
    A. cachexia
    B. morbidity
    C. mortality
    D. deficit
    E. prognosis

91. The term patency means
    A. the state of being freely open
    B. the state of being firmly attached
    C. the state of being closed
    D. the state of being occluded
    E. protected by a patent

92. A term commonly used to describe a depressed immune system is
    A. decreased
    B. exacerbated
    C. compromised
    D. flaccid
    E. compliant

93. Which of the following noun forms is spelled correctly?
    A. mucous
    B. aerobe
    C. ecchimosis
    D. culpitis
    E. diabetes mellitus

94. An abnormal growth that is well-defined, fluid-filled, and noncancerous is termed a
    A. polyp
    B. cyst
    C. tumor
    D. nodule
    E. wen

95. The study of the cause of disease is known as
    A. pathogenesis
    B. epidemiology
    C. pathology
    D. prognosis
    E. etiology

96. Which of the following conditions is a dermatophytosis?
    A. histoplasmosis
    B. *Tinea cruris*
    C. moniliasis
    D. nocardiosis
    E. *Herpes zoster*

97. Dyspareunia means the occurrence of
    A. painful urination
    B. vaginal itching or burning
    C. testicular swelling with acute pain
    D. pain in women during sexual intercourse
    E. painful ejaculation in men

98. A chemical that can cause unconsciousness by suffocation is termed a(n)
    A. asphyxiant
    B. corrosive
    C. oxidizer
    D. ingestant
    E. inhalant

99. A predisposing factor is defined as a
    A. disease that is inherited
    B. tendency toward a disease
    C. direct cause of disease
    D. secondary cause of disease
    E. spontaneous cause of disease

100. Infections that occur only under special circumstances and are caused by a microorganism that is usually harmless are termed
    A. endemic
    B. opportunistic
    C. communicable
    D. allergic
    E. self-limited

SIMULATION TEST 2

Part 2—Administrative Procedures

Directions: *Each of the following questions or incomplete statements precedes five suggested answers or completions. Select the ONE answer or completion that is BEST in each case, and fill in the circle containing the corresponding letter on the answer sheet.*

101. The appointment system that combines one long appointment with two or more shorter procedures and has the patients arrive at the same time of the hour is known as the
    A. stream system
    B. time-allotted system
    C. wave system
    D. modified wave system
    E. grouping system

102. In the preceding appointment system, each of the following statements is true EXCEPT
    A. The patients can be seen in an order chosen by the physician.
    B. The system is well suited for offices with more than one medical assistant.
    C. The system is well suited for scheduling more than one physician at the same time.
    D. All rooms can be filled at the beginning of the office visit session.
    E. Patients may object when they realize several of them have the same appointment time.

103. If a patient is covered under a health maintenance plan or independent practice association, what is required before the plan will allow coverage of a hospital admission for necessary but not urgent care?
    A. authorization of services
    B. preadmission certification
    C. benefits verification
    D. a second surgical opinion
    E. a referral authorization

104. During a hospital stay under the service of a specialist, a patient insured by a network plan does not respond to treatment and needs to remain hospitalized beyond the proposed hospitalization. In this situation, what form must be completed?
    A. continued stay review
    B. assignment of benefits
    C. authorization to release records
    D. extension of benefits
    E. explanation of benefits

105. In the situation just described, where should the required form be submitted?
    A. hospital admission department
    B. hospital billing department
    C. Health Care Financing Administration
    D. primary care facility
    E. insurance carrier

106. In this same situation, when should the required form be filed?
    A. before the patient's last certified day
    B. on the patient's last certified day
    C. after the patient's last certified day
    D. before discharge
    E. after discharge

107. In the foregoing situation, who should file the required form?
    A. hospital admission department
    B. hospital billing department
    C. primary care facility
    D. the attending physician
    E. the nursing unit

108. A patient calls to cancel his appointment. The medical assistant should
    A. write "cancel" in the appointment book and initial it
    B. write the date and "canceled" on the patient's chart
    C. both A and B
    D. send a letter to the patient confirming the cancellation
    E. both A and D

109. A patient calls and cancels a nonessential appointment. When the medical assistant offers a new time, the patient states he cannot predict the next time he can take off from work and that he will get back with the office as soon as he can. The medical assistant should notate the appointment as
    A. canceled
    B. C
    C. w/c
    D. C, w/c
    E. recall

110. Although one is not required by an insurance carrier, a patient wishes to have a second surgical opinion. What type of coverage is offered by most insurance carriers for this type of second opinion?
    A. no coverage
    B. coverage at 50%
    C. copay coverage at 70%
    D. copay coverage at 80%
    E. 100% coverage

111. All appointment "no shows" should be handled by
    A. calling the patient immediately
    B. documenting the medical record
    C. both A and B
    D. sending the patient a letter
    E. both A and D

112. The physician calls at the beginning of the morning appointments and says she will be delayed on hospital rounds for another hour. One patient was not able to be contacted and shows up for his 6-month check-up. The medical assistant should
    A. make arrangements for another physician to see the patient
    B. ask the patient to leave and come back when the physician is expected back
    C. say nothing to the patient, then move him into the examining room after 30 minutes
    D. tell the patient the physician will be delayed and offer him magazines to read
    E. offer to reschedule the patient

113. Which of the following is important if a practice stops accepting new patients?
    A. To provide patients with a written statement of this policy
    B. To complete a patient mailing with an update of this policy
    C. To provide patients with numbers of local medical societies for referral
    D. To provide patients with the names of other physicians who take referrals
    E. To mail a policy statement to other physicians in the area

114. For elective surgical procedures involving large self-pay fees, office policies should include
    A. lump-sum payments prior to the surgeries
    B. credit rating reports from credit bureaus
    C. cash only payments
    D. additional finance fees for long-term installment plans
    E. bank references concerning the patient's financial status

115. The form of appointment scheduling that is the LEAST time efficient for the physician is scheduling
    A. patients in a steady stream
    B. all patients for a session at the same time
    C. by double booking
    D. the same procedures together
    E. on a first-come, first-served basis

116. Which of the following is true concerning the use of a patient database?
    A. Computer data are not easily accessed or changed.
    B. Only designated persons should be authorized to make changes.
    C. Completed consent forms should be stored on the computer.
    D. Data changes should be made at any time by authorized persons.
    E. Data should never be purged.

117. For which of the following functions is a database the program of choice?
    A. budget projections
    B. tracking monthly expenses
    C. processing insurance claims
    D. tracking insurance payments
    E. creating correspondence

118. When submitting a medical manuscript, which of the following printer fonts will produce uniform character size and spacing?
    A. Times Roman
    B. Universal
    C. CG Times
    D. Courier
    E. Helvetica

119. Mass-produced letters, such as for invitations or announcements, can be produced in WordPerfect 5.1 by merging a mailing list with a form letter. The letter is retrieved when the program screen asks for the
    A. primary merge file
    B. secondary merge file
    C. index
    D. macro file
    E. document

120. On the WordPerfect 5.1 menu bar, right and left margins can be changed under the menu
    A. File
    B. Edit
    C. Tools
    D. Fonts
    E. Format (Layout)

121. Which of the following is required to receive information concerning laboratory reports, insurance claims, and memos from other facilities over telephone wires?
    A. local area network (LAN)
    B. AB switch box
    C. modem
    D. server
    E. bulletin board system (BBS)

122. If you type "\m" at the end of a backup command, the computer will back up
    A. the entire hard disk
    B. one subdirectory
    C. all files beginning with "m"
    D. files worked on since the last backup
    E. macro files

123. Which of the following statements is a correct response to protect against loss of information on a computer?
    A. alternating between two separate sets of backup disks
    B. making backup data files monthly
    C. making backup copies of programs daily
    D. making backup copies of the disk daily
    E. making each backup run as large as possible

124. A system of computers connected by wires in the same office or office building is called a
    A. LAN system
    B. Compuserve
    C. bulletin board system
    D. e-mail system
    E. Internet

125. On an envelope with a four-line address, the room, suite, and building numbers should be
    A. omitted
    B. typed alone on the second line
    C. typed on the same line as the street address
    D. typed on a new line directly below the street line
    E. typed on a separate line directly above the city, state, and zip code

126. Correctly addressing an envelope includes
    A. periods after all abbreviations
    B. periods after middle initials
    C. a comma between the street and building numbers
    D. a comma between city and state
    E. omitting all punctuation

127. In which letter style may the complimentary close be omitted?
    A. Simplified
    B. Block
    C. Modified block
    D. Semiblock
    E. Open punctuation

128. The continuation page of a medical report should begin with
    A. patient name, page number, date
    B. sender name, page number, date
    C. patient name, case number, page number
    D. date, page number
    E. page number only

129. Correspondence styles to avoid with mixed or standard punctuation include
    A. memos
    B. modified block
    C. semiblock
    D. hanging indentation
    E. simplified

130. Correspondence that can be signed by the medical assistant includes
    A. patient letters dictated by the physician
    B. referral letters
    C. consultation reports
    D. notes to the medical file
    E. nonmedical insurance paperwork

131. When addressing an envelope, the last line of the address should not exceed
    A. 18 spaces
    B. 26 spaces
    C. 36 spaces
    D. 50 spaces
    E. 60 spaces

132. When preparing outgoing mail to a company, the company's address should
    A. include as many lines as necessary for punctual delivery
    B. include as many lines as printed on the company's stationery
    C. be limited to three lines
    D. be limited to four lines
    E. not exceed five lines

133. Which of the following abbreviation usages is discouraged on outgoing correspondence?
    A. bcc:
    B. xc:
    C. Attn:
    D. RE:
    E. encl

134. A proofreader's mark that means insert a space is
    A. /
    B. #
    C. ^
    D. =
    E. [ ]

135. The physician is to submit a medical manuscript for publication. The final manuscript should be submitted with
    A. single spacing
    B. page numbers centered at the bottom of the page
    C. both A and B
    D. half-inch margins at the right and left
    E. both A and D

136. When preparing a manuscript, legends to illustrations are typed
    A. as they occur on the manuscript pages
    B. as footnotes at the bottom of the manuscript pages
    C. indented and in smaller-sized type on the manuscript pages
    D. on a separate sheet of paper
    E. each on a separate sheet on which the illustration is mounted

137. In the bibliography entry "Author, AA: Title of the article. Journal Title, 1994, 9(3):33," the number "33" indicates
    A. volume
    B. page
    C. chapter
    D. issue
    E. edition

138. A master list of equipment items would include each of the following EXCEPT
    A. date of purchase
    B. cost
    C. operating manuals
    D. description of equipment
    E. estimated life

139. On the physician's vitae, presentations are listed
   A. alphabetically by title
   B. alphabetically by organization
   C. chronologically
   D. geographically
   E. by subject

140. On the physician's vitae, publications are listed first by year, then
   A. alphabetically by title
   B. alphabetically by journal
   C. alphabetically by subject
   D. alphabetically by author
   E. by month of publication

141. The best method of filing medical journal reprints is
   A. by journal name
   B. chronologically
   C. by subject
   D. by author
   E. alphabetically by title

142. Records of the physician's association activities, such as committees, recommendations, presentations, and meeting attendance, would be filed best
   A. by terminal digit coding
   B. numerically
   C. chronologically by subject
   D. geographically by subject
   E. alphabetically by subject

143. Numeric filing is preferred if
   A. documents refer to the names of organizations
   B. retrieval is likely to be by subject rather than alphabetically
   C. documents may be reasonably grouped by activities or products
   D. many subdivisions are necessary
   E. documents refer to ongoing contract or research project numbers

144. "For deposit only, Jane Doe" is an example of what kind of check endorsement?
   A. open
   B. blank
   C. special
   D. limited
   E. restricted

145. With which billing document should the first collection notice be included?
   A. superbill at the time of the visit
   B. first statement
   C. second statement
   D. third statement
   E. fourth statement

146. Which of the following is usually a situation in which a "write-off" is recommended?
   A. $1000 balance of a patient without medical insurance
   B. $15 account balance; patient does not respond to notices
   C. both A and B
   D. an insurance indemnity plan that reduces a fee to 80% of an allowed charge
   E. both A and D

147. The collection of an overdue account is limited by statutes of limitation. The time of an "open book" account runs from
   A. the first time the patient is seen
   B. the last entry for a specific illness
   C. the last payment for a specific illness
   D. the date of the last payment due
   E. the first collection notice

148. The collection of an overdue account is limited by statutes of limitation. The time of a "single entry" account based on a written contract runs from the date of
   A. the last single payment due
   B. the last installment
   C. both A and B
   D. filing a collection suit
   E. both A and D

149. Which of the following adjustments is meant to be final with no collection reinstatement expected?
   A. accounts written off as uncollectible
   B. accounts turned over to a collection agency
   C. both A and C
   D. accounts written off as bad debt
   E. both A and D

150. Checks that are unacceptable for payment of services include
   A. counter checks
   B. blank checks
   C. checks with two endorsements
   D. money orders
   E. travelers' checks

151. The aging of accounts should be performed
  A. daily
  B. monthly
  C. before sending out statements
  D. as deposits are made
  E. annually

152. A record that is particular to the one-write system only is the
  A. day sheet
  B. patient ledger card
  C. petty cash journal
  D. transaction slip
  E. patient receipt

153. A debit balance on a patient ledger card represents
  A. charge
  B. payment
  C. income
  D. overpayment
  E. accounts receivable

154. A patient fee of $150 was collected by a collection agency, which in turn kept 50% and forwarded the balance to the physician. The entry on the patient's account card would be
  A. an adjustment posted in the amount of $75
  B. a payment posted in the amount of $150
  C. both A and B
  D. a payment posted in the amount of $75
  E. both A and D

155. A Medicare payment allows only $35 of a $55 fee charged to a patient. The $20 balance determined by Medicare to be above the allowable charge is
  A. written off in the adjustment column
  B. written off in the payment column
  C. added to the insurance payment and then written off
  D. subtracted from the original charge in the payment column
  E. brought down to the next ledger card line for next month's patient billing

156. A trial balance is a comparison of
  A. daily charges and payments
  B. assets, liabilities, and owner's equity
  C. ledger card totals and the accounts receivable month end balance
  D. the balance sheet and the income statement
  E. cash on hand and total cash received

157. Which of the following is correctly written without a hyphen?
  A. tetralogy of Fallot
  B. iodine 131
  C. Epstein Barr virus
  D. soft tissue lesion
  E. xradiation

158. Select the sentence with the correct use of an abbreviation
  A. Fig. 11 illustrates the histologic changes under ×250 magnification.
  B. The lesion (Fig. 11) was 10 microns in diameter.
  C. Nearly 90% of the patients with this size lesion recover fully.
  D. The patients were each instructed to take the medication p.r.n.
  E. Fever, headache, etc., were present in all the cases.

159. Each of the following should be italicized (underlined) EXCEPT
  A. in-situ
  B. The Merck Manual
  C. The Professional Medical Assistant
  D. Staphylococcus aureus
  E. V-shaped

160. The medical assistant can ensure a patient's eligibility for medical assistance payments by checking
  A. "From-Thru" eligibility dates on the medical assistance card
  B. that "Call EVS" is embossed on the medical assistance card
  C. that "Federal" is written on the medical assistance card
  D. calling the Eligibility Verification System
  E. calling the patient's primary care provider

161. "Call EVS" is embossed on a new patient's Medicaid card. On verification, the patient is reported as an "invalid recipient." This could mean
    A. the patient's ID number was incorrectly entered by the medical assistant
    B. the patient is not eligible for funds
    C. both A and B
    D. the patient is eligible for services but restricted to chosen providers
    E. both A and D

162. A Medicare patient being treated by a participating physician will be financially responsible for the
    A. difference between the Medicare Fee Schedule and the 80% Medicare payment
    B. difference between the participating physician's charge and the 80% Medicare payment
    C. the participating physician's charge and the Medicare Fee Schedule
    D. the deductible amount only
    E. noncovered charges only

163. The participating physician charges $160 for a service to a Medicare patient. The Medicare Fee Schedule amount is $125. The patient's responsibility is
    A. $0
    B. $25
    C. $32
    D. $45
    E. $60

164. Examples of a primary insurance program include
    A. Blue Shield Major Medical
    B. Blue Shield Supplemental
    C. both A and B
    D. Medicare
    E. both A and D

165. Enrollees in a straight HMO who go outside of the network to receive services without a referral
    A. do not have any additional out-of-pocket expenses
    B. will pay deductibles
    C. will pay copayments
    D. will pay deductibles and copayments
    E. will pay the total expenses

166. In an HMO plan, an elective referral is
    A. a self-referral
    B. a referral from a managed-care organization (MCO)
    C. both A and B
    D. a referral from a primary care physician (PCP)
    E. both A and D

167. An HMO patient obtains a referral from her primary provider and receives covered services from an in-plan consulting physician. The consultant's fee is greater than the benefit paid by the plan. The consultant collects from the patient
    A. no fee
    B. the difference between the charge and the plan fee only
    C. copayment from the patient up to the original amount charged
    D. deductible, if applicable, and copayment based on plan fee
    E. the copayment only, based on the plan fee

168. Which of the following is a group of physicians that contract with an HMO or managed-care plan to provide services, usually on a per-patient, fee-for-service basis?
    A. group model HMO
    B. staff model HMO
    C. network model HMO
    D. independent practice association (IPA)
    E. point of service managed care plan

169. When completing a Doctor's First Report of Occupational Injury or Illness claim, the form must include the
    A. name of the employer's compensation insurance carrier
    B. name of the patient's insurance carrier
    C. both A and B
    D. employer's ID number
    E. both A and D

170. Which of the following statements is true concerning coordination of benefits?
A. The man's insurance is primary to the woman's.
B. A self-purchased policy is primary over an employer-provided policy.
C. Medicare is always the insurance of last resort.
D. Medicare is primary to medical assistance.
E. If a patient has group coverage and also is covered by her husband, the husband's insurance is billed first.

171. Which of the following patient individual ID numbers will begin with the letter "R"?
A. BS Major Medical
B. BS Supplemental
C. BS Reciprocity
D. BS Federal Employee Plan
E. BS National Account Plan

172. When a patient has reciprocity Blue Shield coverage, services rendered are billed to the
A. Blue Shield National Account
B. local Blue Shield plan
C. either A and B
D. out-of-state Blue Shield plan
E. either A and D

173. When a 65-year-old female spouse of a wage earner, drawing social security benefits because of her husband's contribution, becomes a widow, the widow's Medicare eligibility is
A. reclassified and the Medicare card suffix code changed to a B
B. reclassified and the Medicare card suffix code changed to a D
C. limited to part A only
D. limited to part B only
E. discontinued

174. Which of the following is true if the physician chooses not to participate in Medicare?
A. The physician is not able to bill the patient for the entire amount.
B. The fee schedule is based on 100% of the participating fee schedule amount.
C. Charges cannot exceed 120% of the nonparticipant fee schedule.
D. Charges cannot exceed 115% of the nonparticipant fee schedule.
E. Nonparticipating physician claims are processed within 10 days.

175. A medical practice has grown so large that there is no more room for the storage of medical records. The medical assistant should
A. discard records of patients who have died
B. discard records of patients who have had records transferred to a new physician
C. transfer all records to another rented location
D. transfer active records to one file cabinet
E. transfer inactive records to another rented location

176. The disadvantage of alphabetic filing include
A. misfiling of common names
B. difficulty in classifying records
C. difficulty in retrieving miscellaneous records
D. cumbersome indexing
E. incompatibility with color coding

177. When filing "U.S. Department of the Air Force" alphabetically, which is the first indexing unit?
A. Govt.
B. United States
C. Air Force
D. U.S.
E. Department

178. In the POMR system, the physical examination results are recorded under the entry of
A. objective data
B. assessment
C. subjective data
D. plan
E. problem list

179. Under which of the following circumstances is the need for a written release of records waived?
A. subpoena
B. requests for records from other medical offices
C. insurance company requests
D. attorney requests
E. hospital requests

180. Which of the following hospital records can be released by an attending surgeon's authorization alone?
    A. billing information
    B. nursing notes
    C. radiology reports
    D. laboratory reports
    E. operative notes

181. Medical records may be released without a formal consent form to
    A. government agencies
    B. Medicare and medical assistance
    C. both A and B
    D. research agencies
    E. both A and D

182. After setting a patient appointment by telephone, the medical assistant should close the conversation by saying:
    A. "Thank you for calling. Goodbye."
    B. "We look forward to seeing you next week. Goodbye."
    C. "Call me if you cannot keep this appointment. Thank you."
    D. "I'll see you on Wednesday the 29th at 10:30. Goodbye."
    E. "Your appointment is now scheduled for next Wednesday at 10:30 am. Goodbye."

183. A patient calls during office hours and complains that his bill is incorrect. The medical assistant examines the ledger card, which appears accurate. The medical assistant should respond:
    A. "I'll discuss your charges with Dr. Jones and call you back this afternoon."
    B. "All bills are accurately generated by computer. I'll call you back if it is incorrect."
    C. "I'll need you to write a letter explaining what you think is wrong. Then our bookkeeper will look into your complaint."
    D. "Why don't you call back this afternoon when I can give you more time?"
    E. "We could have made a mistake. Let's go over your charges together."

184. Which of the following calls can the medical assistant handle without additional documentation in the patient record? The medical assistant
    A. gives the patient a name of a physician in another specialty
    B. cancels the patient's appointment for the third time
    C. confirms an appointment
    D. gives continued reassurance concerning an illness
    E. clarifies directions about a treatment

185. A repeated caller, who talks on and on, calls for reassurance that she does not need to come in to see the physician. The medical assistant should
    A. talk if the office is not busy
    B. set limits on time after recording the patient's message
    C. tell the caller that she will call her after work
    D. tell the patient that new policy will result in a charge
    E. tell the patient that now is not a good time to talk

186. A patient caller is extremely agitated that he cannot have the appointment he wants and demands to speak to the physician. The physician will be at teaching rounds when the patient wants to schedule. The medical assistant should
    A. transfer the call to the physician
    B. tell the patient not to talk that way
    C. ask the patient to call back the day he wants to come in, to see if there is an opening
    D. tell the patient the physician does want to see him and his name will be given priority on the recall list
    E. tell the patient the physician will call him back at the end of office hours

187. A patient asks to speak to the physician who has left instruction that she not be disturbed during patient hours except in an emergency. What should be the medical assistant's FIRST response?
    A. "The doctor cannot be disturbed during patient hours."
    B. "Dr. Smith left instructions that she not be disturbed during patient hours."
    C. "Dr. Smith is with a patient."
    D. "Dr. Smith is busy now."
    E. "Is this an emergency?"

188. A business solicitor calls and asks to speak to the physician. What should the medical assistant respond?
    A. "Please send literature for the doctor to review."
    B. "The doctor is busy now."
    C. "I'll take your number and have the doctor return your call."
    D. "We're not interested at this time."
    E. "The doctor is not in."

189. An appointment system needs modification if
    A. examination rooms are empty
    B. patients are waiting more than 15 minutes in the examining room
    C. both A and B
    D. patients are waiting more than 30 minutes in the waiting room
    E. both A and D

190. During which of the following appointment cancellations could the medical assistant feel comfortable terminating the telephone conversation without setting another appointment for the patient?
    A. when the appointment follows an extensive procedure
    B. when a patient who just moved to the area is seeking a new physician
    C. when a patient is being monitored for a new medication
    D. when a patient has been taking a pain medication
    E. when an appointment follows a serious illness

191. Methods by which CPT-4 modifiers may be reported include being entered
    A. using the 09900 series
    B. using the 99200 series
    C. both A and B
    D. using a two-digit number after the five-digit CPT-HCPCS code
    E. both A and D

192. A patient specimen is sent to a reference lab for analysis; however, the physician wishes to bill the carrier for the test. The claim form must contain the CPT-4 code with
    A. the modifier -90
    B. name of the lab and the lab charges to the physician
    C. both A and B
    D. the charge for the specimen collection
    E. both A and D

193. Under major surgery global package policies, separate charges for office visits are permitted in which of the following cases?
    A. preoperative evaluation the same day as minor surgery
    B. preoperative evaluation the same day as a proctoscopy
    C. one postoperative visit following a gastroscopy
    D. six-month examination following major surgery
    E. one-week postoperative visit following minor surgery

194. A second attending surgeon can be reimbursed, with the use of a CPT modifier, in each of the following circumstances EXCEPT
    A. preoperative and postoperative care only
    B. postoperative care only
    C. assisting in a surgical procedure as a specialist with a different skill
    D. assisting in a surgical procedure in a nonteaching hospital
    E. replacing an available resident in a surgical procedure

195. A patient is seen in the office the same day following a chemodenervation of a facial nerve (64612, 10-day global fee period) caused by hemifacial spasms. During the visit the patient reports moderate weakness in the upper extremities. The physician obtains a history of when the symptoms began, examines the patient, and recommends further testing to determine the cause of the weakness (99213). The physician then performs another chemodenervation of the facial nerve, injecting 15 units of Botox (J0585). The claim should be coded as follows:
    A. 99213-25, 64612, J0585
    B. 99213, 64612-25, J0585
    C. 99213, 64612, J0585-25
    D. 99213-25, 64612-25, J0585
    E. 99213-25, J0585

196. The same patient returns in 7 days because of a spasmodic torticollis. The same physician performs additional chemodenervation of the cervical spinal muscles (64613), injecting 30 units of Botox (J0585). The claim should be coded as follows (a modifier may be used if appropriate):
    -24 Postoperative E&M service unrelated to surgery
    -51 Multiple surgery
    -79 Postoperative unrelated surgical procedure
    A. 64613-79, J0585
    B. 64613, J0585-79
    C. 64613, J0585-51
    D. 64613-24, 64613, J0585
    E. 99213, 64613-51, J0585

197. A patient undergoes a laminectomy with decompression of nerve roots, including partial facetectomy and foraminotomy, and/or excision of herniated intervertebral disk involving C1, C2, and C3 cervical interspaces. The claim should be coded as follows (the multiple surgery modifier -51 may be used if appropriate):
    A. 63020, 63035, 63035
    B. 63020 (C1), 63035 (C2), 63035 (C3)
    C. 63020 (C1), 63035-51 (C2), 63035-51 (C3)
    D. 63020-51, 63035-51, 63035-51
    E. 63020-51 (C1), 63035-51 (C2), 63035-51 (C3)

198. The same patient returns to the office 2 months later complaining of facial spasm, unrelated to the foregoing surgery. The physician performs a level III E&M established patient office visit (99213). The claim should be coded as follows (one or more modifiers may be used, if appropriate):
    -24 Postoperative E&M service unrelated to surgery
    -79 Unrelated postoperative surgical procedure
    -55 Postoperative care only
    A. 99213
    B. 99213-24
    C. 99213-79
    D. 99213-55
    E. 63020, 99213-51

199. A surgeon examines a patient with acute abdominal pain, performing an initial consultation (99243) requested by the patient's family physician. After consultation and testing, the surgeon determines (-57) acute appendicitis, and the patients undergoes surgery (44950) the same day. How would this claim be coded?
    A. 44950-57
    B. 99243-57
    C. 99243, 44950
    D. 99243, 44950-57
    E. 99243-57, 44950

200. A patient undergoes surgery that has a 90-day postoperative global fee period. The patient returns for a follow-up visit and complains of a rash of the upper extremities. The condition is unrelated to surgery, but the physician takes 10 minutes to obtain a brief history of when the symptoms began, examines the patient, and provides a recommended course of treatment. The physician bills a level II E&M service. The claim should be coded
    A. 99212-24
    B. 99212-25
    C. 99272
    D. 99272-24
    E. 99272-25

SIMULATION TEST 2

Part 3—Clinical Procedures

Directions: *Each of the following questions or incomplete statements precedes five suggested answers or completions. Select the ONE answer or completion that is BEST in each case, and fill in the circle containing the corresponding letter on the answer sheet.*

201. Which is the marking code for V₁?
    A. - - -
    B. - - - - - -
    C. - - - -
    D. - - - - - - -
    E. - - - - - - - - - - - -

202. Which is the marking code for V₄?
    A. - - -
    B. - - - - - -
    C. - - - -
    D. - - - - - - -
    E. - - - - - - - - - - - -

Use the diagram below to answer the next two questions.

203. Which of the following ECG artifacts is represented in the diagram?
    A. muscle artifact
    B. wandering baseline
    C. somatic tremor
    D. alternating current
    E. interrupted baseline

204. If this diagram occurred, what is the reasonable next step?
    A. Cover the patient with a blanket.
    B. Reposition the patient's left arm.
    C. Rearrange the lead wires.
    D. Check the contacts between the skin and the electrodes.
    E. Move the patient to a new location away from the wall.

205. A small U wave seen after a T wave may be an indication of
    A. arrhythmia
    B. heart damage following a myocardial infarction
    C. digitalis overdose
    D. rheumatic fever
    E. slow recovery of the Purkinje fibers

206. The electrode connection on the patient's right arm should be checked if there is interference in lead
    A. I
    B. II
    C. both A and B
    D. III
    E. both A and D

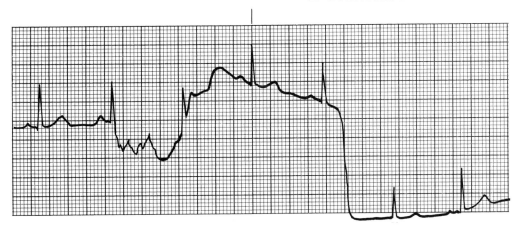

207. Which of the following actions would result in inaccurate ECG results when hooking up the equipment?
    A. grounding a metal examining table
    B. pointing the power cord toward the patient
    C. pointing the lead connectors toward the patient's feet
    D. arranging the lead wires to follow the body contour
    E. supporting the patient cable on the patient's abdomen

208. Which of the following artifacts can be caused by unequal amounts of electrolyte gel?
    A. wandering baseline
    B. somatic tremor
    C. voluntary muscle movement
    D. alternating current
    E. interrupted baseline

209. When counting the heart rate, the medical assistant starts at one R wave and counts the number of lines to the next R wave. If the second R wave falls on the fifth line, the patient's heart rate is
    A. 150
    B. 100
    C. 75
    D. 60
    E. 50

210. Each of the following statements about a normal electrocardiogram pattern is correct EXCEPT
    A. The P wave should be upright in lead I.
    B. The P wave should be inverted in lead aVR.
    C. The PR interval should remain constant.
    D. Sinus rhythm should be present.
    E. As leads move from V_1 to V_6, the R wave should decrease in height.

211. Each of the following statements about electrocardiogram patterns is correct EXCEPT
    A. The normal QRS wave in V_1 should have a small R wave and a large S wave.
    B. An old infarction is recognized by significant Q waves.
    C. An old infarction is recognized by abnormal ST and T waves.
    D. A PR greater than 0.20 second demonstrates first-degree AV block.
    E. A QRS interval of 0.12 second or greater signifies a bundle branch block.

212. Which of the following is true about sponging for fever?
    A. Relief is long-term, making antipyretic medication unnecessary.
    B. Sponging should be for at least 30 minutes.
    C. Sponging should be discontinued if shivering occurs.
    D. Alcohol, cold water, or ice water are methods of choice.
    E. The body should be immersed or covered with washcloths.

213. Finish the statement for the formula estimating the duration of a pregnancy: "From the first day of the last period, _____."
    A. subtract 3 months, add 1 year
    B. subtract 3 months and 7 days, add 1 year
    C. add nine months, subtract 7 days
    D. add 7 days, subtract 3 months, add 1 year
    E. subtract 7 days, add 9 months

214. A patient who is breast-feeding develops tenderness in the right breast. The patient should be advised to
    A. continue to breast-feed, and discontinue the breast pump for 2 to 3 days
    B. use only the breast pump for 2 to 3 days on the right side
    C. continue to breast-feed and empty the right breast with a breast pump
    D. discontinue both breast-feeding and use of the breast pump on the right side
    E. see the doctor immediately

215. Which of the following is the most accurate adjunct to early detection of breast cancer?
    A. mammography
    B. manual examination by a health professional
    C. self-examination before menstruation
    D. self-examination during menstruation
    E. self-examination after menstruation

216. Each of the following can be used to prevent "swimmer's ear" EXCEPT
    A. using ear plugs while swimming
    B. dislodging water with a sudden tap on the side of the head above the ear
    C. introducing a large wisp of cotton to draw out water by capillary attraction
    D. instilling a few drops of 70% alcohol after each swimming session
    E. lying on the affected side with a towel beneath the ear after swimming

217. Where does the infrared thermometer record body temperature?
    A. in the oral cavity
    B. in the ear
    C. on the fingertip
    D. in the rectum
    E. in the axillary region

218. What is the industry code for a rectal thermometer?
    A. red calibrations
    B. security bulb shape
    C. long, slender bulb
    D. red tip
    E. blue tip

219. After recording a right arm blood pressure of 180/110, the medical assistant should
    A. check the blood pressure in the left arm
    B. check the blood pressure with the patient prone
    C. recheck the blood pressure in the same arm immediately
    D. recheck the pressure after 2 minutes
    E. immediately alert the physician

220. The position of choice for the routine collection of stool for occult blood from a male patient is
    A. prone
    B. lithotomy
    C. jack-knife
    D. Sims
    E. dorsal recumbent

221. When handing the patient a cup to cover one eye to test for visual acuity, the patient asks if he can just close one eye and not use the cup. The medical assistant would explain that closing one eye
    A. allows a patient to cheat on the examination
    B. is too uncomfortable for the time it takes to complete the test
    C. may cause watering of the eyes
    D. decreases his ability to see the chart
    E. increases his ability to see the chart

222. During application of a 4×4 dressing with antibiotic cream to a thigh wound, it slips off the would onto an adjacent area of cleaned skin. The medical assistant should
    A. discard the dressing and prepare a new one
    B. gently slip the dressing back in place
    C. apply fresh antibiotic to the same dressing
    D. apply a second medicated dressing underneath the first
    E. apply antibiotic cream to the other side of the dressing and reapply the first side away from the skin

223. A pulse that is rated 3+ is called
    A. thready
    B. full
    C. rapid
    D. formicant
    E. bigeminal

224. Prior to CO_2 laser surgery, the patient's skin is prepared with
    A. sterile water
    B. Betadyne
    C. both A and B
    D. alcohol
    E. both A and D

225. Precautions during electrosurgery include
    A. avoiding the use of alcohol products whenever possible
    B. keeping the patient's skin flat on the grounding plate
    C. both A and B
    D. avoiding paper products
    E. both A and D

226. Following a dressing change, the medical assistant records sanguineous drainage on the patient's chart. This type of drainage is characterized by
   A. serum
   B. blood
   C. both A and B
   D. pus
   E. both A and D

227. Positive diagnostic signs of pregnancy include
   A. absence of expected menses greater than 1 month
   B. breast tenderness and enlargement
   C. fetal heartbeat
   D. enlarged, pigmented nipples
   E. nausea and vomiting

228. When bandaging fingers or toes, it is important to separate digits with layers of roller gauze to prevent
   A. uneven support
   B. uneven pressure
   C. movement without loosening the bandage
   D. severe skin infection
   E. loss of circulation

229. During a dressing change, the patient is lying prone on an examining table. The patient states he feels faint. The medical assistant would
   A. loosen any tight clothing
   B. administer spirits of ammonia
   C. administer small sips of water
   D. roll the patient onto his side
   E. sit the patient up and place his head between his knees

230. Immediate at-home care for a child who has ingested a small amount of drain cleaner (alkali) includes
   A. Ipecac
   B. large amount of water by mouth
   C. vinegar
   D. lemon juice
   E. nothing by mouth

231. A patient enters the office with a ruptured varicose vein of the leg and profuse bleeding from the bony prominence of the lower shin. Immediate control of blood loss would include applying
   A. pressure with fingers between the chin and the heart
   B. digital pressure above the chin until the bleeding stops
   C. a large compact bandage held firmly against the shin bone
   D. a coin or similar disklike object held firmly against the vein
   E. a tourniquet

232. If a patient is lying unconscious on the floor of the examining room, the medical assistant should
   A. keep the patient's head motionless and ask, "Are you OK?"
   B. open the airway by raising the chin and tilting the head backward
   C. turn the patient's head to one side to prevent the tongue from occluding the airway
   D. arouse the patient, then help the patient to the examination table
   E. raise the patient's legs and administer spirits of ammonia

Using the following Vacutainer stopper colors, answer the next six questions:
   A. yellow SPS
   B. red
   C. red-and-gray mottled top
   D. blue
   E. lavender

233. Which of the tubes is used for HIV testing?

234. Which of the tubes is used for emergency chemistries or stat serum determinations?

235. Which of the tubes requires no tube inversions after filling?

236. Which of the tubes is used for erythrocyte sedimentation determinations as well as coagulation studies?

237. When blood is added to Vacutainer tubes from a syringe venipuncture, which tube is filled last?

238. If all of the tubes listed previously were used in a multiple draw, which one would be used last?

239. Of the following types of pipettes, which type is the Unopette?
     A. volumetric pipette
     B. graduated pipette
     C. capillary pipette
     D. micropipette
     E. transfer pipette

240. For which of the following reasons is white bandage tape placed in a centrifuge?
     A. blood splatter detection
     B. as a balancing load
     C. to create a better rim seal
     D. as a tube cushion
     E. to soak up any specimen spills

241. A throat culture is ordered on a 7-year-old child suspected to have strep throat. Acceptable swabs to use include
     A. Dacron
     B. cotton
     C. both A and B
     D. calcium alginate
     E. both A and D

242. If a throat culture is to be grown on generic, nonselective media, the medical assistant would choose
     A. group A–selective streptococci agar
     B. blood agar
     C. Thayer-Martin agar
     D. eosin-methylene blue (EMB) agar
     E. chocolate agar

243. In the previous situation, colony characteristics indicating the presence of B-hemolytic streptococci organisms include
     A. green discoloration of the media
     B. incomplete hemolysis surrounding the colonies
     C. clear zones of hemolysis surrounding the colonies
     D. metallic sheen across the media
     E. colonies with purple centers

244. Extreme caution must be taken with blood samples that indicate hepatitis. This type of blood specimen would most likely contain serum that appears
     A. frothy
     B. bright red
     C. brownish-yellow
     D. milky white
     E. dark maroon

245. When screening for group A streptococci, which of the following would be an interpretable negative enzyme immunoassay?
     A. colored symbols in the test circle; colored symbol in the QC area
     B. no color in the test circle; colored symbol in the QC area
     C. colored symbol in the test circle; no color in the QC area
     D. no color in the test circle; no color in the QC area
     E. no agglutination occurs

246. The request slip for an alpha-fetoprotein test for fetal abnormalities must include
     A. the mother's blood type
     B. an accurate statement of gestation weeks
     C. both A and B
     D. the mother's Rh factor
     E. both A and D

247. In a chain of custody specimen transport, how must the completed paperwork be transported?
     A. in a separate enveloped, sealed
     B. stapled to the specimen bag
     C. written on the specimen bag
     D. in a sealed envelope in the specimen bag
     E. folded in the bag with the patient's name showing through the bag

248. In serum pregnancy testing, hCG levels will be lower in
     A. a tubal pregnancy
     B. the first trimester of a pregnancy
     C. both A and B
     D. hydatidiform mole
     E. both A and D

249. During the determination of a hematocrit using the microhematocrit system, which of the following situations would result in a false-low result?
     A. if blood is left standing too long
     B. if clots are rimmed from the inside of the Vacutainer opening
     C. if blood left on the outside of the capillary tube seeps inside
     D. if centrifuge time is cut short
     E. if the capillary tube is not fully sealed

250. Once opened, urine reagent strips should be used or discarded
   A. within 7 days
   B. within 14 days
   C. within 1 month
   D. within 2 months
   E. according to the expiration date on the label

251. During pregnancy, which of the following is expected to rise?
   A. white blood cell count
   B. sedimentation rate
   C. both A and B
   D. hemoglobin
   E. both A and D

252. When one is counting cells in the hemacytometer, sources of error resulting in a low count include
   A. failing to expel several drops of blood cell dilution onto gauze
   B. flooding the chamber with too much fluid from the Unopette
   C. both A and B
   D. using too little fluid from the Unopette
   E. both A and D

253. Diluted blood prepared with the Thoma pipette or the Unopette for WBC counting must be allowed to sit before charging the hemacytometer to allow
   A. the RBCs to lyse
   B. the WBCs to lyse
   C. the RBCs to settle
   D. the WBCs to settle
   E. even cell distribution

254. The critical step to keeping cells intact on a blood smear examination is
   A. speed of spreading
   B. angle of the spreader slide
   C. feathering
   D. amount of stain used
   E. speed of drying

255. During preparation of a blood smear, feathering is important to
   A. ensure monolayer cell distribution
   B. prevent cell distortion
   C. ensure cell coloration
   D. observe erythrocytes
   E. observe leukocytes

256. The critical step to making a blood smear wide enough for proper examination is
   A. centering the drop of blood on the slide
   B. holding the spreader slide at a 20-degree angle
   C. holding the spreader slide at a 45-degree angle
   D. waiting for blood to travel the width of the spreader slide
   E. applying pressure to the spreader slide

257. An ammonia-smelling urine is usually caused by
   A. fat metabolism in starvation
   B. diabetes mellitus
   C. dehydration
   D. excessive exercise
   E. urinary tract infection

258. The physician orders Liquid Elixir given to an 8-year-old child. The bottle is labeled 120 mg/tsp. The physician orders 8 ml. How many teaspoons should be administered?
   A. 1/2 tsp
   B. 3/4 tsp
   C. 1 tsp
   D. 2 tsp
   E. 4 tsp

259. In the previous question, what strength medication did the child receive?
   A. 4 ml
   B. 8 ml
   C. 16 ml
   D. 120 mg
   E. 240 mg

260. The mid-deltoid intramuscular injection site is bounded on the bottom by
   A. the deltoid tuberosity
   B. a point opposite the armpit
   C. the head of the humerus
   D. the upper edge of the acromion process
   E. the lower edge of the acromion process

261. The mid-deltoid intramuscular injection site is bounded on the top by
   A. the deltoid tuberosity
   B. a point opposite the armpit
   C. the head of the humerus
   D. the upper edge of the acromion process
   E. the lower edge of the acromion process

262. When injecting a medication into the right ventrogluteal area intramuscular injection site, a "V" is formed at the site with the medical assistant's left-hand fingers. The middle left finger must rest on the
    A. anterior superior iliac spine
    B. iliac crest
    C. greater trochanter
    D. gluteus medius muscle
    E. gluteus maximus muscle

263. When injecting a medication into the right ventrogluteal area intramuscular injection site, a "V" is formed at the site with the medical assistant's left-hand fingers. In relation to the "V," the injection is made
    A. at the base between the thumb and the index finger
    B. in the center between the thumb and the index finger
    C. at a point to the right of the index finger opposite the tip of the thumb
    D. at the base between the index and middle finger
    E. in the center between the middle finger and the index finger

264. When injecting a medication into the right ventrogluteal area intramuscular injection site, the needle is directed
    A. slightly toward the anterior superior iliac spine
    B. slightly toward the crest of the ilium
    C. slight toward the greater trochanter
    D. anteriorly
    E. downward

265. In which of the following situations is a liquid medication for instillation into the ear canal contraindicated?
    A. foreign body in the ear canal
    B. presence of cerumen
    C. pain or tenderness in the front of the ear
    D. pain or tenderness in the back of the ear
    E. appearance of a tear in the tympanic membrane

266. Which of the following disinfectants is permitted for use on human tissues?
    A. Gamophen
    B. pHisoHex
    C. Wescodyne
    D. Zephiran Chloride 17%
    E. Betadine

267. Which of the following immunizations is administered subcutaneously?
    A. hepatitis B
    B. *Haemophilus influenzae* b conjugated
    C. influenza
    D. rubella
    E. tetanus

268. A first appointment is scheduled for an 11-month-old child not immunized at the recommended time in early infancy. The mother asks if the child can be immunized for anything. The medical assistant could reply that
    A. DPT immunizations can be started immediately
    B. the polio vaccine schedule can be started immediately
    C. both A and B
    D. MMR can be administered
    E. both A and D

269. Which of the following vaccines is usually given to children older than 12 months of age?
    A. MMR
    B. DPT #2
    C. DPT #3
    D. OPV #1
    E. OPV #2

270. The physician orders Sudafed Syrup 30 mg/5 mL, taken 1/2 tsp tid for 5 days. What size bottle will have to be dispensed?
    A. 1 oz
    B. 2 oz
    C. 3 oz
    D. 4 oz
    E. 5 oz

271. The physician orders 120 mL of cough syrup. A patient asks how much medication that is in lay terms. The medical assistant would reply
    A. 2 tsp
    B. 1 tsp
    C. 2 fl dr
    D. 4 oz
    E. 1 pt

272. The physician orders Tylenol drops given to a 3-month-old child. The bottle is labeled 80 mg/0.8 mL. The physician orders 1/2 dropper. How many milliliters would be administered?
    A. 0.4 mL
    B. 0.8 mL
    C. 1.5 mL
    D. 40 mg
    E. 80 mg

273. The physician orders Tylenol drops given to an 3-year-old child. The bottle is labeled 80 mg/0.8 mL. The physician orders 120 mg. How much should be administered?
    A. 0.4 mL
    B. 0.8 mL
    C. 1.5 mL
    D. 1 dropper
    E. 1½ droppers

274. The physician orders Liquiprin Drops given to a 6-month-old infant. The bottle is labeled 60 mg/1.2 mL. The physician orders 30 mg. How many drops should be administered?
    A. 1/2 drop
    B. 0.6 drop
    C. 9 drops
    D. 18 drops
    E. 30 drops

275. Transdermal medications are applied to the
    A. upper arm
    B. upper torso
    C. both A and B
    D. gluteus muscle
    E. both A and D

276. Which of the following needle sizes is correct for administering a long-acting penicillin to a 24-month-old child?
    A. 26-gauge, 3/8"
    B. 24-gauge, 5/8"
    C. 25-gauge, 5/8"
    D. 22-gauge, 1"
    E. 22-gauge, 1½"

277. An injection of iron is given by the Z-track method because this technique will
    A. allow faster absorption of the drug
    B. allow slower absorption of the drug
    C. prevent irritation to the skin and tissues
    D. decrease pain during the injection
    E. allow the use of a shorter-length needle

278. At the proximal end, the vastus lateralis intramuscular injection site is bounded
    A. by the greater trochanter
    B. two fingers' breadth below the greater trochanter
    C. one hand's breadth below the greater trochanter
    D. two fingers' breadth above the patella
    E. two hands' breadth above the patella

279. Because measles-mumps-rubella live virus vaccine may reduce tuberculin test skin reactions, a tuberculin test should be administered
    A. before the MMR vaccine
    B. at the same time as the MMR vaccine
    C. either A or B
    D. later than the MMR vaccine
    E. either A or D

280. Which of the following vaccines must be stored in a freezer?
    A. polio virus vaccine, live, trivalent
    B. hepatitis B surface antigen, recombinant
    C. hepatitis B surface antigen
    D. influenza vaccine
    E. pneumococcal vaccine, polyvalent

281. A medication that is enteric-coated should be
    A. taken with a full glass of water
    B. diluted in water before administration
    C. dissolved under the tongue
    D. chewed and followed with a full glass of water
    E. scored before it is taken

282. To avoid a systemic reaction following the administration of eyedrops in a young child, the medical assistant should
    A. apply pressure to the nasolacrimal duct while administering the medication
    B. apply pressure to the inner canthus after administering the medication
    C. drop the medication under the upper lid
    D. use multiple applications of smaller amounts
    E. tilt back the child's head during the administration

283. When teaching a hypertensive patient about a low-sodium diet, the correct condiment to suggest for seasoning foods is
   A. dry dressing
   B. catsup
   C. soy sauce
   D. garlic salt
   E. lemon juice

284. Which of the following standards is required for biohazard bags?
   A. leak proof
   B. puncture resistant
   C. both A and B
   D. orange or orange-red color coding
   E. both A and D

285. According to OSHA standards, regulated waste includes
   A. items caked with dried blood
   B. empty vaccine containers
   C. both A and B
   D. dry paper products used in the examining room
   E. both A and D

286. In compliance with the universal blood and body fluid precautions, the correct barrier protection when giving an intramuscular injection includes
   A. gown
   B. gloves
   C. gown and gloves
   D. mask
   E. clean bare hands, washed thoroughly before and after the injection

287. Which of the following is a limitation of autoclaving?
   A. expensive to operate
   B. ineffective at certain pH values
   C. does not remove all organisms
   D. some materials not permeated by moisture
   E. probably not effective against hepatitis virus

288. Which of the following skin disinfectants stops the growth of bacteria rather than kills bacteria?
   A. 70% alcohol
   B. 2%–3% germicidal soaps (hexachlorophene)
   C. 2% tincture of iodine
   D. 0.1% quaternary ammonia compounds, tincture
   E. 0.1% mercurials

289. During CPR, what should be standard procedure to prevent transmission of disease from the patient to those administering CPR ventilations?
   A. limiting the number of rescuers who perform the ventilations
   B. wearing disposal gloves
   C. using disposal airway bags
   D. using an endotracheal tube
   E. cleaning the victim's mouth with an antiseptic solution

290. A laboratory ventilation system consisting of a hood and fan
   A. dilutes contaminants
   B. removes contaminants
   C. redirects contaminants
   D. mixes contaminants with fresh air
   E. neutralizes contaminants

291. To protect from accidental exposure to HBV or HIV, persons transporting specimen containers should wear
   A. masks and gloves
   B. masks and goggles
   C. gloves and goggles
   D. gowns
   E. gloves

292. Which of the following reprocessing methods is required for medical equipment that comes into contact only with the patient's mucous membranes (e.g., laryngoscope blades, endotracheal tubes)?
   A. environmental disinfection
   B. low-level disinfection
   C. intermediate disinfection
   D. high-level disinfection
   E. sterilization

293. To be used as a disinfectant of medical equipment coming into contact with the patient's intact skin rather than as a routine housekeeping disinfectant, a disinfectant must be able to destroy
   A. all forms of microbial life
   B. high numbers of bacterial spores
   C. tuberculocidal activity
   D. most viruses
   E. fungi

294. A liquid that has a flash point below 100°F
is considered
    A. combustible
    B. flammable
    C. ignitable
    D. corrosive
    E. unstable

295. For commercial products such as hand
lotion, the hazardous and toxic substances
laws require which of the following?
    A. chemical information list on file
    B. Material Safety Data Sheets on file
    C. both A and B
    D. a hazard label on all secondary
       containers
    E. both A and D

296. On a Material Safety Data Sheet, a special
fire hazard would be indicated by a
    A. low evaporation rate
    B. high flash point
    C. low reactivity
    D. low boiling point
    E. high boiling point

297. A procedure that requires an intravenous
injection is
    A. cardiac ultrasound
    B. chest MRI
    C. chest CT
    D. spine MRI
    E. spine CT

298. To be eligible for an MRI, the patient must
be screened for
    A. allergy to iodine
    B. allergy to contrast media
    C. the amount of x-radiation in the past
    D. metal implants
    E. prescription medications

299. Routine patient preparation for an MRI
scan (not pelvis) includes
    A. oral preparations
    B. laxatives
    C. refraining from caffeine
    D. no food 6 hours before the
       examination
    E. refraining from medications the day of
       the examination

300. Which of the following is a noninvasive
diagnostic test to image heart chamber size
and valvular function?
    A. Holter monitoring
    B. Exercise stress test
    C. CT chest
    D. Echocadiography
    E. Angiography

ANSWER KEY FOR SIMULATION TEST 2

1. **B.** Children in the 1- to 5-year age group may experience febrile convulsions. Evidence indicates that these seizures are set off by the rate of temperature rise (sudden, fast rise) rather than the degree of fever (how high). A febrile convulsion usually occurs very early in an illness and before it is known that a fever is present. *Frew, Lane, and Frew, p. 346.*

2. **B.** Pulse readings may be obtained anywhere on the body where the artery is near the body surface and lies over a bone. The popliteal artery lies behind the knee and is easily palpated for measuring pulse and even blood pressure. *Frew, Lane, and Frew, pp. 352–354.*

3. **C.** The testes secrete androgen, a hormone that promotes maleness—androgens develop and maintain secondary sex characteristics and influence adult male sexual behavior. *Gylys and Wedding, p. 298; Sheldon, p. 470.*

4. **C.** Supine hypotension in the pregnant woman occurs when the patient near term lies in a supine position. The patient's arterial blood pressure drops owing to fetal pressure on the abdominal aorta, which reduces blood flow back to the heart. *Lane, Keenon, Coleman (eds.), p. 471.*

5. **A.** The total electrolyte concentration is essentially the same in all three phases of body fluid (plasma, interstitial fluid, and intracellular fluid), but the relative amounts of the different electrolytes vary widely. In the extracellular fluid (plasma and interstitial fluid), the principal basic electrolyte is sodium; in the intracellular fluid the chief electrolyte is potassium. *Sheldon, p. 104.*

6. **E.** Hormonal imbalances such as increased prostaglandin secretions have been associated with primary dysmenorrhea, the pain associated with menstruation without any identifiable pathologic disorder. In general, pain is a primary defense mechanism, and all structures of the body respond to inflammation by signaling pain. In addition to prostaglandin secretion, other substances credited with the perception of pain include histamine, acetylcholine, and bradykinin, all known as mediators of inflammation. Endorphins, on the other hand, are substances that reduce the perception of pain. *Sheldon, p. 119; Tamparo and Lewis, pp. 121, 355.*

7. **B.** This newly recognized tick-borne disease is caused by a spirochete. Although this spirochete may involve the nervous system of patients in the same way as the spirochetes of syphilis, most of the cases involve arthritis in patients who are not treated early in the disease. The arthritis usually involves the knees and other large joints. Most broad-spectrum antibiotics easily treat the disease. *Sheldon, pp. 180–181.*

8. **B.** Pus is the liquefactive remains following digestion of cells by leukocytic enzymes. It commonly forms focal bacterial lesions called abscesses. It is part of the inflammatory reaction and repair process. *Sheldon, p. 22.*

9. **E.** Hormones, produced by the endocrine glands, are among the most important structures in the body, for they control metabolism and regulate personality. The difference between endocrine health and disease can mean the difference between the finest mental power and severe mental deficit. The principal endocrine glands are the pituitary, the thyroid and parathyroids, the adrenals, the islets of Langerhans in the pancreas, and the gonads. *Sheldon, p. 30.*

10. **A.** The prostate is a gland about the size of a horse chestnut situated at the neck of the bladder, surrounding the urethra. Although it belongs to the male reproductive system, when diseased, it produces symptoms associated with the urinary system on account of its position at the outlet of the bladder. ***Sheldon, p. 434.***

11. **C.** At the end of the previous menstrual cycle, estrogen levels are low, which in turn triggers the hypothalamus to issue orders to the anterior pituitary to release follicle-stimulating hormone. As follicles grow, the cells around them produce estrogen, which acts on the main target organ, the endometrium (inner lining of the uterus). The endometrium responds by growth of tissue in preparation for a fertilized ovum that will eventually be released from one of the growing follicles. ***Sheldon, p. 443.***

12. **B.** At approximately the 14th day of the menstrual cycle, a sudden increase in estrogen and follicle-stimulating hormone stimulates the hypothalamus to release a surge of luteinizing hormone (LH) from the anterior pituitary, called ovulation. LH travels to the ovary and releases a mature ovum into the fallopian tube. In women taking the contraceptive pill, this surge does not occur. Follicle-stimulating hormone is released from the anterior pituitary during the proliferative phase, under which the ovarian follicle which contains the ovum begins to grow. Estrogen and progesterone are produced in the ovaries. HCG is produced in a portion of the placenta following fertilization. The detection of hCG is the basis of pregnancy tests. ***Sheldon, pp. 443–445.***

13. **E.** The placenta is a temporary organ that transfers nutrients and oxygen to the fetus and passes metabolic waste products back to the mother for excretion, although not all chemicals are filtered out. The blood of the mother and the fetus pass close to each other but usually do not mix. The umbilicus connects the arteries and veins to the fetus, and amniotic fluid bathes the fetus. ***Sheldon, p. 457.***

14. **A.** Each time the baby nurses, oxytocin is released, which facilitates uterine involution. Breast-feeding is not an effective method of birth control, as ovulation is difficult to detect. Breast-fed babies can develop colic. ***Sheldon, p. 461.***

15. **D.** Heparin (antithrombin), present in minute quantities in the blood, prevents blood clotting in the normal vessel. When blood escapes from a broken vessel, blood platelets are activated and liberate thromboplastin, which neutralizes heparin. Once heparin is eliminated, the complex clotting of blood (coagulation) takes place: prothrombin and calcium form thrombin, then thrombin combines fibrinogen to form fibrin. Fibrin threads seal over the vessel opening, like a spider web, and a plug is formed by platelets that aggregate and form a sticky mass that eventually dries and becomes a scab. ***Sheldon, p. 88.***

16. **D.** In placenta previa, the placenta is implanted abnormally low in the uterus so that it covers all or part of the internal cervical os or opening. This condition is dangerous because the placenta may prematurely separate from the uterus, causing maternal hemorrhaging and an interruption of oxygen to the fetus. ***Tamparo and Lewis, p. 130; Lane, Medications, p. 471.***

17. **D.** Glucose, formed from the digestion of carbohydrates, is stored in the liver in the form of glycogen. Glucagon stimulates the liver to convert glycogen to glucose and raises the blood glucose level. Insulin promotes the movement of glucose through the cell membranes, lowering the blood glucose level. ***Tamparo and Lewis, p. 268; Wedding and Toenjes, p. 133.***

18. **B.** Orchitis typically arises as a consequence of infection from the mumps virus or injury. Mumps orchitis is usually unilateral and may follow or precede the enlargement of the parotid gland, which is characteristic of mumps. Sterility or impotence resulting from mumps orchitis is unusual. Prostatitis may be bacterial, nonbacterial, or a chronic condition in men over 50 years old. Cryptorchidism is an undescended testicle. ***Tamparo and Lewis, pp. 115–116; Sheldon, p. 438.***

19. **E.** Urticaria, also known as hives, is an inflammatory reaction of the capillaries beneath a localized area of the skin. It is characterized by the eruption of pale raised wheals on the skin, possibly surrounded by redness (erythema). The lesions form, then resolve rapidly, and are usually accompanied by intense itching. Contact dermatitis is any acute skin inflammation caused by irritants coming into contact with the skin. It is characterized by erythema and the appearance of small vesicles that ooze, scale, itch, burn, or sting. *Tamparo and Lewis, pp. 315–316.*

20. **D.** Psoriasis is characterized by discrete pink or dull-red skin lesions with silvery scaling. A high rate of skin cell turnover produces thick, flaky scaling, with the affected areas appearing dry, cracked, and encrusted. *Tamparo and Lewis, pp. 314–315.*

21. **B.** Premenstrual syndrome is a cluster of symptoms that regularly recur several days before the onset of menstruation. PMS appears more frequently in females during their 30s and 40s. Its cause is not clearly understood, although some theories suggest water retention, estrogen-progesterone imbalance, psychologic factors, or dietary deficiencies. Diagnosis depends on the timing of symptoms rather than any specific set of symptoms. *Tamparo and Lewis, pp. 118–119.*

22. **C.** High-density lipoprotein (HDL) seems to protect against atherosclerosis. Two other types, low-density (LDL) and very low–density lipoprotein (VLDL) are thought to be responsible in the development of atherosclerosis. The higher the ratio of HDL to LDL and VLDL, the better for the patient. *Wedding and Toenjes, p. 133.*

23. **C.** If both the recipient's antigen and its corresponding antibody are present in the donor, the antibody will unite with the antigen in an agglutinating reaction and is an incomplete cross match. Type O lacks both the A and B antigens and, therefore, will not be agglutinated by any other blood type. O is therefore the universal donor blood type. Conversely, type AB blood plasma contains no antibodies to agglutinate with any other blood type and, therefore, is considered the universal recipient blood type. *Wedding and Toenjes, p. 305.*

24. **C.** Urine formation involves three processes: filtration, reabsorption, and secretion. Filtration occurs in the Bowman's capsule, reabsorption in the proximal tubule, and secretion in the distal tubule. *Wedding and Toenjes, p. 60.*

25. **A.** Oliguria is a decrease in urine volume. Severe diarrhea, vomiting, or severe burns result in a negative water balance and a state of dehydration. Decrease of body water from whatever cause is first seen in the intravascular compartment with a reduction in blood volume, carrying with it a decreased urinary output, and, if unchecked, shock. Polyuria is increased urine flow; anuria, the absence of urine flow; nocturia, excessive urination at night; and diuresis, the passage of abnormally large amounts of urine. *Wedding and Toenjes, p. 60; Sheldon, p. 100.*

26. **E.** The kidneys, along with the lungs, are responsible for maintaining blood and extracellular fluids at a stable pH. The lungs excrete the volatile gas carbon dioxide, and the kidneys excrete many of the nonvolatile substances associated with the metabolic process. When blood or extracellular fluids change in pH, even slightly, a correction must be made by the lungs and/or the kidneys in order to establish a normal blood pH of 7.35 to 7.45. *Wedding and Toenjes, p. 98; Sheldon, p. 105.*

27. **D.** At present, a physician refusing the patient access to the medical record would have to prove that he or she is exercising the Doctrine of Professional Discretion in doing so. Under this doctrine, the physician may determine that the patient's emotional health would be adversely affected if access is granted. The Doctrine of Professional Discretion is usually applied by physicians treating patients who are mentally or emotionally ill. *Frew, Lane, and Frew, p. 338.*

28. **D.** Physicians are now subject to record-keeping requirements for all recordable occupational injuries and illnesses. OSHA requires that a log, known as OSHA Form 200, be maintained and retained for 5 years. *Frew, Lane, and Frew, pp. 692–694.*

29. **B.** Recordable injuries and illnesses include every occupational death; every nonfatal occupational illness; and those nonfatal occupational injuries that involve one or more of the following: loss of consciousness, restriction of work or motion, transfer to another job, or medical treatment (other than first aid). *Frew, Lane, and Frew, p. 693.*

30. **C.** CLIA quality control regulations require the use of FDA-approved testing methods and test kits whenever possible. Modified methods should also be approved by the FDA. In addition, the law requires the medical assistant to follow manufacturer directions for specimen collection and the operation of the instruments and the kits. Annual training sessions and evaluations are also required by OSHA. *Frew, Lane, and Frew, pp. 711, 717.*

31. **E.** The OSHA Hazard Communication Program consists of the OSHA: Access to Information About Hazardous and Toxic Substances Act, 29 CFR 1910.122, and the OSHA: Occupational Exposure to Bloodborne Pathogens Act, 29 CFR 1910.1030. These laws outline procedures for flammable and toxic chemicals, infectious materials, and electrical equipment. Fire extinguisher maintenance is regulated by fire marshals and is within local government jurisdiction. *Frew, Lane, and Frew, pp. 712, 716.*

32. **A.** Each container of hazardous material used or shipped from a workplace must have a hazard warning label with the following information: name of the chemical; appropriate hazard warning; and name and address of the manufacturer. Dispensers and portable containers must be labeled the same way. *Frew, Lane, and Frew, p. 713.*

33. **D.** State statutes indicate the minimum length of time medical records have to be retained. This length of time runs from the last entry. *Lane, Keenon, Coleman (eds.), p. 24.*

34. **D.** Urine specimens may be collected by the medical assistant or the physician. The patient must sign a preprinted consent for drug screening on which he or she lists any drugs or alcohol ingested over the last 10 days. The consent must be witnessed by the person performing the specimen collection procedure. Drug testing must be conducted in laboratories. All steps for sealing the specimen and preparing the specimen for transport must be done in view of the patient. *Lane, Keenon, Coleman (eds.), pp. 258–259.*

35. **C.** A signature, either handwritten or typed, is required on all notes by audit agencies as proof of service rendered. If a signature is absent, repayment to the insurance company of any funds reimbursed for services provided may be necessary. *Lane, Keenon, Coleman (eds.), p. 26.*

36. **C.** Medical assistants are not licensed as members of an occupation in any state. Most states grant physicians the right to delegate certain clinical tasks to qualified medical assistants by a clause in state medical practice acts. *Lane, Keenon, Coleman (eds.), p. 279.*

37. **A.** The Living Will is a document in which a person essentially states that if he or she became terminally ill, he or she would want no heroic or extraordinary measures taken to prolong his or her life. The durable power of attorney allows a broader scope of power than the Living Will. In this document, a person appoints someone to act for him or her in the event the person becomes unable to act for himself or herself. This can cover financial as well as medical decisions. The withdrawal of life support is currently being challenged in court cases. *Lane, Medications, p. 294; Frew, Lane, and Frew, p. 59; Lewis and Tamparo, pp. 101–102.*

38. **D.** A patient may be expected to make an appointment to obtain a personal copy of his or her medical record and pay reproduction fees. Usual requests for records should be honored free of charge for transfer to a new physician, in the form of a photostatic copy of the complete or partial record or the physician's summary. When patients are referred to other physicians, the continuance of the patient's medical history is paramount to the process, and the history should be released without additional charge. *Lewis and Tamparo, p. 113.*

39. **D.** Regulation Z requires the completion of a Truth in Lending agreement that includes information about finance charges whenever medical bills will be paid in more than four installments, whether or not there is a finance charge. If, however, the office sends a statement for the fee in full or a patient unilaterally decides to pay partial payments not agreed on with the physician, a Truth in Lending agreement in not necessary. *Lewis and Tamparo, p. 120.*

40. **D.** Patients should be provided the opportunity to pay before leaving the office. A written bill should be presented to the patient, and the medical assistant should be ready to itemize the charges and explain each fee. Billing at the conclusion of each office visit results in better month-end receipts than mailing out statements at the end of the month. *Lewis and Tamparo, p. 123.*

41. **D.** The Federal Trade Commission has specific regulations that prohibit misrepresenting who you are or why you are contacting a person or violating the patient's privacy and reputation by discussing his or her debts with relatives, friends, employers, or coworkers. *Lewis and Tamparo, p. 123.*

42. **E.** If an office denies credit on the basis of a poor credit rating from a credit bureau, the Fair Credit Reporting Act makes it law that the office volunteer the name and address of the agency providing the information, even if the patient does not ask. Couching the denial of credit by citing other office policies that may or may not exist is deceitful and illegal. The patient should be sent a formal letter of denial and a copy kept for office record. *Lewis and Tamparo, p. 123.*

43. **C.** Age and birth date may be requested on an application, provided the information is not used for preferential treatment. Citizenship is valid when determining the applicant's legal work status. No inquiries may be made concerning the applicant's race or color, which includes inquiries regarding skin, eye, and hair color and nationality. Although no inquiries can be made concerning the applicant's marital status or number of children, an employer has the right to request assurances from the applicant that he or she is able to work regular hours without chronic absenteeism or lateness. *Lewis and Tamparo, p. 134.*

44. **B.** In sexual harassment cases, an employer must make it easy and safe for the harassed to seek help. When harassment is allowed to continue and an employer does not correct the situation, the employer is liable under Title VII of the Civil Rights Act of 1964. *Lewis and Tamparo, p. 135.*

45. **A.** The Office of Equal Employment Opportunities administrates the Civil Rights Act of 1964 and can make the employer strictly liable for the acts of supervisory employees as well as for some acts of harassment by coworkers and clients of the business. *Lewis and Tamparo, p. 135.*

46. **E.** Generally, the best way to end harassment is to tell the harasser to stop the behavior. Less effective is threatening to tell or telling someone else. The worst solution is to ignore the behavior; this does not work. *Lewis and Tamparo, p. 136.*

47. **D.** The consent form should include a time limitation, usually not more than 90 days; otherwise it could be construed as a "blanket" consent and not valid. Parts of the informed consent forms must be completed in the presence of the patient. Blanket consent forms that are not specific must be avoided. Informed consent should be obtained as soon as possible after the need is identified. Usually a waiting period between consent and treatment is allowed: consent signed the day of surgery could be construed as having been obtained without patient autonomy. *Lewis and Tamparo, pp. 97–104.*

48. **B.** Restatement can be annoying if not timed appropriately or if used too much. When used, it assures the patient that you are a listener, but the real purpose of restatement is to help the patient to continue speaking and should be used only in the initial phases of active listening. *Davis p. 104.*

49. **A.** Reflecting the words, feelings, and attitudes of the patient indicates the MA is hearing more than just words, which helps the patient clarify her own thoughts and feelings. The most unhelpful response is indifference: to not listen means an inability or unwillingness to help. Offering reassurances is but a pretense of attention before trying to get away as soon as possible. Judgmental responses reveal, appropriately or inappropriately, personal feelings and pay little attention to the patient. Defensiveness indicates a personalization and refusal to listen carefully to what the patient is saying and does nothing to solve the patient's problems. *Davis, pp. 104–105.*

50. **A.** Using "I" statements takes a risk. It bares feelings to the other person who may not respond with helpfulness and concern, but it does tell the other person that you are owning your upset, and that both you and the other person are worthy and capable of solving the problem with appropriate, clear, and respectful conversation. "You" messages, as in "You don't give me credit for what I do," risk placing the other person on the defensive. *Davis, p. 106.*

51. **E.** "I" messages clearly place the ownership of a problem with the one who is upset. Then it is up to the other person to respond, hopefully with concern or active listening, although that is never a guarantee. What "I" statements guarantee is that your feelings will be expressed and you take responsibility for the upset, rather than blaming someone else. *Davis, p. 106.*

52. **D.** Communication that is helpful resists the need to respond impulsively or to offer quick advice or a quick solution to the problem. Therapeutic communication strives to clarify the problem and to assist the patient to solve it for himself or herself. *Davis, p. 107.*

53. **B.** Nonassertive behavior is failing to get your point across by remaining quiet and passive. Saying no and being confrontive are assertive responses that express what commonly appear to be negative emotions. Expressing an opinion is an assertive response that is task-specific and neutral, and expressing affection is an assertive response that expresses a positive emotion. *Davis, pp. 121–123.*

54. **A.** The Development of Trust or Mistrust is the first emotional job in life. This first stage lasts from birth to approximately 24 months of age. The feeling of physical comfort accompanied by minimal fear and uncertainty of being alone results in a sense of trust for the infant. Food and love demonstrations provide the foundations for psychological trust throughout life. *Davis, p. 19.*

55. **C.** During the 4th and 5th years, motor skills have developed sufficient to permit the development of the child's imagination. The child in this stage is "into everything" and seeks verbal and physical attention. Sexual curiosity and stimulation are apparent. Adult reinforcement of curiosity helps to resolve some of the child's guilt problems. Adult suppression of curiosity, sexual or otherwise, may result in the child feeling guilty for mere thoughts or actions not observed by adults. The more a child's thoughts are perceived as worthy, the more a child learns it is all right to self-initiate imagination and activities. *Davis, p. 19.*

56. **B.** During the 2nd through the 4th years, the child begins to discover his or her behavior can bring about certain results: behavior can bring about autonomy, but it also can cause conflicts about asserting oneself or remaining dependent on parents. During this time, it is difficult for the child to remain in a confined place, and the child becomes more and more occupied with activities involving retaining and releasing—objects, words, and bodily functions. The degree to which the child will allow others to control him or her is constantly tested, leading to a greater sense of self and responsibility. On the other hand, early potty training (when evacuation muscle controls are not yet developed) is considered overcontrol by the adult, leading to shame and doubt. *Davis, pp. 21–22.*

57. **A.** Piaget first determined that young children are unable to handle abstract logic. Erikson is known for his "Stages of Man." Abraham Maslow developed the "Hierarchy of Needs of Man." Carl Jung, a student of Freud, first described the psychologic types "introverted" and "extroverted." Penelope Leach is a well-known childhood development personality who has written many books on the subject of parenting. *Davis, p. 19.*

58. **D.** If a child is born to parents who have little love to give and smother or beat the child because they cannot stand to hear the child cry, the child learns that the world is a very hostile place without love and comfort and will mistrust from the first days of life. This situation is the genesis of violent adolescents and adults who in turn abuse their spouses and children when they grow up. *Davis, p. 21.*

59. **C.** Codependence has been defined as an exaggerated dependent pattern of learned behaviors, beliefs, and feelings that make life painful. These are leftover fragments, memories of immature needs from our totally dependent infant. *Davis, p. 27.*

60. **E.** Sympathy is fellow-feeling, side by side; pity is sympathy with superior feeling; identification is the projection of personal values onto another, making the patient less important; and self-transposal—thinking of oneself in the position of the other—although it sets the stage for empathy to occur, is the cognitive attending to another and stops just short of empathy. Empathy occurs just a millisecond after self-transposal, when the listener "crosses over" into the world of the speaker and is at one with him or her. This represents the momentary merging with another person in a unique moment of shared meaning, before jumping back into one's "own skin." *Davis, pp. 88–90.*

61. **D.** In therapeutic communication the medical assistant is fully present and totally focused on and interested in the patient. The medical assistant must listen and resist quick advice, categorizing, or projecting personal beliefs. Sympathy is pity with superior feelings; the most unhelpful response is remaining neutral or indifferent. *Frew, Lane, and Frew, pp. 53, 331; Davis, pp. 87, 102.*

62. **E.** Displacement of free-floating anger is a defensive response toward objects or persons that have no significance to the emotion. Compensation is replacing an attitude or feeling with its opposite; rationalization is justifying feelings to avoid truthful self-confrontation. Dissociation is disconnecting emotional significance from specific ideas or events. Projection is imagining that another person is displaying one's own feelings. *Frew, Lane, and Frew, p. 57.*

63. **C.** Correct communication requires listening to the patient, clarifying or asking what the patient means, and never assuming or making quick judgments when trying to identify the problem. Offering false reassurances is unhelpful, as this stems from the medical assistant's desire to "quick-fix" it. Because the incorrect responses minimize the patient's concerns and do not encourage him to elaborate on his "worries," further communication is blocked and could even solicit legal problems because it comes very close to promising a cure. *Frew, Lane, and Frew, p. 57; Davis, p. 88.*

64. **A.** The word is derived from the Greek for "divided mind" and connotes a disconnection between thoughts and feeling on the one hand and actions on the other. It involves the fragmentation of all the processes of thought and feeling that enable a healthy person to remain in touch with the world. *Sheldon, p. 318.*

65. **E.** When a temperature reading does not make sense in relation to the situation, it must be considered that the patient has either tampered with or interfered with the reading. In this case, the patient may have heated the thermometer to feign a fever. A different thermometer should be used, to eliminate equipment failure as the cause and to avoid insulting the patient; but the medical assistant should also stay in the room to monitor the patient during the time the thermometer is registering. Changing the body area used would add another variable because temperature differs in each body area. *Taber's, p. 724.*

66. **D.** Alzheimer's disease is a chronic organic brain syndrome characterized by progressive intellectual impairment. The disease progresses through three stages: the first stage is characterized by mild mental impairment; the second by increased forgetfulness, agitation, irritability, and extreme restlessness; and the third by an inability to care for oneself, incontinence, and an inability to communicate. *Tamparo and Lewis, p. 258.*

67. **A.** "R." usually represents respiration; "R" within a circle, right; "ROS," review of systems; and "(R)" immediately following the body temperature reading, rectal. *Frew, Lane, and Frew, p. 333.*

68. **B.** Defervescence. *Frew, Lane, and Frew, p. 347.*

69. **A.** Mastitis. *Frew, Lane, and Frew, p. 490.*

70. **B.** Dysphagia is the inability to swallow or difficulty in swallowing. Dysphasia is difficulty speaking (speech). *Gylys and Wedding, p. 101.*

71. **E.** The surgical repair suffix for suture is "rrhaphy." *Gylys and Wedding, p. 12.*

72. **B.** "Carcino" is the combining form for cancer, and "gen" is the suffix meaning "to produce." The "ic" ending is an adjectival ending meaning "pertaining to." *Gylys and Wedding, p. 13.*

73. **B.** A blood clot (embolus) may be removed directly by excision (embolectomy) or indirectly by means of a balloon catheter (angioplasty). In extreme cases the a vein is tied (ligated) and removed (stripped). *Gylys and Wedding, p. 156; Taber's, p. 107.*

74. **B.** Rachicentesis. Hematopoiesis, diarrhea, parenchyma, hemiplegia. *Taber's, pp. 347, 1660.*

75. **A.** Ultrasonography is a noninvasive ultrasound technique used to evaluate the female genital tract and the fetus in the obstetric patient. Hysterosalpingography and uterotography are radiographic visualizations following an injection of contrast medium. Culdoscopy is performed through an incision made in the posterior vaginal cul-de-sac to permit direct visualization of the uterus and other organs with an endoscope. Colposcopy is the use of optical instruments to view three-dimensionally the external cervical epithelium. *Gylys and Wedding, p. 277.*

76. **B.** Epiphysis, epiphyses. For words ending in "is," the "is" is dropped and "es" added. *Gylys and Wedding, pp. 29, 205.*

77. **C.** Phacoemulsification is a method of treating cataracts by using ultrasonic waves to disintegrate the cataract, which is then aspirated and removed. *Gylys and Wedding, p. 355.*

78. **B.** The word element for softening is *malacia*, as in osteomalacia, softening of the bone. *Gylys and Wedding, p. 411.*

79. **A.** Alopecia. *Gylys and Wedding, p. 73.*

80. **A.** Stertor. *Lane, Keenon, Coleman (eds.), p. 313.*

81. **A.** Nulligravida. *Lane, Keenon, Coleman (eds.), p. 467.*

82. **C.** Risk management. *Lane, Keenon, Coleman (eds.), p. 68.*

83. **A.** āā. *Lane, Keenon, Coleman (eds.), p. 696.*

84. **E.** Symptom. *Lane, Keenon, Coleman (eds.), p. 698.*

85. **A.** Medical informatics is the basic science of computers in medicine and deals with the exchange of computer-based information. Medical informatics has developed into a new specialty and includes computer technology for patient history taking and monitoring, test result retrieval, insurance and financial management, medical education, and research. *Lewis and Tamparo, p. 112.*

86. **B.** In situ. *Sheldon, p. 449.*

87. **A.** A hydrosalpinx is distention of the fallopian tube by a clear fluid. *Sheldon, p. 454.*

88. **B.** A new method using gamma cameras and computer analysis is called PET scanning. It makes possible the visualization and localization of small amounts of isotopes in organs of the body. For example, radioactive glucose can be injected into the arteries of the brain and then the patient is asked to view a strong emotional image, a gamma computer can show the increased concentration of the isotope in the part of the brain that is working to read the image. The technique has real promise for locating small brain tumors before they invade and destroy normal tissue. *Sheldon, p. 82.*

89. **D.** Larva, larvae. For singular words ending in "um," the "um" is dropped and an "a" added. For singular words ending in "a," the "a" is retained and an "e" added. ***Taber's, p. 1080.***

90. **B.** Morbidity. ***Taber's, p. 1236.***

91. **A.** Patency is the state of being freely open, evident, accessible. ***Taber's, p. 1444.***

92. **C.** Compromised. ***Taber's, p. 430.***

93. **B.** Aerobe. ***Taber's, p. 48.***

94. **B.** Cyst. ***Taber's, p. 483.***

95. **E.** Etiology. ***Taber's, p. 681.***

96. **B.** A dermatophytosis is a superficial fungal infection of the skin. Tinea is a term used for any fungal skin disease. Tinea capitis (head), tinea corporis (body), tinea cruris (jock-itch), tinea pedis (athlete's foot) are examples of superficial fungal infections of the skin. Histoplasmosis, moniliasis, and nocardiosis are systemic fungal conditions. Herpes zoster, also known as shingles, is a condition caused by the varicella-zoster virus. ***Tamparo and Lewis, p. 320.***

97. **D.** Dyspareunia is the occurrence of pain in women during sexual intercourse. Vaginal burning or itching may also occur. ***Tamparo and Lewis, p. 104.***

98. **A.** Asphyxiant. ***Tamparo and Lewis, p. 15.***

99. **B.** The term "predisposing" indicates a tendency to, or susceptibility to, disease in the presence of specific environmental stimuli. ***Tamparo and Lewis, p. 3.***

100. **B.** Opportunistic infections. ***Tamparo and Lewis, p. 388; Gylys and Wedding, p. 186.***

101. **D.** The modified wave system allows for the scheduling of certain blocks of time with predictable activities. At the same time that a physical examination is scheduled for one examining room, three or four other patients requiring less time can be scheduled in other examination rooms. ***Lane, Keenon, Coleman (eds.), p. 8.***

102. **C.** The modified wave system is best suited when one physician and multiple assistants use multiple examining rooms. The system is limited by space and personnel. It is not necessary for the physician to see the patients in the order they arrive. The medical assistant might place one patient in the physician's office, a second to undress, a third at the vital signs stations, and so on. Patients often object when they see a waiting room suddenly fill at one time. ***Lane, Keenon, Coleman (eds.), p. 8.***

103. **B.** If a patient is to be admitted to the hospital, the reasons for and planned length of stay must be reviewed and certified by the patient's insurance plan. ***Frew, Lane, and Frew, p. 199.***

104. **A.** If medical complications prolong the patient's stay beyond the certified period, a continued stay review must be filed with the insurance carrier. ***Frew, Lane, and Frew, p. 199.***

105. **E.** The continued length of stay review should be submitted to the insurance carrier. ***Frew, Lane, and Frew, p. 199.***

106. **A.** A continued stay review must be submitted for recertification before the patient's last certified day. ***Frew, Lane, and Frew, p. 199.***

107. **C.** For network plan coverage, the participating primary care facility is responsible for initiating precertification and continued stay reviews. ***Frew, Lane, and Frew, p. 199.***

108. **C.** Cancellations are noted as "canceled" in the appointment book and recorded in the progress notes section of the patient record. ***Frew, Lane, and Frew, p. 198.***

109. **D.** If a patient's appointment is not rescheduled and the patient prefers to reschedule at another time, the notation "C, w/c" should be written in the appointment book. ***Frew, Lane, and Frew, p. 198.***

110. **E.** Most insurance carriers now encourage patients to seek second opinions, and pay 100% of the cost. ***Frew, Lane, and Frew, p. 199.***

111. **C.** All no-shows should be called and the medical record documented according to office policy. *Lane, Keenon, Coleman (eds.), p. 11.*

112. **E.** If there is time, nonurgent patients should be called and rescheduled. If the patient shows up at the appointed time and the reason for the visit is nonurgent, one should politely explain the situation and offer to reschedule. *Lane, Keenon, Coleman (eds.), p. 12.*

113. **D.** Physicians who are not accepting new patients should make available the names, addresses, and phone numbers of other physicians for referral. This protects the physician from any unethical charges if a new patient is unknowingly seriously ill or suffers harm from not receiving medical care. *Lane, Keenon, Coleman (eds.), p. 12.*

114. **B.** When collecting large sums of money from the patient without insurance coverage, the office policy of choice here is obtaining a credit rating, which is a history of the patient's ability and willingness to pay on an installment basis. Very few patients can pay a large fee in one lump sum or in cash prior to surgery, although a down-payment is appropriate. Few physicians will charge a finance fee, although to do so is both legal and ethical, and a patient's financial status should have no bearing on the kind of treatment they should receive: the physician's decision to accept the patient's credit should be based on the patient's ability to pay, not his or her net worth. *Lewis and Tamparo, p. 120–123.*

115. **E.** The first-come, first-served schedule is not ideal for the physician because of the difficulty in using his or her time efficiently. Without appointing patients to specific times, there can be downtime, with the patients controlling the practice more than the physician. It is also difficult to limit the day without risk of turning away patients at closing time. Scheduling all patients together or double booking is advantageous to the physician, but it is unfair to the patients to have to wait for long periods. Scheduling like procedures in a steady stream with time-allotted slots is an efficient system, as long as patients show up and are punctual. *Lane, Keenon, Coleman (eds.), p. 9.*

116. **B.** Computer data are easily accessed and changed. For this reason, untrained persons should not be permitted freedom of access and confidential information should not be entered onto the computer. Written procedures should be established identifying who is authorized to make changes to the database or the data itself, when those changes can be made, and who should be notified of changes. Data must be purged on a regular basis. Written procedures are necessary for when data are purged, what data are purged, and whether purged data are stored elsewhere or destroyed. *Lewis and Tamparo, p. 113.*

117. **C.** A database program is a program that manipulates facts. It can store information about patients and insurers. It allows the retrieval of data for completing forms and mail merging. *Walter, p. 148.*

118. **D.** The most popular monospaced font is Courier. *Walter, pp. 34–35.*

119. **A.** The operator should press Control-F9, "Merge/sort," and then "Merge" (M). Then the name of the form letter is typed as the "primary merge file," then the mailing list as the "secondary merge file." *Walter, p. 139.*

120. **E.** Margins are changed under "Format-Line," Shift-F8 then L. *Walter, p. 58.*

121. **C.** A modem allows the computers to communicate through a telephone line. E-mail (electronic mail) depends on equipment that can modulate computer signals into telephone signals and then demodulate telephone signals back into computer signals. Modulation-demodulation is accomplished with a modem. A local area network (LAN) runs wires between computers in the same office using one main computer, called a server. A bulletin board system is part of a more extensive on-line service, although it may include e-mail service. It first requires buying a modem. An AB switch is used when two or more computers share one local printer. *Walter, pp. 222–227.*

122. **D.** The "m" stands for modified files. If you say "\m" at the end of a backup command, the computer will back up just the files that "need" to be backed up. These files would include those that had been modified, that is, edited or created since the last backup. *Walter, p. 556.*

123. **A.** It is preferable to alternate between two or more sets of backup disks. That way, if something is wrong with today's data, one can go back to a good data set. Most businesses back up data files daily, program files monthly, and the entire hard disk weekly or monthly. Backups should be made as small as practical, usually by subdirectory. This way, if one floppy gets ruined, you lose just one subdirectory instead of the whole hard disk. *Walter, pp. 556–557.*

124. **A.** If wires are run between computers that are in the same office building, a LAN is created. Each computer in the LAN is called a node and is coordinated by a server. *Walter, pp. 225–227.*

125. **C.** For optical character reading, the mailing address should be limited to four lines. In long addresses, the apartment or suite number is placed after the street address. *Fordney and Diehl, p. 116.*

126. **E.** Single spacing, abbreviations, all caps, and no punctuation are used. *Fordney and Diehl, p. 119.*

127. **A.** The complimentary close may be omitted in a simplified letter. *Fordney and Diehl, p. 189.*

128. **C.** The continuation page of a medical report would contain, at the left-hand margin in horizontal format, the name of the patient, the case or history number, and the page number. *Fordney and Diehl, p. 233.*

129. **E.** Simplified and full block letters are often used with open punctuation. Mixed or standard punctuation is most common in medical practice and is used appropriately with full block, modified block, and semiblock letter styles. *Frew, Lane, and Frew, p. 125.*

130. **E.** The physician should personally sign all letters dictated or handwritten regarding patient medical care. Except for claim forms, the medical assistant may sign letters to insurance carriers and other vendors. *Frew, Lane, and Frew, p. 133.*

131. **B.** The number of characters in the last line is limited to 26 for optical character reader processing by the post office. *Frew, Lane, and Frew, p. 138.*

132. **D.** For optical character recognition, the mailing address should be limited to four lines. *Frew, Lane, and Frew, p. 138.*

133. **A.** The use of the blind carbon copy is discouraged. *Lane, Keenon, Coleman (eds.), p. 35.*

134. **B.** The symbol for insert a space is the pound sign, #. *Fordney and Diehl, p. 361.*

135. **B.** The body of the manuscript is always double-spaced with the page numbers centered at the bottom. The left margin should be 1 inch or 1.5 inches and the right margin should be 1 inch. *Fordney and Diehl, pp. 218–220.*

136. **D.** Legends are typed on a separate sheet, double-spaced, and numbered to correspond with each figure in the manuscript. *Fordney and Diehl, p. 219.*

137. **B.** Use a colon and no extra space between the volume number and the page number. *Fordney and Diehl, p. 56.*

138. **C.** A master list of equipment items includes description, date of purchase, purchase cost, and estimated actual life. A separate file should be maintained for operating manuals, guarantees, and repair records. *Frew, Lane, and Frew, p. 100.*

139. **C.** Meeting presentations are listed chronologically by month and year. *Fordney and Diehl, p. 472.*

140. **D.** Publications are listed first by year, then alphabetically by authors' names in the same order as they appear in the publication. *Fordney and Diehl, p. 473.*

141. **C.** Medical articles will most likely be retrieved by topic rather than when or where they appeared or by whom they were written. Subject filing facilitates retrieval by topic better than alphabetic or date referencing. *Frew, Lane, and Frew, p. 106.*

142. **E.** Filing alphabetically by subject is advisable when records might otherwise become minutely subdivided. *Lane, Keenon, Coleman (eds.), p. 20.*

143. E. Numeric systems are best maintained for record retention by case history number, contract, or project for an indefinite period. Numeric retrieval is indirect because the user must refer to an alphabetized code to find the number assigned to a document name or subject. A numeric system requiring many subdivisions would require a cumbersome index. *Frew, Lane, and Frew, pp. 106–107.*

144. E. A restrictive endorsement includes the words "For deposit only," making it impossible for anyone other than the bank to cash the check. *Frew, Lane, and Frew, p. 234.*

145. C. If payment is not received, the second statement should initiate the collection process. *Frew, Lane, and Frew, p. 256.*

146. B. Write-offs are usually acceptable when the costs of collecting an account exceed the amount owed and the amount is minimum. Collection attempts should be made for the other two examples. *Frew, Lane, and Frew, p. 258.*

147. B. The time of an open book account runs from the date of the last entry (charge) for a specific illness. *Frew, Lane, and Frew, p. 258.*

148. C. When a written contract exists, the time runs from the date of the last installment or the single due date, if payment was not made, whichever is the case. *Frew, Lane, and Frew, p. 258.*

149. D. For tax purposes, an account written off as bad debt is final once it is claimed on a tax return. Collection practices should be discontinued. Delinquent accounts turned over to a collection agency or labeled uncollectible may be reinstated if any amounts are recovered. *Lane, Keenon, Coleman (eds.), p. 87.*

150. C. Checks with two endorsements are unacceptable for payment. Such checks often require that change be paid back to the patient or the acceptance of a check from an unknown person or company. *Lane, Keenon, Coleman (eds.), p. 101.*

151. C. Aging once a month just before sending out statements ensures that all accounts are present and accounted for. *Lane, Keenon, Coleman (eds.), p. 129.*

152. D. A transaction slip, with or without a receipt, is a component particular only to the one-write systems. *Lane, Keenon, Coleman (eds.), p. 79.*

153. E. The accounts receivable balance usually represents the debit balance. If an overpayment occurs, the balance is a credit balance. *Lane, Keenon, Coleman (eds.), p. 84.*

154. E. When this account was turned over to the collection agency, the amount due on the account card was written off as a deduction in the adjustment column (−$150). Following recovery by the collection agency, the $75 received is recorded in the payment column and the $75 kept by the agency is recorded in the adjustment column, still leaving a zero balance (75.00 [75.00] = 0). *Lane, Keenon, Coleman (eds.), pp. 87–88.*

155. A. Because the $20 deduction is not in the form of a payment, the deduction should be taken in the adjustment column. The amount paid by the insurance company is entered in the payment column and the nonallowed amount in the adjustment column. *Lane, Keenon, Coleman (eds.), p. 90.*

156. C. A trial balance, performed at the close of each month, compares the total accounts receivable from the ledger cards to the end-of-month accounts receivable balance. *Lane, Keenon, Coleman (eds.), p. 92.*

157. A. Hyphens are used with letters or words describing chemical elements (unless superscripts or subscripts are used), with compounded surnames, to join two or more words used to describe a noun when clarity is required, and to join a single letter to a word to form a coined compound (e.g., x-ray). *Fordney and Diehl, pp. 79, 84, 158, 159.*

158. B. Words placed in parentheses may be abbreviated. Beginning a sentence with an abbreviation should be avoided. The use of "etc." should be avoided in sentences and lists. Percent is spelled out unless it appears in parentheses or tables. Current practice favors excluding periods from abbreviations. *Frew, Lane, and Frew, p. 148.*

159. **E.** Words that are italicized include foreign words or phrases; titles of books and journals; Latin scientific name of genera, species, and subspecies; or a word spoken of as a word, a phrase as a phrase, and a letter as a letter, except when the letter is used to indicate shape. *Fordney and Diehl, pp. 456–461.*

160. **D.** Medicaid patients are given some means of identifying themselves as being eligible for the program. The medical assistant must check eligibility each time the patient is provided with care. Since July of 1992, the Eligibility Verification System (EVS) superseded the "From-Thru" dated card system. Verification is processed by calling the EVS 800 number or local number. *Department of Health and Human Resources, EVS Hotline Bulletin.*

161. **C.** Medicare's Eligibility Verification System (EVS) issues eligibility statuses, depending on the recipient's entitled benefits. A invalid message may mean either the recipient number was entered incorrectly or the recipient is not eligible. Re-enter to check the data. *Department of Health and Human Resources, EVS Hotline Bulletin.*

162. **A.** Patients seen by Medicare-participating physicians pay only the annual deductible fee and the 20% copayment of the charges allowed to the physician. *Frew, Lane, and Frew, p. 288.*

163. **B.** The participating physician payment is based on the fee schedule amount. Medicare pays 80% of the fee schedule amount, whereas the patient is responsible for 20%. The difference between the Medicare fee schedule amount and the participating physician's charge is the contractual adjustment. *Frew, Lane, and Frew, p. 289.*

164. **D.** Medicare is a primary two-part program covering inpatient hospital services and services furnished by the physician. Blue Shield Supplemental is a type of Medi-Gap insurance that is secondary to Medicare. Blue Shield Major Medical is additional insurance purchased to cover catastrophic coverage for costs of illness and injury beyond those covered in the basic medical plan. *Frew, Lane, and Frew, p. 300.*

165. **E.** All routine medical care must be provided by in-plan members. HMO enrollees who elect to go "out of plan" without prior authorization are responsible for payment of all services. *Frew, Lane, and Frew, p. 301.*

166. **A.** Referrals outside of the HMO require prior approval from the HMO. An elective referral is the self or "out of plan" referral of a member who requests covered services without presenting a managed care organization (MCO) or primary care physician (PCP) referral authorizing the delivery of specific covered services. *Frew, Lane, and Frew, p. 301.*

167. **D.** Because the patient is following procedure by staying within the plan, getting a referral, and receiving covered services, the "hold harmless" law states that the patient is only responsible for the copayment or deductible amount. The consultant should not bill the patient for any differences between the charge and the plan allowance. *Gylys, p. 202.*

168. **D.** An entity consisting of physicians or groups of physicians for the purpose of contracting with managed care plans on a per-patient, fee-for-service basis is the Individual Practice Association (IPA) or Individual Profession Plan (IPP) *Gylys, p. 203.*

169. **A.** The workers' compensation form must include the name and address of the employer's compensation insurance carrier and the name and address of the employer. Including the name of the patient's insurance carrier is not necessary. *Gylys, p. 205.*

170. **D.** Medicare is billed as a primary payer only when the patient's other coverage is Medicare supplemental (Medi-Gap). *Gylys, p. 211.*

171. **D.** The Federal Employee Program (FEP) is a unique national account. FEP cards begin with the letter "R." *Lane, Keenon, Coleman (eds.), p. 160.*

172. **B.** The bill should be sent to the local Blue Shield plan, which will pay the provider directly. The local plan will then bill the out-of-state BS plan for reimbursement. In other words, the patient with reciprocity should be registered as a local BS recipient. *Lane, Keenon, Coleman (eds.), p. 161.*

173. **B.** When a female spouse of a wage earner, drawing social security benefits because of her husband's contribution, becomes a widow, her Medicare suffix may change from a B (wife not dependent or having child in her care) to D (widow, at least age 60). *Lane, Keenon, Coleman (eds.), p. 162.*

174. **D.** Beginning in 1993, the limiting charges could not exceed 115% of the nonparticipant fee schedule, which is based on 95% of the participating physician fee schedule. *Lane, Keenon, Coleman (eds.), pp. 172–173.*

175. **E.** Inactive files of patients who have not been seen in the last few years, who have moved away, or have died can be purged and stored in a separate place, in the office building or a rented space. Active records should be filed on site for ready access. Records should not be discarded based on active or inactive status, but according to the end of the statute of limitations period on a case-by-case review, if they are discarded at all. Transferring active records from one place to another in the office will not relieve the overcrowded situation; inactive records should be purged on a regular basis, preferably annually. Color-coded year labels can make the process easier. *Lewis and Tamparo, p. 114.*

176. **A.** One major disadvantage is the common misfiling of common names. *Frew, Lane, and Frew, p. 106.*

177. **D.** The first indexing unit is United States. *Frew, Lane, and Frew, p. 111.*

178. **A.** Objective data include the physical examination and laboratory findings. *Frew, Lane, and Frew, p. 323.*

179. **A.** A signed authorization is not required for subpoena. *Frew, Lane, and Frew, p. 89.*

180. **E.** Records dictated by the physicians but generated by a hospital, such as operative notes are usually considered part of the physician's records and can be released by the physician. *Lane, Keenon, Coleman (eds.), p. 31.*

181. **C.** The federal government generally has the power to override conflicting state rules regarding the release of medical records. There is a mandatory duty to report cases to government agencies that keep vital statistics, monitor abuse cases, and monitor communicable diseases. Medicare and Medicaid agencies have the right under the law to obtain the medical records of a patient with prior consent. Patients must sign a release before being included in any research project. *Lane, Keenon, Coleman (eds.), p. 32.*

182. **D.** The conversation may be closed by restating the major points of the conversation—in this case, the setting of an appointment. *Frew, Lane, and Frew, pp. 164, 169.*

183. **E.** One should acknowledge the caller's viewpoint, then direct the communication to problem solving as quickly as possible. *Frew, Lane, and Frew, p. 167.*

184. **C.** Medically significant or legally significant calls should be documented in the medical record. Written notes ensure accurate message interpretation and avoids having the caller repeat the message when the physician calls back. The medical assistant should record the information in the record or attach the notation to the patient record for the physician's attention and return call. *Frew, Lane, and Frew, pp. 167, 178.*

185. **B.** For patients who call the office repeatedly to ask questions concerning an illness or treatment, one should acknowledge the patient's need for reassurance, identify any patient needs such as instructions or clarifications, then take some action such as setting an appointment or telling the patient the message will be given to the physician. Any comment suggesting the termination of the call is inappropriate and solutions should be considerate of the patient's needs with regard to medical law and ethics. *Frew, Lane, and Frew, pp. 167–168.*

186. **D.** Perhaps the most difficult patient is the one who disregards the practice's schedule. One must be patient and acknowledge that the patient is important to the physician, and try to gain control of the conversation. The communication should be directed to problem solving as quickly as possible ("Let's solve the problem"). Closure and follow-up technique may be used to reinforce resolution of the conflict. *Frew, Lane, and Frew, p. 167; Lane, Keenon, Coleman (eds.), p. 12.*

187. **C.** The response should convey the message that the doctor is interested in talking with the patient but is, at the moment, unable to stop what he or she is doing. Saying the physician is with a patient or in surgery or on another line with a patient is more acceptable than saying he or she is "busy" or making any other general statement. *Frew, Lane, and Frew, p. 168.*

188. **A.** The medical assistant should handle nonmedical business independently. One appropriate response is to ask for written information with the promise that the physician will be given the literature for review. *Frew, Lane, and Frew, p. 168.*

189. **E.** The appointment flow needs to be reduced if patients are waiting more than 30 minutes either in the waiting room or in the examination room when there are no emergencies. If the physician feels the pace is too slow or examination rooms are not being used to their fullest, the system should be reviewed to increase the number of appointments. *Lane, Keenon, Coleman (eds.), p. 12.*

190. **B.** A new patient seeking health care in general is not considered a patient of the practice until the patient keeps an appointment and sees the physician, unless the patient is a referral from another doctor. Significant illnesses need follow-up. These include follow-up after discharge from a hospital or outpatient facility for each and every outpatient procedure, and patients with serious problems, on new medications, or in pain. *Lane, Keenon, Coleman (eds.), p. 16; Frew, Lane, and Frew, p. 200.*

191. **E.** A modifier may be recorded as a two-digit number placed after the usual procedure number, separated by a hyphen. Alternatively the modifier may be recorded as a separate five-digit code (09900 series) that is used in addition to the procedure code. *CPT-94, p. 70.*

192. **C.** When laboratory procedures are performed by a party other than the treating or reporting physician, the procedure may be identified by adding the modifier -90 to the usual procedure number or by using the separate five-digit modifier code 09990. The name of the laboratory and the laboratory charges to the physician must accompany the code. *CPT-94, p. 75.*

193. **D.** The major surgical global package includes a 1-day preoperative visit, usual and necessary intraoperative services, and follow-up visits for a 90-day postoperative period. *Lane, Keenon, Coleman (eds.), p. 716.*

194. **E.** The unavailability of a qualified resident surgeon is a prerequisite for use of a modified CPT code (-82 or 09982) and payment of a claim. *CPT -94, p. 74.*

195. **A.** The modifier -25 is added to the established patient E and M service code, 99213, to identify the separate service as performed the same day as the procedure, 64612 (chemical denervation). *Lane, Keenon, Coleman (eds.), pp. 717, 721.*

196. **A.** The -79 modifier is required because the second injection procedure rendered by the same physician is within the 10-day global fee period of the first chemodenervation service. *Lane, Keenon, Coleman (eds.), pp. 717, 721.*

197. **C.** The modifier -51 is used on the second and third additional surgical services involving cervical interspaces C2 and C3. One should always indicate the highest value procedure code first without the -51 modifier. The -51 modifier is required only for the subsequent surgical services. *Lane, Keenon, Coleman (eds.), p. 717.*

198. **B.** the -24 modifier is required because the visit and diagnosis are unrelated to the prior surgery. To receive payment for this unrelated E and M visit, the modifier -24 is reported with the visit. *Lane, Keenon, Coleman (eds.), p. 717.*

199. **E.** An E and M code that results in the initial decision to perform surgery may be identified by adding the modifier -57 to the applicable E and M level of service. Adding the modifier to the E and M code indicates that the E and M service is not part of the global surgical procedure. *Lane, Keenon, Coleman (eds.), p. 722.*

200. **A.** The physician bills a level II E and M service, office visit, established patient, problem focused, 10 minutes of time (99212). Postoperative E and M services unrelated to surgery require the surgical modified -24. The claim should be coded as 99212-24. *Lane, Keenon, Coleman (eds.), pp. 717, 721.*

201. **C.** One standard lead code for V_1 is one dash, one dot. *Frew, Lane, and Frew, p. 843.*

202. **D.** One standard code for V_4 is a dash and four dots. *Frew, Lane, and Frew, p. 848.*

203. **B.** The stylus looses its position at the center of the paper and the horizontal axis wanders all over the tracing. *Frew, Lane, and Frew, p. 844.*

204. **D.** A wandering baseline is caused by faulty sensor conditions. The evenness of the application of the electrolyte solution should be checked. The skin and sensors must be dry before electrode attachment. *Frew, Lane, and Frew, p. 844.*

205. **E.** The presence of a U wave that appears after the T wave may be due to slow recovery of the Purkinje fibers or to low serum potassium. *Frew, Lane, and Frew, p. 840.*

206. **C.** If interference is present in both leads I and II, the source of interference is the patient's right arm. *Frew, Lane, and Frew, p. 844.*

207. **B.** The ECG's power cord can be a source of AC interference. The power is positioned away from the patient. *Frew, Lane, and Frew, pp. 844, 847.*

208. **A.** An electrolyte solution that has not been evenly applied can cause a wandering baseline as a result of decreased conduction of the impulses from the skin to the sensor. *Frew, Lane, and Frew, pp. 844, 847.*

209. **D.** Heart rate can be calculated using the "300-150-100-75-60-50" rule. The examiner starts at an R wave that falls on a heavy black line, then counts the heavy black lines using 300 for the first, 150 for the second, 100 for the third, and so on. If in this case the next R wave falls on the fifth line, the heart is 60 beats per minute. *Lane, Keenon, Coleman (eds.), p. 502.*

210. **E.** As the leads move across the chest from V_1 to V_6, the R wave should increase in height and the S wave should decrease in depth. This is called normal R-wave progression. *Lane, Keenon, Coleman (eds.), p. 504.*

211. **C.** If the infarction is acute, the ST segments will be elevated. As the infarction evolves, the ST segments return to baseline and the T waves invert. An old infarction is recognized by significant Q waves and no ST- or T-wave abnormalities. *Lane, Keenon, Coleman (eds.), p. 506.*

212. **C.** Sponging is discontinued if shivering occurs. Sponging provides only temporary relief and is not recommended for most fevers. The principle of sponging is to increase heat loss through evaporation. Sponging should be done for only 15 to 20 minutes, while waiting for the first dose of antifever medication to take effect. *Frew, Lane, and Frew, p. 347.*

213. **D.** Nagele's rule is as follows: From the first day of the last period, add 7 days, subtract 3 months, and add 1 year. *Lane, Keenon, Coleman (eds.), p. 467.*

214. **C.** If breast tenderness or cracking of the nipple occurs, the patient is instructed to discontinue feeding on that side; however, the affected breast must be emptied on the same schedule manually or with a breast pump. *Lane, Keenon, Coleman (eds.), p. 473.*

215. **A.** Even though breast self-examination is an important adjunct to early detection of breast changes, it is not as accurate as mammography. *Taber's, p. 267.*

216. **A.** Ear plugs should not be used while swimming because they may interfere with pressure equalization. *Taber's, pp. 597, 599.*

217. **B.** Infrared thermometers resemble an otoscope and can measure body temperature in seconds in the ear canal. *Frew, Lane, and Frew, p. 248.*

218. **D.** The upper tips of rectal and oral thermometers are color-coded for ease of identification: red for rectal and blue for oral. *Frew, Lane, and Frew, p. 347.*

219. **D.** If the reading is not certain, one should wait 2 minutes to prevent venous congestion and false-high readings, and then recheck using the same arm. *Frew, Lane, and Frew, p. 380.*

220. **D.** In men, the rectum can be easily examined in the Sims position. This position is frequently used to collect a specimen for occult blood. *Frew, Lane, and Frew, p. 389.*

221. **E.** If the eye not being examined is closed, the visual acuity of the open eye is affected. Closing one eye causes squinting in the open eye, which temporarily increases visual acuity. *Frew, Lane, and Frew, p. 441.*

222. **A.** A sterile dressing must be applied without touching the wound or the patient's skin. The patient's skin would contaminate the wound and the medical assistant's gloves during the rest of the procedure. *Frew, Lane, and Frew, p. 644.*

223. **B.** On a scale of 3+ to 0, a 3+ pulse is a full, bounding pulse; 2+, normal; 1+, weak; and 0, absent. *Lane, Keenon, Coleman (eds.), p. 312.*

224. **A.** During CO_2 laser surgery, iodine-based antiseptics can produce "tattoo" marks on the patient's skin. Alcohol can cause flash fire from the laser beam, burning the patient's skin. *Lane, Keenon, Coleman (eds.), p. 388.*

225. **C.** If the unit is to be used with a patient grounding plate, the patient's skin must be flat against the plate to avoid accidental burns to the patient from the electrosurgical unit. Alcohol is flammable and, if used, must be allowed to evaporate completely before using the electrosurgery instrument. *Lane, Keenon, Coleman (eds.), pp. 389–390.*

226. **C.** Drainage is serous (serum), sanguineous (serum and blood), or purulent (containing pus). *Lane, Keenon, Coleman (eds.), p. 390.*

227. **C.** Confirmation of pregnancy is considered the presence of fetal heart tone, detection of fetal movement by the physician, elevated hCG levels or ultrasound detection of an amniotic sac with fetus visualization. *Lane, Keenon, Coleman (eds.), p. 467.*

228. **D.** When bandaging, one should not allow the skin of one part to come into contact with the skin of another part, as severe skin infections can result. *Taber's, p. 198.*

229. **A.** Recovery from fainting or near fainting almost always occurs within minutes if a reclining position is maintained. The best treatment is to comfort the patient and to loosen any clothing that may be making the patient uncomfortable or warm. The patient should be rolled onto the side only if there is vomiting. Water should be given only after the patient has fully recovered. The use of chemicals is unnecessary. *Frew, Lane, and Frew, pp. 672–673.*

230. **B.** Vomiting or gastric lavage should not occur. The patient should drink large quantities of water or milk to dilute the alkali. Demulcents such as olive oil or egg whites should be given. *Lane, Keenon, Coleman (eds.), p. 738.*

231. **D.** If bleeding is over a bony area, a coin held firmly against the vein will provide immediate control of the blood loss. If bleeding is from an area over the soft tissue, a large but compact bandage is held firmly against the bleeding point. A tourniquet should not be used. The patient should be seen by a physician as soon as possible. *Taber's, p. 235.*

232. **A.** If the patient is unconscious or has an injury to the head and upper neck, a spinal injury is assumed. The head of an unconscious patient should not be moved. To do so could cause paralysis. Following the rules of Basic Life Support, the next step is to determine the patient's responsiveness, and if none exists, to call immediately for help. Spirits of ammonia is no longer recommended as a treatment for fainting or loss of consciousness. *Taber's, pp. 59, 317.*

233. **B.** Red-stoppered tubes contain no additive and no anticoagulants. They are used to test serum (most blood chemistries, AIDS, viral studies, serology test, blood banking). *Wedding and Toenjes, p. 144.*

234. **C.** The red-and-gray mottled (speckled) stopper designates a serum separator tube, which is used for emergency chemistry, lipid, and stat serum determinations. *Frew, Lane, and Frew, p. 723.*

235. **B.** Tubes without additives are not inverted, as there is no mixing of the additive with the blood sample. *Frew, Lane, and Frew, p. 723.*

236. **D.** Light blue tubes are used for prothrombin time, partial prothrombin time, and erythrocyte sedimentation rate. *Frew, Lane, and Frew, p. 724.*

237. **B.** When blood is added to tubes from a syringe, tubes with additive tubes precede tubes with no additive. *Frew, Lane, and Frew, p. 728.*

238. **E.** Tubes with additive are used after culture tubes, tubes with no additives, and tubes needed for coagulation studies. *Frew, Lane, and Frew, p. 728.*

239. **D.** The Unopette is a disposable micropipette that consists of a reservoir containing a diluent, a pipette, and a pipette shield. *Frew, Lane, and Frew, p. 732.*

240. **A.** White bandage tape can be placed around the rim of the centrifuge to provide a visible means of detecting splatter of blood during centrifugation. *Frew, Lane, and Frew, p. 732.*

241. **E.** Dacron, rayon, and calcium alginate swabs are used for specimen collection; cotton swabs are not. *Frew, Lane, and Frew, p. 775.*

242. **B.** Sheep blood agar (BA) is a generic medium that supports the growth of many organisms. *Frew, Lane, and Frew, pp. 776, 778.*

243. **C.** β-hemolytic streptococci produce zones of clear hemolysis around each colony. *Frew, Lane, and Frew, p. 778.*

244. **C.** Jaundiced serum or plasma appears either brownish-yellow or bright yellow. This coloring will interfere with test results and should be reported immediately. Extreme caution should be taken in handling the specimen as jaundiced serum is an indication of hepatitis. *Frew, Lane, and Frew, p. 815.*

245. **B.** In the test area, a colored symbol appears only if the test is positive. A separate QC symbol should with both negative and positive results. If the control symbol does not appear, the test is considered not able to be interpreted. *Frew, Lane, and Frew, p. 822.*

246. **B.** The normal level of AFP varies with the week of gestation; therefore, the laboratory request form must include an accurate statement of gestation weeks. *Lane, Keenon, Coleman (eds.), p. 472.*

247. **E.** When completed paperwork is put into the specimen bag, it is important that the name of the patient can be read through the bag. If the paper is placed so that the name could not be read, the bag would have to be opened, which would invalidate the chain of custody. *Lane, Keenon, Coleman (eds.), p. 548.*

248. **E.** HCG is a hormone produced by the placenta 7 to 10 days after fertilization. HCG levels rise rapidly during the first trimester. In abnormal pregnancies and ectopic pregnancy, the levels are much lower. *Lane, Keenon, Coleman (eds.), p. 646.*

249. **E.** If capillary tubes are not sealed properly, more red blood cells than plasma will be lost, resulting in false-low results. Clotting blood, blood on the outside of the tube entering the reservoir (adding more blood to the solution), and inadequate time for the centrifuge to force the red blood cells to become packed on the bottom of the tube give false-high results. ***Lane, Keenon, Coleman (eds.), pp. 824–825.***

250. **D.** Any bottle of reagent strips that has been opened for 2 months must be discarded even though the expiration has not been reached. When a new bottle is opened, the date is written on the label with an indelible marker. ***Wedding and Toenjes, p. 101.***

251. **B.** During pregnancy sedimentation rates and hematocrit levels may be elevated. Hemoglobin levels, if affected, are often decreased. Except in disease states, white blood cell counts are unaffected in pregnancy. ***Wedding and Toenjes, pp. 218, 243.***

252. **E.** A few drops of diluting fluid are expelled before charging the hemacytometer. The tip of the pipette contains only a few cells, and unless discarded, these will produce an erroneously low count. Too little fluid will result in too few cells and a false-low count. ***Wedding and Toenjes, p. 257.***

253. **A.** When using the Thoma or Unopette system for WBC counting, the specimen is allowed to sit so that the diluting fluid has time to lyse the red blood cells. ***Wedding and Toenjes, p. 263.***

254. **E.** Speed-drying minimizes cell distortion and broken cells ***Wedding and Toenjes, p. 273.***

255. **E.** A feathered edge ensures that all of the leukocytes are observable. Without a feathered edge, the smear would be too thick to provide meaningful data. ***Wedding and Toenjes, p. 274.***

256. **D.** The spreader slide is drawn into a drop of blood and the examiner waits until the blood travels almost its entire width. This makes a smear wide enough for proper examination and produces a slight margin the length of the slide. ***Wedding and Toenjes, p. 282.***

257. **E.** Because of the danger associated with biohazardous material and more sophisticated methods of testing, smelling a patient's urine to assess its odor is no longer a part of the urine analysis. If a patient describes urine as ammonia-smelling, an appointment should be made. Ammonia odors in fresh urine may be caused by urinary tract infection. ***Wedding and Toenjes, pp. 80–81.***

258. **D.** 1 tsp = 4 or 5 mL; 8 mL = 2 tsp. ***Lane, Medications, p. 12.***

259. **E.** 120 mL/tsp $\times$ 2 tsp = 240 mL. ***Lane, Medications, p. 12.***

260. **B.** The mid-deltoid area boundaries are located by forming a rectangle bounded by the lower edge of the acromion on the top to a point on the lateral side of the arm opposite the axillar or armpit on the bottom. ***Lane, Medications, p. 203.***

261. **E.** The mid-deltoid area boundaries are located by forming a rectangle bounded by the lower edge of the acromion on the top to a point on the lateral side of the arm opposite the axillar or armpit on the bottom. ***Lane, Medications, p. 203.***

262. **B.** When locating the ventrogluteal area for a right intramuscular injection, the medical assistant places the palm of the left hand on the greater trochanter and the index finger on the anterior superior iliac spine. The middle finger is spread posteriorly away from the index finger as far as possible along the iliac crest. In this way, a "V" space or triangle between the index and middle finger is formed. The injection is made in the center of the triangle with the needle directed slightly upward toward the crest of the ilium. ***Lane, Medications, p. 206.***

263. **E.** When locating the ventrogluteal area for a right intramuscular injection, the medical assistant places the palm of the left hand on the greater trochanter and the index finger on the anterior superior iliac spine. The middle finger is spread posteriorly away from the index finger as far as possible along the iliac crest. In this way, a "V" space or triangle between the index and middle finger is formed. The injection is made in the center of the triangle with the needle directed slightly upward toward the crest of the ilium. *Lane, Medications, p. 206.*

264. **B.** When locating the ventrogluteal area for a right intramuscular injection, the medical assistant places the palm of the left hand on the greater trochanter and the index finger on the anterior superior iliac spine. The middle finger is spread posteriorly away from the index finger as far as possible along the iliac crest. In this way, a "V" space or triangle between the index and middle finger is formed. The injection is made in the center of the triangle with the needle directed slightly upward toward the crest of the ilium. *Lane, Medications, p. 206.*

265. **E.** Medications should never be instilled in the ear canal if the ear is draining or there is a possibility of an eardrum perforation. *Frew, Lane, and Frew, p. 452.*

266. **E.** Betadine is a skin disinfectant; the remaining disinfectants are for general disinfection use only. *Frew, Lane, and Frew, p. 600; Taber's, p. 559.*

267. **D.** Measles, mumps, and rubella vaccines are given subcutaneously. *Lane, Keenon, Coleman (eds.), p. 424.*

268. **C.** If initiated in the first year, DPT and OPV are given according to a time schedule recommended for normal infants and children. MMR is given at 15 months of age. *Lane, Keenon, Coleman (eds.), p. 425.*

269. **A.** MMR should not be given to children under 12 months of age. The effectiveness of immunization is questionable if given too early, when the child's passive immunity is still in effect. *Lane, Keenon, Coleman (eds.), p. 425.*

270. **B.** 5 mL = 1 tsp; 1/2 tsp = 2.5 mL tid × 5 days = 37.5 mL; 30 or 32 mL = 1 oz. A 2-oz bottle should be dispensed. *Lane, Medications, p. 12.*

271. **D.** 30 mL = 1 oz; 120 mL = 4-oz bottle. *Lane, Medications, p. 12.*

272. **A.** 1 dropperful = 0.8 mL. 1/2 dropperful = 0.4 mL. *Lane, Medications, p. 12.*

273. **E.** 1 dropperful = 0.8 mL. 120 mg = 1.2 mL. 1.2 mL = 1.5 dropperful. *Lane, Medications, p. 12.*

274. **C.** 1.2 mL = 18 drops. One half of 18 drops is 9 drops. *Lane, Medications, p. 12.*

275. **C.** Transdermal patches are applied to the upper arms, upper legs, torso, or abdomen. *Lane, Medications, p. 196.*

276. **D.** IM drugs are administered with a 1- to 3-inch, 20- to 23-gauge needle. The 2-year-old child's vastus lateral is small enough to use the minimal 1-inch length; the 1.5-inch needle would be too long. *Lane, Medications, p. 202.*

277. **C.** Iron preparations are extremely irritating to the skin and subcutaneous tissues. Using the Z-tract technique prevents the deposited medication from seeping back into the skin layers. *Lane, Medications, p. 204.*

278. **C.** The vastus lateralis IM injection site is one hand's breadth below the greater trochanter at the proximal end and another hand's breadth above the knee at the distal end. *Lane, Medications, p. 204.*

279. **C.** The tuberculin test is given before or at the same time as the MMR vaccine. Once artificial MMR immunity is active, the tuberculin tine test may yield a false-negative result. *Lane, Medications, p. 262.*

280. **A.** Polio virus, live, trivalent vaccine must be stored frozen. It must be completely thawed before administration. *Lane, Medications, p. 263.*

281. **A.** Enteric-coated tablets are covered with a substance that delays the dissolution of drugs that may cause vomiting or nausea if they come into contact with the stomach lining. Enteric tablets remain intact in the stomach and are dissolved by the alkaline secretions in the upper part of the intestine. *Lane, Medications, p. 61.*

282. **B.** If the physician requests the medical assistant to keep systemic absorption to a minimum, the medical assistant can apply slight pressure to the inner canthus with a sterile cottonball for a few seconds following the administration of eyedrops. *Taber's, p. 699.*

283. **E.** Lemon juice is an excellent alternative to condiments with a high salt content. Avoid salty condiments, including barbecue sauce, catsup, mustard, soy and worcestershire sauce, and commercially prepared foods, such as salad dressings. *Frew, Lane, and Frew, p. 534.*

284. **E.** Biohazard bags must be leak proof and color-coded orange or orange-red. They may or may not have the biohazard label. *Frew, Lane, and Frew, p. 345.*

285. **C.** Regulated, hazardous waste includes items caked with blood or other potentially infected materials, items that would release blood or other potentially infected materials if compressed, pathologic or microbiologic wastes containing them, and contaminated sharps. Although dry paper products may contain large numbers or pathogenic microorganisms, without contamination by blood or body fluids, the actual risk of disease transmission is negligible. *Frew, Lane, and Frew, pp. 383, 387.*

286. **B.** Because an injection is an invasive procedure, there is the possibility of exposure to blood. Wear gloves for every injection, unless facility policy demands otherwise. *Frew, Lane, and Frew, p. 589.*

287. **D.** Autoclaving is used to sterilize instruments not harmed by heat and water pressure. Its disadvantages are that moisture will not permeate some materials and it cannot be used for heat-sensitive items. *Frew, Lane, and Frew, p. 603.*

288. **B.** Germicidal soaps (hexachlorophene) are bacteriostatic rather than bacteriocidal. *Frew, Lane, and Frew, pp. 618–619.*

289. **C.** No transmission of HBV or HIV during mouth-to-mouth resuscitation has been documented, but because of the risk of salivary transmission of other infectious diseases and the theoretical risk of HBV/HIV transmission, OSHA recommends the use of disposable airway equipment during emergency artificial ventilation. *Frew, Lane, and Frew, p. 698.*

290. **B.** Biosafety cabinets can be used to contain and remove air contaminants through an outside exhaust system. *Frew, Lane, and Frew, p. 738.*

291. **E.** If the employee is expected to have hand contact with blood or other potentially infectious materials or contaminated surfaces, he or she must wear gloves. *Frew, Lane, and Frew, p. 750.*

292. **D.** High-level disinfection is required for items coming into contact with the patient's mucous membrane. Hot water pasteurization (80°C to 100°C, 30 min) or exposure to an EPA-registered "sterilant" chemical (6 to 10 hr), except for short exposure time (10 to 45 min or as directed by the manufacturer). High-level disinfection destroys all forms of microbial life except a high number of bacterial spores. *Frew, Lane, and Frew, p. 899.*

293. **C.** EPA-registered germicides that have a label claim for tuberculocidal activity may be used for equipment that comes into contact with the intact skin. *Frew, Lane, and Frew, p. 899.*

294. **B.** A flammable liquid, according to the DOT and NFPA is one that has a flash point below 100°F (37.8°C). Liquids that have a flash point at or above 100°F do not ignite as easily as flammable liquids. *OSHA "Hazard Communication" Rule (29 CFR 1910.1200).*

295. **C.** Although a hazard label is not required on some consumer products used in the office, the physician is required to include a Material Safety Data Sheet on the items and list the items on the office's Chemical Information List. *OSHA "Hazard Communication" Rule (29 CFR 1910.1200).*

296. **D.** The temperature at which the vapor pressure of a liquid equals atmospheric pressure or at which the liquid changes to a vapor is called the boiling point. The boiling point is usually expressed in degrees Fahrenheit. If a flammable material has a low boiling point, it indicates a special fire hazard. Materials and chemical with low evaporation rates, high flash points, low reactivity, or high boiling points are less likely to be a danger. *OSHA "Hazard Communication" Rule (29 CFR 1910.1200).*

297. **C.** Except for the CT spine, most CT examinations require an intravenous injection into the patient's arm or back of the hand. *Frew, Lane, and Frew, p. 862.*

298. **D.** Patient preparation for MRI requires screening for internal metal, such as aneurysm clips, a pacemaker, or bone pins. If internal metal is present, the magnetic force is so strong it could remove metal from the patient. *Frew, Lane, and Frew, p. 864.*

299. **C.** Patients are requested to refrain from caffeine 4 hours before examination. Patients may eat normal meals and take their prescription medications. No laxatives or oral preparations are routinely required. *Frew, Lane, and Frew, pp. 864–865.*

300. **D.** Echocardiography is a noninvasive diagnostic test that uses ultrasound to image internal cardiac structures. Chamber size, valvular function, and general anatomic orientation are assessed. *Lane, Keenon, Coleman (eds.), p. 518.*

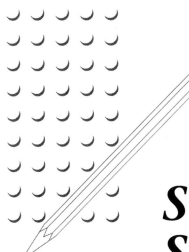

Sample Examination Simulation 3

- The following pages contain 300 test items.

- The examination is divided into

    Part 1—General Medical Knowledge
    Part 2—Administrative Procedures
    Part 3—Clinical Procedures.

- Answer sheets are provided for your use.

- The answer key immediately follows the test items and includes references with page numbers.

- References and suggested readings are at the end of the book.

Directions for Marking Answers

Example

- Use a black lead pencil (No. 2 or softer). Do NOT use pen or a pencil with hard lead.
- Make each mark heavy and black enough to completely obliterate the letter within the circle. Marks should fill the circles.
- Erase clearly any answer you wish to change.
- Make no stray marks on this answer sheet.
- Mark one and only one answer for each question. Multiple answers will be counted as wrong.

WRONG   Ⓐ Ⓑ̸ Ⓒ Ⓓ Ⓔ
WRONG   Ⓐ Ⓑ̷ Ⓒ Ⓓ Ⓔ
WRONG   Ⓐ Ⓑ Ⓒ Ⓓ Ⓔ
RIGHT   Ⓐ Ⓑ Ⓒ ● Ⓔ

1 Ⓐ Ⓑ Ⓒ Ⓓ Ⓔ	26 Ⓐ Ⓑ Ⓒ Ⓓ Ⓔ	51 Ⓐ Ⓑ Ⓒ Ⓓ Ⓔ	76 Ⓐ Ⓑ Ⓒ Ⓓ Ⓔ
2 Ⓐ Ⓑ Ⓒ Ⓓ Ⓔ	27 Ⓐ Ⓑ Ⓒ Ⓓ Ⓔ	52 Ⓐ Ⓑ Ⓒ Ⓓ Ⓔ	77 Ⓐ Ⓑ Ⓒ Ⓓ Ⓔ
3 Ⓐ Ⓑ Ⓒ Ⓓ Ⓔ	28 Ⓐ Ⓑ Ⓒ Ⓓ Ⓔ	53 Ⓐ Ⓑ Ⓒ Ⓓ Ⓔ	78 Ⓐ Ⓑ Ⓒ Ⓓ Ⓔ
4 Ⓐ Ⓑ Ⓒ Ⓓ Ⓔ	29 Ⓐ Ⓑ Ⓒ Ⓓ Ⓔ	54 Ⓐ Ⓑ Ⓒ Ⓓ Ⓔ	79 Ⓐ Ⓑ Ⓒ Ⓓ Ⓔ
5 Ⓐ Ⓑ Ⓒ Ⓓ Ⓔ	30 Ⓐ Ⓑ Ⓒ Ⓓ Ⓔ	55 Ⓐ Ⓑ Ⓒ Ⓓ Ⓔ	80 Ⓐ Ⓑ Ⓒ Ⓓ Ⓔ
6 Ⓐ Ⓑ Ⓒ Ⓓ Ⓔ	31 Ⓐ Ⓑ Ⓒ Ⓓ Ⓔ	56 Ⓐ Ⓑ Ⓒ Ⓓ Ⓔ	81 Ⓐ Ⓑ Ⓒ Ⓓ Ⓔ
7 Ⓐ Ⓑ Ⓒ Ⓓ Ⓔ	32 Ⓐ Ⓑ Ⓒ Ⓓ Ⓔ	57 Ⓐ Ⓑ Ⓒ Ⓓ Ⓔ	82 Ⓐ Ⓑ Ⓒ Ⓓ Ⓔ
8 Ⓐ Ⓑ Ⓒ Ⓓ Ⓔ	33 Ⓐ Ⓑ Ⓒ Ⓓ Ⓔ	58 Ⓐ Ⓑ Ⓒ Ⓓ Ⓔ	83 Ⓐ Ⓑ Ⓒ Ⓓ Ⓔ
9 Ⓐ Ⓑ Ⓒ Ⓓ Ⓔ	34 Ⓐ Ⓑ Ⓒ Ⓓ Ⓔ	59 Ⓐ Ⓑ Ⓒ Ⓓ Ⓔ	84 Ⓐ Ⓑ Ⓒ Ⓓ Ⓔ
10 Ⓐ Ⓑ Ⓒ Ⓓ Ⓔ	35 Ⓐ Ⓑ Ⓒ Ⓓ Ⓔ	60 Ⓐ Ⓑ Ⓒ Ⓓ Ⓔ	85 Ⓐ Ⓑ Ⓒ Ⓓ Ⓔ
11 Ⓐ Ⓑ Ⓒ Ⓓ Ⓔ	36 Ⓐ Ⓑ Ⓒ Ⓓ Ⓔ	61 Ⓐ Ⓑ Ⓒ Ⓓ Ⓔ	86 Ⓐ Ⓑ Ⓒ Ⓓ Ⓔ
12 Ⓐ Ⓑ Ⓒ Ⓓ Ⓔ	37 Ⓐ Ⓑ Ⓒ Ⓓ Ⓔ	62 Ⓐ Ⓑ Ⓒ Ⓓ Ⓔ	87 Ⓐ Ⓑ Ⓒ Ⓓ Ⓔ
13 Ⓐ Ⓑ Ⓒ Ⓓ Ⓔ	38 Ⓐ Ⓑ Ⓒ Ⓓ Ⓔ	63 Ⓐ Ⓑ Ⓒ Ⓓ Ⓔ	88 Ⓐ Ⓑ Ⓒ Ⓓ Ⓔ
14 Ⓐ Ⓑ Ⓒ Ⓓ Ⓔ	39 Ⓐ Ⓑ Ⓒ Ⓓ Ⓔ	64 Ⓐ Ⓑ Ⓒ Ⓓ Ⓔ	89 Ⓐ Ⓑ Ⓒ Ⓓ Ⓔ
15 Ⓐ Ⓑ Ⓒ Ⓓ Ⓔ	40 Ⓐ Ⓑ Ⓒ Ⓓ Ⓔ	65 Ⓐ Ⓑ Ⓒ Ⓓ Ⓔ	90 Ⓐ Ⓑ Ⓒ Ⓓ Ⓔ
16 Ⓐ Ⓑ Ⓒ Ⓓ Ⓔ	41 Ⓐ Ⓑ Ⓒ Ⓓ Ⓔ	66 Ⓐ Ⓑ Ⓒ Ⓓ Ⓔ	91 Ⓐ Ⓑ Ⓒ Ⓓ Ⓔ
17 Ⓐ Ⓑ Ⓒ Ⓓ Ⓔ	42 Ⓐ Ⓑ Ⓒ Ⓓ Ⓔ	67 Ⓐ Ⓑ Ⓒ Ⓓ Ⓔ	92 Ⓐ Ⓑ Ⓒ Ⓓ Ⓔ
18 Ⓐ Ⓑ Ⓒ Ⓓ Ⓔ	43 Ⓐ Ⓑ Ⓒ Ⓓ Ⓔ	68 Ⓐ Ⓑ Ⓒ Ⓓ Ⓔ	93 Ⓐ Ⓑ Ⓒ Ⓓ Ⓔ
19 Ⓐ Ⓑ Ⓒ Ⓓ Ⓔ	44 Ⓐ Ⓑ Ⓒ Ⓓ Ⓔ	69 Ⓐ Ⓑ Ⓒ Ⓓ Ⓔ	94 Ⓐ Ⓑ Ⓒ Ⓓ Ⓔ
20 Ⓐ Ⓑ Ⓒ Ⓓ Ⓔ	45 Ⓐ Ⓑ Ⓒ Ⓓ Ⓔ	70 Ⓐ Ⓑ Ⓒ Ⓓ Ⓔ	95 Ⓐ Ⓑ Ⓒ Ⓓ Ⓔ
21 Ⓐ Ⓑ Ⓒ Ⓓ Ⓔ	46 Ⓐ Ⓑ Ⓒ Ⓓ Ⓔ	71 Ⓐ Ⓑ Ⓒ Ⓓ Ⓔ	96 Ⓐ Ⓑ Ⓒ Ⓓ Ⓔ
22 Ⓐ Ⓑ Ⓒ Ⓓ Ⓔ	47 Ⓐ Ⓑ Ⓒ Ⓓ Ⓔ	72 Ⓐ Ⓑ Ⓒ Ⓓ Ⓔ	97 Ⓐ Ⓑ Ⓒ Ⓓ Ⓔ
23 Ⓐ Ⓑ Ⓒ Ⓓ Ⓔ	48 Ⓐ Ⓑ Ⓒ Ⓓ Ⓔ	73 Ⓐ Ⓑ Ⓒ Ⓓ Ⓔ	98 Ⓐ Ⓑ Ⓒ Ⓓ Ⓔ
24 Ⓐ Ⓑ Ⓒ Ⓓ Ⓔ	49 Ⓐ Ⓑ Ⓒ Ⓓ Ⓔ	74 Ⓐ Ⓑ Ⓒ Ⓓ Ⓔ	99 Ⓐ Ⓑ Ⓒ Ⓓ Ⓔ
25 Ⓐ Ⓑ Ⓒ Ⓓ Ⓔ	50 Ⓐ Ⓑ Ⓒ Ⓓ Ⓔ	75 Ⓐ Ⓑ Ⓒ Ⓓ Ⓔ	100 Ⓐ Ⓑ Ⓒ Ⓓ Ⓔ

Dire Answers

Example

- Use a black lead ter). Do NOT use pen or a
  pencil with har
- Make each mack enough to completely obliterate
  the letter witharks should fill the circles.
- Erase clearlyou wish to change.
- Make no strthis answer sheet.
- Mark one aanswer for each question. Multiple answers
  will be coung.

WRONG   Ⓐ Ⓑ̸ Ⓒ Ⓓ Ⓔ
WRONG   Ⓐ ⓧ Ⓒ Ⓓ Ⓔ
WRONG   Ⓐ Ⓑ Ⓒ̲ Ⓓ Ⓔ
RIGHT   Ⓐ Ⓑ Ⓒ ● Ⓔ

101 Ⓐ Ⓑ Ⓒ Ⓓ	126 Ⓐ Ⓑ Ⓒ Ⓓ Ⓔ	151 Ⓐ Ⓑ Ⓒ Ⓓ Ⓔ	176 Ⓐ Ⓑ Ⓒ Ⓓ Ⓔ
102 Ⓐ Ⓑ Ⓒ Ⓓ	127 Ⓐ Ⓑ Ⓒ Ⓓ Ⓔ	152 Ⓐ Ⓑ Ⓒ Ⓓ Ⓔ	177 Ⓐ Ⓑ Ⓒ Ⓓ Ⓔ
103 Ⓐ Ⓑ Ⓒ Ⓓ	128 Ⓐ Ⓑ Ⓒ Ⓓ Ⓔ	153 Ⓐ Ⓑ Ⓒ Ⓓ Ⓔ	178 Ⓐ Ⓑ Ⓒ Ⓓ Ⓔ
104 Ⓐ Ⓑ Ⓒ Ⓓ	129 Ⓐ Ⓑ Ⓒ Ⓓ Ⓔ	154 Ⓐ Ⓑ Ⓒ Ⓓ Ⓔ	179 Ⓐ Ⓑ Ⓒ Ⓓ Ⓔ
105 Ⓐ Ⓑ Ⓒ Ⓓ	130 Ⓐ Ⓑ Ⓒ Ⓓ Ⓔ	155 Ⓐ Ⓑ Ⓒ Ⓓ Ⓔ	180 Ⓐ Ⓑ Ⓒ Ⓓ Ⓔ
106 Ⓐ Ⓑ Ⓒ Ⓓ	131 Ⓐ Ⓑ Ⓒ Ⓓ Ⓔ	156 Ⓐ Ⓑ Ⓒ Ⓓ Ⓔ	181 Ⓐ Ⓑ Ⓒ Ⓓ Ⓔ
107 Ⓐ Ⓑ Ⓒ Ⓓ	132 Ⓐ Ⓑ Ⓒ Ⓓ Ⓔ	157 Ⓐ Ⓑ Ⓒ Ⓓ Ⓔ	182 Ⓐ Ⓑ Ⓒ Ⓓ Ⓔ
108 Ⓐ Ⓑ Ⓒ Ⓓ	133 Ⓐ Ⓑ Ⓒ Ⓓ Ⓔ	158 Ⓐ Ⓑ Ⓒ Ⓓ Ⓔ	183 Ⓐ Ⓑ Ⓒ Ⓓ Ⓔ
109 Ⓐ Ⓑ Ⓒ Ⓓ	134 Ⓐ Ⓑ Ⓒ Ⓓ Ⓔ	159 Ⓐ Ⓑ Ⓒ Ⓓ Ⓔ	184 Ⓐ Ⓑ Ⓒ Ⓓ Ⓔ
110 Ⓐ Ⓑ Ⓒ Ⓓ	135 Ⓐ Ⓑ Ⓒ Ⓓ Ⓔ	160 Ⓐ Ⓑ Ⓒ Ⓓ Ⓔ	185 Ⓐ Ⓑ Ⓒ Ⓓ Ⓔ
111 Ⓐ Ⓑ Ⓒ Ⓓ	136 Ⓐ Ⓑ Ⓒ Ⓓ Ⓔ	161 Ⓐ Ⓑ Ⓒ Ⓓ Ⓔ	186 Ⓐ Ⓑ Ⓒ Ⓓ Ⓔ
112 Ⓐ Ⓑ Ⓒ Ⓔ	137 Ⓐ Ⓑ Ⓒ Ⓓ Ⓔ	162 Ⓐ Ⓑ Ⓒ Ⓓ Ⓔ	187 Ⓐ Ⓑ Ⓒ Ⓓ Ⓔ
113 Ⓐ Ⓑ Ⓒ Ⓔ	138 Ⓐ Ⓑ Ⓒ Ⓓ Ⓔ	163 Ⓐ Ⓑ Ⓒ Ⓓ Ⓔ	188 Ⓐ Ⓑ Ⓒ Ⓓ Ⓔ
114 Ⓐ Ⓑ Ⓒ Ⓓ	139 Ⓐ Ⓑ Ⓒ Ⓓ Ⓔ	164 Ⓐ Ⓑ Ⓒ Ⓓ Ⓔ	189 Ⓐ Ⓑ Ⓒ Ⓓ Ⓔ
115 Ⓐ Ⓑ Ⓒ Ⓔ	140 Ⓐ Ⓑ Ⓒ Ⓓ Ⓔ	165 Ⓐ Ⓑ Ⓒ Ⓓ Ⓔ	190 Ⓐ Ⓑ Ⓒ Ⓓ Ⓔ
116 Ⓐ Ⓑ Ⓒ Ⓔ	141 Ⓐ Ⓑ Ⓒ Ⓓ Ⓔ	166 Ⓐ Ⓑ Ⓒ Ⓓ Ⓔ	191 Ⓐ Ⓑ Ⓒ Ⓓ Ⓔ
117 Ⓐ Ⓑ Ⓒ Ⓔ	142 Ⓐ Ⓑ Ⓒ Ⓓ Ⓔ	167 Ⓐ Ⓑ Ⓒ Ⓓ Ⓔ	192 Ⓐ Ⓑ Ⓒ Ⓓ Ⓔ
118 Ⓐ Ⓑ Ⓒ Ⓔ	143 Ⓐ Ⓑ Ⓒ Ⓓ Ⓔ	168 Ⓐ Ⓑ Ⓒ Ⓓ Ⓔ	193 Ⓐ Ⓑ Ⓒ Ⓓ Ⓔ
119 Ⓐ Ⓑ Ⓒ Ⓔ	144 Ⓐ Ⓑ Ⓒ Ⓓ Ⓔ	169 Ⓐ Ⓑ Ⓒ Ⓓ Ⓔ	194 Ⓐ Ⓑ Ⓒ Ⓓ Ⓔ
120 Ⓐ Ⓑ Ⓒ Ⓔ	145 Ⓐ Ⓑ Ⓒ Ⓓ Ⓔ	170 Ⓐ Ⓑ Ⓒ Ⓓ Ⓔ	195 Ⓐ Ⓑ Ⓒ Ⓓ Ⓔ
121 Ⓐ Ⓑ Ⓒ Ⓔ	146 Ⓐ Ⓑ Ⓒ Ⓓ Ⓔ	171 Ⓐ Ⓑ Ⓒ Ⓓ Ⓔ	196 Ⓐ Ⓑ Ⓒ Ⓓ Ⓔ
122 Ⓐ Ⓑ Ⓒ Ⓔ	147 Ⓐ Ⓑ Ⓒ Ⓓ Ⓔ	172 Ⓐ Ⓑ Ⓒ Ⓓ Ⓔ	197 Ⓐ Ⓑ Ⓒ Ⓓ Ⓔ
123 Ⓐ Ⓑ Ⓒ Ⓔ	148 Ⓐ Ⓑ Ⓒ Ⓓ Ⓔ	173 Ⓐ Ⓑ Ⓒ Ⓓ Ⓔ	198 Ⓐ Ⓑ Ⓒ Ⓓ Ⓔ
124 Ⓐ Ⓑ Ⓒ Ⓔ	149 Ⓐ Ⓑ Ⓒ Ⓓ Ⓔ	174 Ⓐ Ⓑ Ⓒ Ⓓ Ⓔ	199 Ⓐ Ⓑ Ⓒ Ⓓ Ⓔ
125 Ⓐ Ⓑ Ⓒ Ⓔ	150 Ⓐ Ⓑ Ⓒ Ⓓ Ⓔ	175 Ⓐ Ⓑ Ⓒ Ⓓ Ⓔ	200 Ⓐ Ⓑ Ⓒ Ⓓ Ⓔ

Directions for Marking Answers

- Use a black lead pencil (No. 2 or softer). Do NOT use pen or a pencil with hard lead.
- Make each mark heavy and black enough to completely obliterate the letter within the circle. Marks should fill the circles.
- Erase clearly any answer you wish to change.
- Make no stray marks on this answer sheet.
- Mark one and only one answer for each question. Multiple answers will be counted as wrong.

Example

WRONG   Ⓐ Ⓑ̸ Ⓒ Ⓓ Ⓔ

WRONG   Ⓐ ⓧ Ⓒ Ⓓ Ⓔ

WRONG   Ⓐ Ⓑ Ⓒ Ⓓ Ⓔ

RIGHT   Ⓐ Ⓑ Ⓒ ● Ⓔ

201 Ⓐ Ⓑ Ⓒ Ⓓ Ⓔ   226 Ⓐ Ⓑ Ⓒ Ⓓ Ⓔ   251 Ⓐ Ⓑ Ⓒ Ⓓ Ⓔ   276 Ⓐ Ⓑ Ⓒ Ⓓ Ⓔ

202 Ⓐ Ⓑ Ⓒ Ⓓ Ⓔ   227 Ⓐ Ⓑ Ⓒ Ⓓ Ⓔ   252 Ⓐ Ⓑ Ⓒ Ⓓ Ⓔ   277 Ⓐ Ⓑ Ⓒ Ⓓ Ⓔ

203 Ⓐ Ⓑ Ⓒ Ⓓ Ⓔ   228 Ⓐ Ⓑ Ⓒ Ⓓ Ⓔ   253 Ⓐ Ⓑ Ⓒ Ⓓ Ⓔ   278 Ⓐ Ⓑ Ⓒ Ⓓ Ⓔ

204 Ⓐ Ⓑ Ⓒ Ⓓ Ⓔ   229 Ⓐ Ⓑ Ⓒ Ⓓ Ⓔ   254 Ⓐ Ⓑ Ⓒ Ⓓ Ⓔ   279 Ⓐ Ⓑ Ⓒ Ⓓ Ⓔ

205 Ⓐ Ⓑ Ⓒ Ⓓ Ⓔ   230 Ⓐ Ⓑ Ⓒ Ⓓ Ⓔ   255 Ⓐ Ⓑ Ⓒ Ⓓ Ⓔ   280 Ⓐ Ⓑ Ⓒ Ⓓ Ⓔ

206 Ⓐ Ⓑ Ⓒ Ⓓ Ⓔ   231 Ⓐ Ⓑ Ⓒ Ⓓ Ⓔ   256 Ⓐ Ⓑ Ⓒ Ⓓ Ⓔ   281 Ⓐ Ⓑ Ⓒ Ⓓ Ⓔ

207 Ⓐ Ⓑ Ⓒ Ⓓ Ⓔ   232 Ⓐ Ⓑ Ⓒ Ⓓ Ⓔ   257 Ⓐ Ⓑ Ⓒ Ⓓ Ⓔ   282 Ⓐ Ⓑ Ⓒ Ⓓ Ⓔ

208 Ⓐ Ⓑ Ⓒ Ⓓ Ⓔ   233 Ⓐ Ⓑ Ⓒ Ⓓ Ⓔ   258 Ⓐ Ⓑ Ⓒ Ⓓ Ⓔ   283 Ⓐ Ⓑ Ⓒ Ⓓ Ⓔ

209 Ⓐ Ⓑ Ⓒ Ⓓ Ⓔ   234 Ⓐ Ⓑ Ⓒ Ⓓ Ⓔ   259 Ⓐ Ⓑ Ⓒ Ⓓ Ⓔ   284 Ⓐ Ⓑ Ⓒ Ⓓ Ⓔ

210 Ⓐ Ⓑ Ⓒ Ⓓ Ⓔ   235 Ⓐ Ⓑ Ⓒ Ⓓ Ⓔ   260 Ⓐ Ⓑ Ⓒ Ⓓ Ⓔ   285 Ⓐ Ⓑ Ⓒ Ⓓ Ⓔ

211 Ⓐ Ⓑ Ⓒ Ⓓ Ⓔ   236 Ⓐ Ⓑ Ⓒ Ⓓ Ⓔ   261 Ⓐ Ⓑ Ⓒ Ⓓ Ⓔ   286 Ⓐ Ⓑ Ⓒ Ⓓ Ⓔ

212 Ⓐ Ⓑ Ⓒ Ⓓ Ⓔ   237 Ⓐ Ⓑ Ⓒ Ⓓ Ⓔ   262 Ⓐ Ⓑ Ⓒ Ⓓ Ⓔ   287 Ⓐ Ⓑ Ⓒ Ⓓ Ⓔ

213 Ⓐ Ⓑ Ⓒ Ⓓ Ⓔ   238 Ⓐ Ⓑ Ⓒ Ⓓ Ⓔ   263 Ⓐ Ⓑ Ⓒ Ⓓ Ⓔ   288 Ⓐ Ⓑ Ⓒ Ⓓ Ⓔ

214 Ⓐ Ⓑ Ⓒ Ⓓ Ⓔ   239 Ⓐ Ⓑ Ⓒ Ⓓ Ⓔ   264 Ⓐ Ⓑ Ⓒ Ⓓ Ⓔ   289 Ⓐ Ⓑ Ⓒ Ⓓ Ⓔ

215 Ⓐ Ⓑ Ⓒ Ⓓ Ⓔ   240 Ⓐ Ⓑ Ⓒ Ⓓ Ⓔ   265 Ⓐ Ⓑ Ⓒ Ⓓ Ⓔ   290 Ⓐ Ⓑ Ⓒ Ⓓ Ⓔ

216 Ⓐ Ⓑ Ⓒ Ⓓ Ⓔ   241 Ⓐ Ⓑ Ⓒ Ⓓ Ⓔ   266 Ⓐ Ⓑ Ⓒ Ⓓ Ⓔ   291 Ⓐ Ⓑ Ⓒ Ⓓ Ⓔ

217 Ⓐ Ⓑ Ⓒ Ⓓ Ⓔ   242 Ⓐ Ⓑ Ⓒ Ⓓ Ⓔ   267 Ⓐ Ⓑ Ⓒ Ⓓ Ⓔ   292 Ⓐ Ⓑ Ⓒ Ⓓ Ⓔ

218 Ⓐ Ⓑ Ⓒ Ⓓ Ⓔ   243 Ⓐ Ⓑ Ⓒ Ⓓ Ⓔ   268 Ⓐ Ⓑ Ⓒ Ⓓ Ⓔ   293 Ⓐ Ⓑ Ⓒ Ⓓ Ⓔ

219 Ⓐ Ⓑ Ⓒ Ⓓ Ⓔ   244 Ⓐ Ⓑ Ⓒ Ⓓ Ⓔ   269 Ⓐ Ⓑ Ⓒ Ⓓ Ⓔ   294 Ⓐ Ⓑ Ⓒ Ⓓ Ⓔ

220 Ⓐ Ⓑ Ⓒ Ⓓ Ⓔ   245 Ⓐ Ⓑ Ⓒ Ⓓ Ⓔ   270 Ⓐ Ⓑ Ⓒ Ⓓ Ⓔ   295 Ⓐ Ⓑ Ⓒ Ⓓ Ⓔ

221 Ⓐ Ⓑ Ⓒ Ⓓ Ⓔ   246 Ⓐ Ⓑ Ⓒ Ⓓ Ⓔ   271 Ⓐ Ⓑ Ⓒ Ⓓ Ⓔ   296 Ⓐ Ⓑ Ⓒ Ⓓ Ⓔ

222 Ⓐ Ⓑ Ⓒ Ⓓ Ⓔ   247 Ⓐ Ⓑ Ⓒ Ⓓ Ⓔ   272 Ⓐ Ⓑ Ⓒ Ⓓ Ⓔ   297 Ⓐ Ⓑ Ⓒ Ⓓ Ⓔ

223 Ⓐ Ⓑ Ⓒ Ⓓ Ⓔ   248 Ⓐ Ⓑ Ⓒ Ⓓ Ⓔ   273 Ⓐ Ⓑ Ⓒ Ⓓ Ⓔ   298 Ⓐ Ⓑ Ⓒ Ⓓ Ⓔ

224 Ⓐ Ⓑ Ⓒ Ⓓ Ⓔ   249 Ⓐ Ⓑ Ⓒ Ⓓ Ⓔ   274 Ⓐ Ⓑ Ⓒ Ⓓ Ⓔ   299 Ⓐ Ⓑ Ⓒ Ⓓ Ⓔ

225 Ⓐ Ⓑ Ⓒ Ⓓ Ⓔ   250 Ⓐ Ⓑ Ⓒ Ⓓ Ⓔ   275 Ⓐ Ⓑ Ⓒ Ⓓ Ⓔ   300 Ⓐ Ⓑ Ⓒ Ⓓ Ⓔ

Name _____ **Date** _____

Last   First   Middle

Directions for Marking Answers

- Use a black lead pencil (No. 2 or softer). Do NOT use pen or a pencil with hard lead.
- Make each mark heavy and black enough to completely obliterate the letter within the circle. Marks should fill the circles.
- Erase clearly any answer you wish to change.
- Make no stray marks on this answer sheet.
- Mark one and only one answer for each question. Multiple answers will be counted as wrong.

Example

WRONG   Ⓐ Ⓑ Ⓒ Ⓓ Ⓔ

WRONG   Ⓐ Ⓧ Ⓒ Ⓓ Ⓔ

WRONG   Ⓐ Ⓑ Ⓒ Ⓓ Ⓔ

RIGHT   Ⓐ Ⓑ Ⓒ ● Ⓔ

1 Ⓐ Ⓑ Ⓒ Ⓓ Ⓔ   26 Ⓐ Ⓑ Ⓒ Ⓓ Ⓔ   51 Ⓐ Ⓑ Ⓒ Ⓓ Ⓔ   76 Ⓐ Ⓑ Ⓒ Ⓓ Ⓔ

2 Ⓐ Ⓑ Ⓒ Ⓓ Ⓔ   27 Ⓐ Ⓑ Ⓒ Ⓓ Ⓔ   52 Ⓐ Ⓑ Ⓒ Ⓓ Ⓔ   77 Ⓐ Ⓑ Ⓒ Ⓓ Ⓔ

3 Ⓐ Ⓑ Ⓒ Ⓓ Ⓔ   28 Ⓐ Ⓑ Ⓒ Ⓓ Ⓔ   53 Ⓐ Ⓑ Ⓒ Ⓓ Ⓔ   78 Ⓐ Ⓑ Ⓒ Ⓓ Ⓔ

4 Ⓐ Ⓑ Ⓒ Ⓓ Ⓔ   29 Ⓐ Ⓑ Ⓒ Ⓓ Ⓔ   54 Ⓐ Ⓑ Ⓒ Ⓓ Ⓔ   79 Ⓐ Ⓑ Ⓒ Ⓓ Ⓔ

5 Ⓐ Ⓑ Ⓒ Ⓓ Ⓔ   30 Ⓐ Ⓑ Ⓒ Ⓓ Ⓔ   55 Ⓐ Ⓑ Ⓒ Ⓓ Ⓔ   80 Ⓐ Ⓑ Ⓒ Ⓓ Ⓔ

6 Ⓐ Ⓑ Ⓒ Ⓓ Ⓔ   31 Ⓐ Ⓑ Ⓒ Ⓓ Ⓔ   56 Ⓐ Ⓑ Ⓒ Ⓓ Ⓔ   81 Ⓐ Ⓑ Ⓒ Ⓓ Ⓔ

7 Ⓐ Ⓑ Ⓒ Ⓓ Ⓔ   32 Ⓐ Ⓑ Ⓒ Ⓓ Ⓔ   57 Ⓐ Ⓑ Ⓒ Ⓓ Ⓔ   82 Ⓐ Ⓑ Ⓒ Ⓓ Ⓔ

8 Ⓐ Ⓑ Ⓒ Ⓓ Ⓔ   33 Ⓐ Ⓑ Ⓒ Ⓓ Ⓔ   58 Ⓐ Ⓑ Ⓒ Ⓓ Ⓔ   83 Ⓐ Ⓑ Ⓒ Ⓓ Ⓔ

9 Ⓐ Ⓑ Ⓒ Ⓓ Ⓔ   34 Ⓐ Ⓑ Ⓒ Ⓓ Ⓔ   59 Ⓐ Ⓑ Ⓒ Ⓓ Ⓔ   84 Ⓐ Ⓑ Ⓒ Ⓓ Ⓔ

10 Ⓐ Ⓑ Ⓒ Ⓓ Ⓔ   35 Ⓐ Ⓑ Ⓒ Ⓓ Ⓔ   60 Ⓐ Ⓑ Ⓒ Ⓓ Ⓔ   85 Ⓐ Ⓑ Ⓒ Ⓓ Ⓔ

11 Ⓐ Ⓑ Ⓒ Ⓓ Ⓔ   36 Ⓐ Ⓑ Ⓒ Ⓓ Ⓔ   61 Ⓐ Ⓑ Ⓒ Ⓓ Ⓔ   86 Ⓐ Ⓑ Ⓒ Ⓓ Ⓔ

12 Ⓐ Ⓑ Ⓒ Ⓓ Ⓔ   37 Ⓐ Ⓑ Ⓒ Ⓓ Ⓔ   62 Ⓐ Ⓑ Ⓒ Ⓓ Ⓔ   87 Ⓐ Ⓑ Ⓒ Ⓓ Ⓔ

13 Ⓐ Ⓑ Ⓒ Ⓓ Ⓔ   38 Ⓐ Ⓑ Ⓒ Ⓓ Ⓔ   63 Ⓐ Ⓑ Ⓒ Ⓓ Ⓔ   88 Ⓐ Ⓑ Ⓒ Ⓓ Ⓔ

14 Ⓐ Ⓑ Ⓒ Ⓓ Ⓔ   39 Ⓐ Ⓑ Ⓒ Ⓓ Ⓔ   64 Ⓐ Ⓑ Ⓒ Ⓓ Ⓔ   89 Ⓐ Ⓑ Ⓒ Ⓓ Ⓔ

15 Ⓐ Ⓑ Ⓒ Ⓓ Ⓔ   40 Ⓐ Ⓑ Ⓒ Ⓓ Ⓔ   65 Ⓐ Ⓑ Ⓒ Ⓓ Ⓔ   90 Ⓐ Ⓑ Ⓒ Ⓓ Ⓔ

16 Ⓐ Ⓑ Ⓒ Ⓓ Ⓔ   41 Ⓐ Ⓑ Ⓒ Ⓓ Ⓔ   66 Ⓐ Ⓑ Ⓒ Ⓓ Ⓔ   91 Ⓐ Ⓑ Ⓒ Ⓓ Ⓔ

17 Ⓐ Ⓑ Ⓒ Ⓓ Ⓔ   42 Ⓐ Ⓑ Ⓒ Ⓓ Ⓔ   67 Ⓐ Ⓑ Ⓒ Ⓓ Ⓔ   92 Ⓐ Ⓑ Ⓒ Ⓓ Ⓔ

18 Ⓐ Ⓑ Ⓒ Ⓓ Ⓔ   43 Ⓐ Ⓑ Ⓒ Ⓓ Ⓔ   68 Ⓐ Ⓑ Ⓒ Ⓓ Ⓔ   93 Ⓐ Ⓑ Ⓒ Ⓓ Ⓔ

19 Ⓐ Ⓑ Ⓒ Ⓓ Ⓔ   44 Ⓐ Ⓑ Ⓒ Ⓓ Ⓔ   69 Ⓐ Ⓑ Ⓒ Ⓓ Ⓔ   94 Ⓐ Ⓑ Ⓒ Ⓓ Ⓔ

20 Ⓐ Ⓑ Ⓒ Ⓓ Ⓔ   45 Ⓐ Ⓑ Ⓒ Ⓓ Ⓔ   70 Ⓐ Ⓑ Ⓒ Ⓓ Ⓔ   95 Ⓐ Ⓑ Ⓒ Ⓓ Ⓔ

21 Ⓐ Ⓑ Ⓒ Ⓓ Ⓔ   46 Ⓐ Ⓑ Ⓒ Ⓓ Ⓔ   71 Ⓐ Ⓑ Ⓒ Ⓓ Ⓔ   96 Ⓐ Ⓑ Ⓒ Ⓓ Ⓔ

22 Ⓐ Ⓑ Ⓒ Ⓓ Ⓔ   47 Ⓐ Ⓑ Ⓒ Ⓓ Ⓔ   72 Ⓐ Ⓑ Ⓒ Ⓓ Ⓔ   97 Ⓐ Ⓑ Ⓒ Ⓓ Ⓔ

23 Ⓐ Ⓑ Ⓒ Ⓓ Ⓔ   48 Ⓐ Ⓑ Ⓒ Ⓓ Ⓔ   73 Ⓐ Ⓑ Ⓒ Ⓓ Ⓔ   98 Ⓐ Ⓑ Ⓒ Ⓓ Ⓔ

24 Ⓐ Ⓑ Ⓒ Ⓓ Ⓔ   49 Ⓐ Ⓑ Ⓒ Ⓓ Ⓔ   74 Ⓐ Ⓑ Ⓒ Ⓓ Ⓔ   99 Ⓐ Ⓑ Ⓒ Ⓓ Ⓔ

25 Ⓐ Ⓑ Ⓒ Ⓓ Ⓔ   50 Ⓐ Ⓑ Ⓒ Ⓓ Ⓔ   75 Ⓐ Ⓑ Ⓒ Ⓓ Ⓔ   100 Ⓐ Ⓑ Ⓒ Ⓓ Ⓔ

Last   First   Middle

Directions for Marking Answers

- Use a black lead pencil (No. 2 or softer). Do NOT use pen or a pencil with hard lead.
- Make each mark heavy and black enough to completely obliterate the letter within the circle. Marks should fill the circles.
- Erase clearly any answer you wish to change.
- Make no stray marks on this answer sheet.
- Mark one and only one answer for each question. Multiple answers will be counted as wrong.

Example

WRONG (A) (B̸) (C) (D) (E)

WRONG (A) (X̸) (C) (D) (E)

WRONG (A) (B) (©) (D) (E)

RIGHT (A) (B) (C) (●) (E)

101 (A) (B) (C) (D) (E)   126 (A) (B) (C) (D) (E)   151 (A) (B) (C) (D) (E)   176 (A) (B) (C) (D) (E)
102 (A) (B) (C) (D) (E)   127 (A) (B) (C) (D) (E)   152 (A) (B) (C) (D) (E)   177 (A) (B) (C) (D) (E)
103 (A) (B) (C) (D) (E)   128 (A) (B) (C) (D) (E)   153 (A) (B) (C) (D) (E)   178 (A) (B) (C) (D) (E)
104 (A) (B) (C) (D) (E)   129 (A) (B) (C) (D) (E)   154 (A) (B) (C) (D) (E)   179 (A) (B) (C) (D) (E)
105 (A) (B) (C) (D) (E)   130 (A) (B) (C) (D) (E)   155 (A) (B) (C) (D) (E)   180 (A) (B) (C) (D) (E)
106 (A) (B) (C) (D) (E)   131 (A) (B) (C) (D) (E)   156 (A) (B) (C) (D) (E)   181 (A) (B) (C) (D) (E)
107 (A) (B) (C) (D) (E)   132 (A) (B) (C) (D) (E)   157 (A) (B) (C) (D) (E)   182 (A) (B) (C) (D) (E)
108 (A) (B) (C) (D) (E)   133 (A) (B) (C) (D) (E)   158 (A) (B) (C) (D) (E)   183 (A) (B) (C) (D) (E)
109 (A) (B) (C) (D) (E)   134 (A) (B) (C) (D) (E)   159 (A) (B) (C) (D) (E)   184 (A) (B) (C) (D) (E)
110 (A) (B) (C) (D) (E)   135 (A) (B) (C) (D) (E)   160 (A) (B) (C) (D) (E)   185 (A) (B) (C) (D) (E)
111 (A) (B) (C) (D) (E)   136 (A) (B) (C) (D) (E)   161 (A) (B) (C) (D) (E)   186 (A) (B) (C) (D) (E)
112 (A) (B) (C) (D) (E)   137 (A) (B) (C) (D) (E)   162 (A) (B) (C) (D) (E)   187 (A) (B) (C) (D) (E)
113 (A) (B) (C) (D) (E)   138 (A) (B) (C) (D) (E)   163 (A) (B) (C) (D) (E)   188 (A) (B) (C) (D) (E)
114 (A) (B) (C) (D) (E)   139 (A) (B) (C) (D) (E)   164 (A) (B) (C) (D) (E)   189 (A) (B) (C) (D) (E)
115 (A) (B) (C) (D) (E)   140 (A) (B) (C) (D) (E)   165 (A) (B) (C) (D) (E)   190 (A) (B) (C) (D) (E)
116 (A) (B) (C) (D) (E)   141 (A) (B) (C) (D) (E)   166 (A) (B) (C) (D) (E)   191 (A) (B) (C) (D) (E)
117 (A) (B) (C) (D) (E)   142 (A) (B) (C) (D) (E)   167 (A) (B) (C) (D) (E)   192 (A) (B) (C) (D) (E)
118 (A) (B) (C) (D) (E)   143 (A) (B) (C) (D) (E)   168 (A) (B) (C) (D) (E)   193 (A) (B) (C) (D) (E)
119 (A) (B) (C) (D) (E)   144 (A) (B) (C) (D) (E)   169 (A) (B) (C) (D) (E)   194 (A) (B) (C) (D) (E)
120 (A) (B) (C) (D) (E)   145 (A) (B) (C) (D) (E)   170 (A) (B) (C) (D) (E)   195 (A) (B) (C) (D) (E)
121 (A) (B) (C) (D) (E)   146 (A) (B) (C) (D) (E)   171 (A) (B) (C) (D) (E)   196 (A) (B) (C) (D) (E)
122 (A) (B) (C) (D) (E)   147 (A) (B) (C) (D) (E)   172 (A) (B) (C) (D) (E)   197 (A) (B) (C) (D) (E)
123 (A) (B) (C) (D) (E)   148 (A) (B) (C) (D) (E)   173 (A) (B) (C) (D) (E)   198 (A) (B) (C) (D) (E)
124 (A) (B) (C) (D) (E)   149 (A) (B) (C) (D) (E)   174 (A) (B) (C) (D) (E)   199 (A) (B) (C) (D) (E)
125 (A) (B) (C) (D) (E)   150 (A) (B) (C) (D) (E)   175 (A) (B) (C) (D) (E)   200 (A) (B) (C) (D) (E)

Name _____ **Date** _____
                 Last   First   Middle

<table>
<tr><td colspan="2">

Directions for Marking Answers

- Use a black lead pencil (No. 2 or softer). Do NOT use pen or a pencil with hard lead.
- Make each mark heavy and black enough to completely obliterate the letter within the circle. Marks should fill the circles.
- Erase clearly any answer you wish to change.
- Make no stray marks on this answer sheet.
- Mark one and only one answer for each question. Multiple answers will be counted as wrong.

</td><td>

Example

WRONG Ⓐ Ⓑ̸ Ⓒ Ⓓ Ⓔ

WRONG Ⓐ ⊠ Ⓒ Ⓓ Ⓔ

WRONG Ⓐ Ⓑ Ⓒ Ⓓ Ⓔ

RIGHT Ⓐ Ⓑ Ⓒ ● Ⓔ

</td></tr>
</table>

201 Ⓐ Ⓑ Ⓒ Ⓓ Ⓔ	226 Ⓐ Ⓑ Ⓒ Ⓓ Ⓔ	251 Ⓐ Ⓑ Ⓒ Ⓓ Ⓔ	276 Ⓐ Ⓑ Ⓒ Ⓓ Ⓔ
202 Ⓐ Ⓑ Ⓒ Ⓓ Ⓔ	227 Ⓐ Ⓑ Ⓒ Ⓓ Ⓔ	252 Ⓐ Ⓑ Ⓒ Ⓓ Ⓔ	277 Ⓐ Ⓑ Ⓒ Ⓓ Ⓔ
203 Ⓐ Ⓑ Ⓒ Ⓓ Ⓔ	228 Ⓐ Ⓑ Ⓒ Ⓓ Ⓔ	253 Ⓐ Ⓑ Ⓒ Ⓓ Ⓔ	278 Ⓐ Ⓑ Ⓒ Ⓓ Ⓔ
204 Ⓐ Ⓑ Ⓒ Ⓓ Ⓔ	229 Ⓐ Ⓑ Ⓒ Ⓓ Ⓔ	254 Ⓐ Ⓑ Ⓒ Ⓓ Ⓔ	279 Ⓐ Ⓑ Ⓒ Ⓓ Ⓔ
205 Ⓐ Ⓑ Ⓒ Ⓓ Ⓔ	230 Ⓐ Ⓑ Ⓒ Ⓓ Ⓔ	255 Ⓐ Ⓑ Ⓒ Ⓓ Ⓔ	280 Ⓐ Ⓑ Ⓒ Ⓓ Ⓔ
206 Ⓐ Ⓑ Ⓒ Ⓓ Ⓔ	231 Ⓐ Ⓑ Ⓒ Ⓓ Ⓔ	256 Ⓐ Ⓑ Ⓒ Ⓓ Ⓔ	281 Ⓐ Ⓑ Ⓒ Ⓓ Ⓔ
207 Ⓐ Ⓑ Ⓒ Ⓓ Ⓔ	232 Ⓐ Ⓑ Ⓒ Ⓓ Ⓔ	257 Ⓐ Ⓑ Ⓒ Ⓓ Ⓔ	282 Ⓐ Ⓑ Ⓒ Ⓓ Ⓔ
208 Ⓐ Ⓑ Ⓒ Ⓓ Ⓔ	233 Ⓐ Ⓑ Ⓒ Ⓓ Ⓔ	258 Ⓐ Ⓑ Ⓒ Ⓓ Ⓔ	283 Ⓐ Ⓑ Ⓒ Ⓓ Ⓔ
209 Ⓐ Ⓑ Ⓒ Ⓓ Ⓔ	234 Ⓐ Ⓑ Ⓒ Ⓓ Ⓔ	259 Ⓐ Ⓑ Ⓒ Ⓓ Ⓔ	284 Ⓐ Ⓑ Ⓒ Ⓓ Ⓔ
210 Ⓐ Ⓑ Ⓒ Ⓓ Ⓔ	235 Ⓐ Ⓑ Ⓒ Ⓓ Ⓔ	260 Ⓐ Ⓑ Ⓒ Ⓓ Ⓔ	285 Ⓐ Ⓑ Ⓒ Ⓓ Ⓔ
211 Ⓐ Ⓑ Ⓒ Ⓓ Ⓔ	236 Ⓐ Ⓑ Ⓒ Ⓓ Ⓔ	261 Ⓐ Ⓑ Ⓒ Ⓓ Ⓔ	286 Ⓐ Ⓑ Ⓒ Ⓓ Ⓔ
212 Ⓐ Ⓑ Ⓒ Ⓓ Ⓔ	237 Ⓐ Ⓑ Ⓒ Ⓓ Ⓔ	262 Ⓐ Ⓑ Ⓒ Ⓓ Ⓔ	287 Ⓐ Ⓑ Ⓒ Ⓓ Ⓔ
213 Ⓐ Ⓑ Ⓒ Ⓓ Ⓔ	238 Ⓐ Ⓑ Ⓒ Ⓓ Ⓔ	263 Ⓐ Ⓑ Ⓒ Ⓓ Ⓔ	288 Ⓐ Ⓑ Ⓒ Ⓓ Ⓔ
214 Ⓐ Ⓑ Ⓒ Ⓓ Ⓔ	239 Ⓐ Ⓑ Ⓒ Ⓓ Ⓔ	264 Ⓐ Ⓑ Ⓒ Ⓓ Ⓔ	289 Ⓐ Ⓑ Ⓒ Ⓓ Ⓔ
215 Ⓐ Ⓑ Ⓒ Ⓓ Ⓔ	240 Ⓐ Ⓑ Ⓒ Ⓓ Ⓔ	265 Ⓐ Ⓑ Ⓒ Ⓓ Ⓔ	290 Ⓐ Ⓑ Ⓒ Ⓓ Ⓔ
216 Ⓐ Ⓑ Ⓒ Ⓓ Ⓔ	241 Ⓐ Ⓑ Ⓒ Ⓓ Ⓔ	266 Ⓐ Ⓑ Ⓒ Ⓓ Ⓔ	291 Ⓐ Ⓑ Ⓒ Ⓓ Ⓔ
217 Ⓐ Ⓑ Ⓒ Ⓓ Ⓔ	242 Ⓐ Ⓑ Ⓒ Ⓓ Ⓔ	267 Ⓐ Ⓑ Ⓒ Ⓓ Ⓔ	292 Ⓐ Ⓑ Ⓒ Ⓓ Ⓔ
218 Ⓐ Ⓑ Ⓒ Ⓓ Ⓔ	243 Ⓐ Ⓑ Ⓒ Ⓓ Ⓔ	268 Ⓐ Ⓑ Ⓒ Ⓓ Ⓔ	293 Ⓐ Ⓑ Ⓒ Ⓓ Ⓔ
219 Ⓐ Ⓑ Ⓒ Ⓓ Ⓔ	244 Ⓐ Ⓑ Ⓒ Ⓓ Ⓔ	269 Ⓐ Ⓑ Ⓒ Ⓓ Ⓔ	294 Ⓐ Ⓑ Ⓒ Ⓓ Ⓔ
220 Ⓐ Ⓑ Ⓒ Ⓓ Ⓔ	245 Ⓐ Ⓑ Ⓒ Ⓓ Ⓔ	270 Ⓐ Ⓑ Ⓒ Ⓓ Ⓔ	295 Ⓐ Ⓑ Ⓒ Ⓓ Ⓔ
221 Ⓐ Ⓑ Ⓒ Ⓓ Ⓔ	246 Ⓐ Ⓑ Ⓒ Ⓓ Ⓔ	271 Ⓐ Ⓑ Ⓒ Ⓓ Ⓔ	296 Ⓐ Ⓑ Ⓒ Ⓓ Ⓔ
222 Ⓐ Ⓑ Ⓒ Ⓓ Ⓔ	247 Ⓐ Ⓑ Ⓒ Ⓓ Ⓔ	272 Ⓐ Ⓑ Ⓒ Ⓓ Ⓔ	297 Ⓐ Ⓑ Ⓒ Ⓓ Ⓔ
223 Ⓐ Ⓑ Ⓒ Ⓓ Ⓔ	248 Ⓐ Ⓑ Ⓒ Ⓓ Ⓔ	273 Ⓐ Ⓑ Ⓒ Ⓓ Ⓔ	298 Ⓐ Ⓑ Ⓒ Ⓓ Ⓔ
224 Ⓐ Ⓑ Ⓒ Ⓓ Ⓔ	249 Ⓐ Ⓑ Ⓒ Ⓓ Ⓔ	274 Ⓐ Ⓑ Ⓒ Ⓓ Ⓔ	299 Ⓐ Ⓑ Ⓒ Ⓓ Ⓔ
225 Ⓐ Ⓑ Ⓒ Ⓓ Ⓔ	250 Ⓐ Ⓑ Ⓒ Ⓓ Ⓔ	275 Ⓐ Ⓑ Ⓒ Ⓓ Ⓔ	300 Ⓐ Ⓑ Ⓒ Ⓓ Ⓔ

SIMULATION TEST 3

Part 1—General Medical Knowledge

Directions: *Each of the following questions or incomplete statements precedes five suggested answers or completions. Select the ONE answer or completion that is BEST in each case and fill in the circle containing the corresponding letter on the answer sheet.*

1. A sebaceous cyst commonly occurs
   A. within a sweat gland
   B. on the scalp
   C. on the soles of the feet
   D. on the palms of the hand
   E. around the fingernail bed

2. The joints of the cranial bones are called
   A. sutures
   B. fontanels
   C. processes
   D. pivots
   E. hinges

3. Which of the following regulates the activity of cardiac muscle, smooth muscle, and glands?
   A. central nervous system
   B. peripheral nervous system
   C. autonomic nervous system
   D. cranial nerves
   E. somatic nerves

4. As you travel down the spine, the vertebrae become
   A. progressively fused
   B. progressively smaller
   C. progressively larger, then fused
   D. progressively smaller, then successively larger
   E. progressively larger, then successively smaller

5. The bone that forms the base of the cranium is the
   A. occipital
   B. parietal
   C. temporal
   D. sphenoid
   E. frontal

6. The proximal attachment of muscle to bone is called the muscle's
   A. junction
   B. prime mover
   C. proximity
   D. insertion
   E. origin

7. A group of organs working together for a specific function is termed
   A. membrane
   B. gland
   C. system
   D. body cavity
   E. viscera

8. Interference with nerve conduction or disease leads to muscle
   A. contracture
   B. paralysis
   C. dystrophy
   D. myopathy
   E. atrophy

9. The "white of the eye" is properly called the
   A. cornea
   B. sclera
   C. conjunctiva
   D. iris
   E. lens

10. The diagnostic test used to determine brain tissue activity is
    A. neurography
    B. neuroencephalography
    C. ventriculography
    D. myelography
    E. electroencephalography

11. The part of the brain that controls the skeletal muscles is the
    A. cerebrum
    B. cerebellum
    C. medulla oblongata
    D. pons
    E. brain stem

12. Nearsightedness (myopia) is the result of an eye that is
    A. too short from front to back
    B. too long from front to back
    C. irregular in the curvature of the cornea
    D. irregular in the curvature of the lens
    E. limited in ocular mobility

13. An increase in intraocular pressure is
    A. cataracts
    B. strabismus
    C. glaucoma
    D. ambylopia
    E. presbyopia

14. The normal number of spinal curves is
    A. one
    B. two
    C. three
    D. four
    E. none

15. The "shin bone" is another name for the
    A. femur
    B. tibia
    C. fibula
    D. patella
    E. tarsus

16. A tap on which tendon produces the ankle jerk?
    A. extensor carpi
    B. adductor tendon
    C. Achilles tendon
    D. peroneus longus
    E. sartorius

17. When one is counting a pulse at the wrist, the bone used to trap the artery is called the
    A. ulna
    B. radius
    C. humerous
    D. lunate
    E. scaphoid

18. Decreasing the angle of a joint is called
    A. flexion
    B. extension
    C. circumduction
    D. rotation
    E. supination

19. The cranial nerves consist of how many pairs?
    A. 3
    B. 4
    C. 6
    D. 12
    E. 24

20. The membrane covering a joint is termed
    A. periosteal
    B. cartilagenous
    C. fibrous
    D. synovial
    E. hyaline

21. The bony projection of the ulna behind the elbow joint and forming the bony prominence of the elbow is the
    A. sphenoid process
    B. acromion process
    C. coracoid process
    D. olecranon process
    E. glenoid process

22. Folds in the cerebral cortex may be called
    A. gyri
    B. sulci
    C. gyri or sulci
    D. convolutions
    E. gyri or convolutions

23. Bone growth is dependent on which vitamin?
    A. vitamin A
    B. vitamin B
    C. vitamin C
    D. vitamin D
    E. niacin

24. The point of entrance of a nerve into a muscle is called the
    A. origin
    B. insertion
    C. denervation
    D. prime mover
    E. motor point

25. Fluids that surround the cells are called
    A. lymph
    B. blood
    C. serum
    D. interstitial
    E. intracellular

26. The name for the bones in the ear is
    A. auditory meatus
    B. auricles
    C. tympanics
    D. phalanges
    E. ossicles

27. Compared with men, the true pelvis in women is
    A. narrower
    B. deeper
    C. both A and B
    D. shallower
    E. both A and D

28. In anatomy, the term "ventral aspect" refers to
    A. above
    B. below
    C. between
    D. front
    E. back

29. Of the following, the most common type of cell division, where one cell divides into two cells, is
    A. meiosis
    B. mitosis
    C. phagocytosis
    D. osmosis
    E. symbiosis

30. Most blood cells are manufactured in the
    A. spleen
    B. liver
    C. red bone marrow
    D. yellow bone marrow
    E. lymph nodes

31. The knee joint is an example of a
    A. condylar joint
    B. pivot joint
    C. gliding joint
    D. ball-and-socket joint
    E. saddle joint

32. The external intercostal muscles
    A. elevate the ribs on inspiration
    B. decrease the thoracic cavity on inspiration
    C. decrease the thoracic cavity on expiration
    D. increase the thoracic cavity on expiration
    E. increase the thoracic cavity by extending the diaphragm on expiration

33. The anatomic name for the "voice box" is
    A. larynx
    B. pharynx
    C. trachea
    D. epiglottis
    E. glottis

34. "Swimmer's ear" is also called otitis
    A. media
    B. externa
    C. interna
    D. aqua
    E. tympani

35. On the spirogram, the average volume of air entering or leaving the respiratory passages with each breath is
    A. 100–200 mL
    B. 300–400 mL
    C. 500–600 mL
    D. 700–800 mL
    E. 900–1000 mL

36. The exchange of oxygen and carbon dioxide between the blood capillaries and the outside air takes place in the
    A. main bronchi
    B. lobar bronchi
    C. segmental bronchi
    D. alveoli
    E. pleura

37. The three posterior muscles of the thigh are often referred to as the
    A. gluteus muscles
    B. hamstrings
    C. quadriceps group
    D. gastrocnemius
    E. vastus lateralis

38. The thickest heart walls are found in the
    A. right atrium
    B. left atrium
    C. right ventricle
    D. left ventricle
    E. interatrial septum

39. A lateral curvature of the spine is called
    A. spondylolisthesis
    B. spondylitis
    C. kyphosis
    D. lordosis
    E. scoliosis

40. The flat bone that forms the mid-anterior portion of the thorax is termed the
    A. xiphoid
    B. clavicle
    C. floating rib
    D. sternum
    E. scapula

41. The basic functioning unit of the central nervous system is the
    A. plexus
    B. dendrite
    C. axon
    D. ganglion
    E. neuron

42. Nerves that carry impulses from peripheral receptors to the brain and spinal cord are
    A. afferent nerves
    B. efferent nerves
    C. motor nerves
    D. cranial nerves
    E. spinal nerves

43. The hepatic vein carries blood to the
    A. superior vena cava
    B. inferior vena cava
    C. liver
    D. gallbladder
    E. pancreas

44. The tympanic membrane separates the
    A. auditory tube and the tympanic cavity
    B. external acoustic meatus and the tympanic cavity
    C. tympanic cavity and the labyrinth
    D. malleus and the stapes
    E. stapes and the incus

45. Exchange of nutrients and wastes takes place in the
    A. arteries
    B. arterioles
    C. capillaries
    D. venules
    E. veins

46. The joint that has greater range of movement than any other joint is the
    A. wrist
    B. elbow
    C. shoulder
    D. hip
    E. ankle

47. How many lumbar vertebrae are there?
    A. two
    B. four
    C. five
    D. seven
    E. twenty-four

48. Compared with the female urethra, the male urethra is
    A. longer
    B. shorter
    C. more sensitive to injury
    D. more subject to infection
    E. more dilatable

49. Cerebrospinal fluid is formed in the
    A. brain stem
    B. ventral ganglia
    C. dorsal ganglia
    D. meninges
    E. ventricles of the brain

50. The floating ribs are the
    A. first two ribs
    B. first seven or eight ribs
    C. last five ribs
    D. eighth, ninth, and tenth ribs
    E. last two ribs

51. The purpose of red blood cells is to
    A. maintain the fluid consistency of the blood
    B. filter blood
    C. combat pathologic conditions
    D. develop antibodies and immune reactions
    E. carry oxygen to the cells

52. A patient suffering from mitral stenosis would have a defect of the
    A. pulmonary valve
    B. bicuspid valve
    C. tricuspid valve
    D. aortic valve
    E. semilunar valve

53. A middle ear infection can be the cause of a nasal infection by way of the
    A. sinuses
    B. oropharynx
    C. eustachian tube
    D. internal ear
    E. external meatus

54. In negligence, the concept of liability is based on
    A. mere negligent conduct
    B. negligent conduct resulting in injury
    C. deceit based on misrepresentation
    D. intent
    E. outrageous misconduct

55. The correct word for a lawsuit is
    A. trial
    B. charge
    C. conviction
    D. litigation
    E. judgment

56. The term for a person's failure to act in a reasonable and prudent manner is
    A. malfeasance
    B. malpractice
    C. unethical conduct ·
    D. negligence
    E. breach of contract

57. The doctrine that refers to the "law of agency" is
    A. res ipsa loquitur
    B. respondeat superior
    C. eminent domain
    D. last clear chance
    E. proximate cause

58. A patient's legally witnessed signature on a consent form is required for
    A. a stress test
    B. a glucose tolerance test
    C. both A and B
    D. an HIV antibody test
    E. both A and D

59. The medical assistant's credential is kept up-to-date every 5 years by
    A. state registration
    B. retesting
    C. state registration and testing
    D. continuing education
    E. retesting or continuing education

60. If a physician promises a cure and the subsequent treatment does not result in a cure, the physician may be liable for
    A. invasion of privacy
    B. assault
    C. fraud
    D. breach of contract
    E. battery

61. A patient whose brachial nerve was injured as a result of a venipuncture performed by a medical assistant would most likely sue
    A. the physician
    B. the medical assistant
    C. the physician and the medical assistant
    D. the entire medical staff
    E. the physician, medical assistant, and the medical assisting school

62. Euphoria is a feeling of
    A. well-being
    B. hopelessness
    C. restlessness
    D. warmth
    E. apathy

63. A characteristic that differentiates a psychosis from other mental disturbances is
    A. anxiety
    B. stress
    C. depression
    D. phobias
    E. loss of reality

64. A terminally ill patient is in the office and speaks to the medical assistant about his impending death. The medical assistant would best respond:
    A. "Why don't we try to talk about something more cheerful?"
    B. "Have you spoken to your minister about your feelings?"
    C. "Are you saying that these thoughts are frightening?"
    D. "You shouldn't be so down with your thoughts."
    E. "Why don't we have this conversation a little later when we are alone?"

65. A patient has just been diagnosed with diabetes mellitus. The medical assistant is helping her to dress and she is sullen and about to cry. The medical assistant should
    A. teach the patient about dietary control of the disease
    B. comfort the patient that at least she does not have to take insulin
    C. explain that others just like her adjust to the disease
    D. ask the patient to talk about what she is feeling
    E. change the subject and talk about something neutral

66. Schizophrenia often develops
    A. in childhood
    B. in the middle-aged adult
    C. in the elderly
    D. after brain damage
    E. at any age after severe emotional trauma

67. In treating a patient, the viewpoint that the patient's mind and body are interrelated in both health and disease is called
    A. health promotion medicine
    B. stay-well medicine
    C. preventive medicine
    D. holistic medicine
    E. patient advocacy

68. A patient who is responding quite nicely to therapy asks the medical assistant whether or not the assistant thinks her treatments are producing any results. The medical assistant should reply:
    A. "Oh, yes! In fact, you are doing much better than most."
    B. "Most patients respond after the number of treatments you have had."
    C. "How do you think you are responding?"
    D. "It's beyond my experience to give you any definite answers."
    E. "Why don't you ask the doctor that question? That's who you should speak to."

69. Which of the following statements is true concerning health care today?
    A. Disease cures have increased dramatically.
    B. Emphasis today is on stay-well programs.
    C. Patients who are hospitalized tend to be older than in the past.
    D. Patients who are hospitalized are more acutely ill than in the past.
    E. Health promotion is now less important than care of the aging population.

70. Which of the following is correct?
    A. parithyroid
    B. parethyroid
    C. parothyroid
    D. parathyroid
    E. perithyroid

71. Which of the following is correct?
    A. myocardial infraction
    B. myocardiole infarction
    C. miocardial infraction
    D. myocardial infarction
    E. miocardial infarction

72. Which of the following is correct?
    A. seborrheic dermatitis
    B. sebborheic dermatitis
    C. sebborrheic dermatitis
    D. ceborrheic dermatitis
    E. cebborrheic dermatitis

73. Which of the following is correct?
    A. thryotropin
    B. thyotropin
    C. thiotropin
    D. thyrotropin
    E. thryotroppin

74. Which of the following is correct?
    A. opthalmology
    B. opthalmalogy
    C. ophthalmology
    D. ophthalmalogy
    E. ophthamology

75. Which of the following is correct?
    A. luekosite
    B. luekocite
    C. luekocyte
    D. leukacite
    E. leukocyte

76. Which of the following is correct?
    A. uticaria
    B. uticarea
    C. urticaria
    D. urticarea
    E. urturcaria

77. Which of the following is correct?
    A. pernicous anemea
    B. pernicous anemia
    C. pernicious anemea
    D. pernicious anemia
    E. pernitious anemea

78. Which of the following is correct?
    A. anestesia
    B. anisthesia
    C. anesthesia
    D. anistesia
    E. anasthesia

79. A patient with gonorrhea commonly has a urethral discharge containing pus. The term describing this discharge is
    A. mucoid
    B. serous
    C. purulent
    D. pruritic
    E. sanguinous

80. Which of the following is correct?
    A. asitis
    B. asites
    C. ascities
    D. ascites
    E. ascitis

81. The term meaning "difficulty in urinating" is
    A. oliguria
    B. anuresis
    C. diuresis
    D. dysuria
    E. hematuria

82. Another word for joint is
    A. epiphysis
    B. diaphysis
    C. articulation
    D. process
    E. foramen

83. Which of the following is correct?
    A. abcess
    B. absces
    C. abscus
    D. abscess
    E. absess

84. Which of the following is correct?
    A. orthopedac surgery
    B. orthopedic surgery
    C. orthopedic surgury
    D. orthapedic surgury
    E. orthipedic surgury

85. The medical assistant is preparing to publish a patient policy manual. Which of the following charges is the only charge recommended by the AMA Judicial Council?
    A. advice over the telephone
    B. completion of a year-end statement
    C. completion of multiple insurance forms
    D. a missed appointment
    E. interest when extending credit

86. The mucous membranes help to protect against bacterial invasion by
    A. cilia movement
    B. absorbing vitamins
    C. both A and B
    D. secreting mucus
    E. both A and D

87. The optic nerve's function is
    A. miosis
    B. movement of the eye
    C. accommodation
    D. vision
    E. equilibrium

88. Tenderness over the McBurney point may be used as an indication of
    A. cholecystitis
    B. gastric acid reflex
    C. kidney stones
    D. appendicitis
    E. prostatitis

89. The functions of bones include
    A. blood cell production
    B. protein synthesis
    C. both A and B
    D. calcium storage
    E. both A and D

90. The inability of the eye to accommodate nearby objects is
    A. presbyopia
    B. strabismus
    C. glaucoma
    D. ambylopia
    E. myopia

91. Epithelial tissue is found in
    A. skin
    B. muscle
    C. both A and B
    D. blood vessels
    E. both A and D

92. One example of a cancerous condition in which the functional ability of the leukocyte is impaired is
    A. papilloma
    B. Hodgkin's disease
    C. papillocarcinoma
    D. hemangioma
    E. leiomyosarcoma

93. A nasal infection, such as a "head cold," may easily spread to the
    A. external ear
    B. salivary glands
    C. sinuses
    D. lacrimal ducts
    E. tonsils

94. The meninges
    A. filter cerebrospinal fluid
    B. are composed of nervous tissue
    C. are made up of three layers
    D. are involved in many types of headaches
    E. bathe the cells of the brain

95. Each is associated with deafness EXCEPT
    A. inner ear abscess
    B. otosclerosis
    C. Ménière's disease
    D. otitis media
    E. otitis externa

96. Which is a characteristic of veins?
    A. They lack valves.
    B. They spurt blood when bleeding occurs.
    C. Their walls are thinner.
    D. They are less numerous than arteries.
    E. Bleeding is controlled by applying pressure distally to a wound.

97. In which of the following situations would a statute of limitations be extended?
    A. reaching majority
    B. change in the patient's attorneys
    C. both A and B
    D. delay in discovery
    E. both A and D

98. Nonverbal communication may be conveyed by
    A. silence
    B. touch
    C. both A and B
    D. speaking
    E. both A and D

99. Teaching a patient to learn to care for a chronic illness depends on the patient's ability to
    A. set personal goals and objectives
    B. accept family involvement in the care plan
    C. both A and B
    D. differentiate between disease and a state of wellness
    E. both A and D

100. A patient's acceptance of an illness is dependent upon
    A. the individual's perceived or unperceived needs
    B. the individual's physical development
    C. both A and B
    D. the individual's level of education
    E. both A and D

SIMULATION TEST 3

Part 2—Administrative Procedures

Directions: *Each of the following questions or incomplete statements precedes five suggested answers or completions. Select the ONE answer or completion that is BEST in each case and fill in the circle containing the corresponding letter on the answer sheet.*

101. The financial record of daily charges and payments is the
    A. accounts receivable ledger card
    B. cash receipt book
    C. fee schedule
    D. general journal
    E. disbursement journal

102. After retrieving a saved document on a computer, you make major changes in the material. The original document will be permanently altered when you
    A. key in the changes
    B. rename the document
    C. exit the file
    D. save under the same name
    E. turn off the computer

103. The keyed function that prompts the WordPerfect help screen is
    A. ALT-P
    B. ALT-H
    C. F3
    D. F10
    E. CTRL-ALT-DEL

104. After making changes on a saved WordPerfect document, you decide the originally saved document is better. To return to your original document, you would
    A. copy the document, then delete the current document
    B. erase every change on the current document
    C. use the delete command to delete the document you have on screen
    D. escape from the document, then retrieve again
    E. save the document, then retrieve again

105. Before you save a word processed document, typed information is temporarily held in which part of the computer's memory?
    A. read only memory (ROM)
    B. random access memory (RAM)
    C. utilities
    D. disks
    E. macro files

106. In IBM-compatible systems, the operating system diskette is called the
    A. DOS diskette
    B. program diskette
    C. target diskette
    D. source diskette
    E. fixed diskette

107. A partial projection of the expected income for a month can be calculated by totaling the
    A. patient ledger card amounts
    B. patient statements
    C. chart of accounts
    D. current liabilities
    E. fixed assets

108. When one is writing a check, which of the following omissions would make the check nonnegotiable?
    A. date
    B. payee
    C. sum of money
    D. signature
    E. endorsement

117

109. Calculate the simple interest you would have to pay for 1 year if you borrowed $2000 at 18%.
    A. $3
    B. $3.60
    C. $30
    D. $36
    E. $360

110. A medical supplier's invoice reads "1/1/96, $450.00 purchase. Terms 2/10, 1/20, net 30." You would pay
    A. 1% discount if paid within 20 days
    B. 10% discount if paid within 2 days
    C. 5% discount if paid in 1 to 20 days
    D. 20% discount if paid by January 20
    E. 5% discount if paid by February 10

111. Find 15% simple interest of $200.
    A. $3
    B. $13.33
    C. $15
    D. $30
    E. $150

112. When one is reconciling a bank account, outstanding checks are checks
    A. written for sums greater than the amount on deposit
    B. that have not cleared the bank
    C. that have been paid by the bank and returned with the bank statement
    D. that have stop payment orders on them
    E. automatically drawn by a bank without the payer's signature

113. A successful trial balance means
    A. correct charges have been entered on ledger cards
    B. ledger card totals balance with the journal
    C. charges have been entered accurately in the journal
    D. the cash flow statement balances with the checkbook
    E. the assets equal the liabilities plus capital (owners equity)

114. Which is a true statement about a petty cash fund?
    A. It is drawn from money in the cash drawer.
    B. Cash on hand and receipts must balance at all times.
    C. It is drawn from money in the cash drawer and cash on hand and receipts must balance at all times.
    D. It is used to make change for patients.
    E. It is drawn from money in the cash drawer and is used to make change for patients.

115. The accounting system used by most physicians is
    A. cash
    B. accrual
    C. cash/accrual
    D. modified cash
    E. modified accrual

116. Effective credit arrangements are best ensured by
    A. sending a fee schedule in advance of services
    B. a personal interview before services are rendered
    C. a signed agreement or contract before services are rendered
    D. carefully detailed statements
    E. a series of collection letters

117. Which of the following records must always match the business deposits for the month?
    A. accounts receivable
    B. accounts payable
    C. patient charges
    D. patient ledger card totals
    E. received on account

118. Once a patient account has been turned over to a collection agency, the medical assistant should
    A. reduce the bill by the commission fee and continue billing
    B. reduce the bill by the commission fee and forward the bill to the collection agency
    C. forward the full bill to the collection agency and continue billing
    D. forward the full bill to the collection agency and discontinue billing
    E. forward the bill to the collection agency and discontinue future services

119. In insurance terminology, indemnity allowance means
  A. a list of specified amounts to be paid by an insurance company for medical services
  B. an amendment to an insurance policy that increases certain aspects of coverage
  C. the dollar amount of benefits that an insurance company will pay in any one year
  D. specific criteria indicating when benefits may be granted, to whom, and for how long
  E. the fee amount to be paid by the insurance plan (differences less than the physician's fee to paid by the patient)

120. The Resource-Based Relative Value Scale replaces
  A. Medicare's UCR system
  B. ICD-9-CM coding
  C. DRGs
  D. CPT-4 coding
  E. office fee schedules

121. Failure to assign benefits will result in
  A. write-offs
  B. claim rejection
  C. illegal release of information
  D. insurance payments that are lower than expected
  E. insurance payments made to the patient

122. Which of the following is an insurance claim processing error?
  A. entering only one diagnosis per claim
  B. using "no diagnosis established"
  C. stating "continued treatment: see previous report dated ____"
  D. recording one procedure per line
  E. using ICD codes and CPT codes on the same claim

123. A nonduplication of benefits clause may also be called
  A. coordination of benefits
  B. major medical
  C. catastrophic coverage
  D. copayment plan
  E. service benefit plan

124. An example of a patient fee-for-service plan is
  A. closed-panel HMO
  B. open-panel HMO
  C. prospective payment system (PPS)
  D. diagnosis related groups (DRGs)
  E. individual Blue Shield plan

125. Physicians may elect to become participating physicians in CHAMPUS/CHAMPVA by
  A. registering with a local military health facility
  B. signing a claim form on a case-by-case basis
  C. registering on an annual basis with a local fiscal intermediary
  D. contracting with a local military base
  E. registering on a one-time basis with a local fiscal intermediary

126. A period of noncoverage for an illness that existed prior to the issuance of a health insurance policy will be written into the insurance policy under
  A. pre-existing conditions
  B. exclusions
  C. special risk riders
  D. waiting periods
  E. prior authorizations

127. Which of the following is best filed alphabetically?
  A. Hamot Medical Center
  B. M-198-A Drug Trials
  C. Rochester, New York Collaboration
  D. Prescription Forms, Controlled Substances
  E. Treatment Protocols

128. Allergies should be clearly labeled within the patient's medical history because these conditions are
  A. infectious
  B. long-lasting
  C. closely related to drug treatments
  D. unpredictable
  E. dangerous to health care personnel

129. In most states, the physician is legally bound to do which of the following concerning the patient's medical record?
    A. send the original patient record in its entirely to another physician
    B. send a written summary or photocopied excerpts from the patient's record
    C. send a photocopy of a patient record in its entirety to another physician
    D. dispose of medical records by shredding and burning
    E. make available records to mentally ill patients

130. SOAP is an acronym for
    A. source-oriented medical records
    B. problem-oriented progress notes
    C. a copyright pertaining to computerized records
    D. a national society of pathologists
    E. a syndrome of parental child abuse

131. A patient has not been in the office since her annual physical examination 2 years ago. Her medical record would be found in the
    A. active files
    B. inactive files
    C. open files
    D. closed files
    E. dead storage files

132. Which of the following filing systems would be the LEAST advantageous for separating active file storage and inactive file storage?
    A. color-coded alpha
    B. terminal-digit numeric
    C. consecutive numeric
    D. color-coded straight numeric
    E. non–color-coded alpha

133. A medical record that is developed and organized according to the patient's health is called a
    A. case study record
    B. traditional medical record
    C. problem-oriented medical record
    D. source-oriented medical record
    E. terminal-digit medical record

134. The filing of miscellaneous documents is most difficult in which of the following systems?
    A. alphabetic
    B. subjective
    C. descriptive
    D. chronologic
    E. numeric

135. When adding records to the source-oriented medical record, new notes are added
    A. in alphabetical order
    B. chronologically front to back
    C. chronologically back to front
    D. in subject order
    E. by creating a new file

136. The patient's name is Harold Wilson MacDonald, Jr. Which is the third indexing unit?
    A. Harold
    B. Wilson
    C. Mac
    D. Donald
    E. Jr.

137. A patient is diagnosed as having primary (essential) hypertension. Which of the following abbreviations on her medical history is significant?
    A. gravida III
    B. UCDs
    C. FH:HBP
    D. PH:RHD
    E. PI:UTI

138. A filing system made up of monthly and daily dividers is called a
    A. to do file
    B. day-timer file
    C. monthly-minder file
    D. recall file
    E. tickler file

139. Which is the proper inside address for an attorney?
    A. Mr. John D. Smith, Attny.
    B. Mr. John D. Smith, Esq.
    C. Mr. John D. Smith, Esqs.
    D. John D. Smith, JD, Attny.
    E. John D. Smith, Esq.

140. Which of the following is the best way to cue the reader to the purpose of the letter?
    A. Enclosed is the report on Ms. Smith's biopsy.
    B. Enclosed you will find the report on Ms. Smith's biopsy.
    C. Enclosed please find the report on Ms. Smith's biopsy.
    D. I am writing about the report on Ms. Smith's biopsy, which is enclosed.
    E. Please find the report on Ms. Smith's biopsy, which is enclosed.

141. Which of the following is a grammatically correct way to close a letter?
    A. Thanking you in advance, I look forward to hearing your acceptance.
    B. Will you please give every consideration to this invitation?
    C. Your early response to this invitation will be appreciated irregardless of your answer.
    D. I anticipate your acceptance of this invitation.
    E. Should you accept this invitation, please contact me.

142. Which of the following is the proper order for the elements following the signature block?
    A. identification initials, enclosures, carbon copy notation.
    B. identification initials, carbon copy notation, enclosures.
    C. carbon copy notation, identification initials, enclosures.
    D. carbon copy notation, enclosures, identification initials.
    E. enclosures, identification initials, carbon copy notation.

143. Which is the correct composition?
    A. A large growth on the right arm that was left of midline was noted.
    B. Noted was a large growth on the right arm to the left of midline.
    C. A large growth was noted on the right arm, which was to the left of midline.
    D. A large growth, which was to the left of midline, was noted on the right arm.
    E. A large growth to the left of midline was noted on the right arm.

144. Which of the following is a correct opening sentence?
    A. Dr. Jones has asked me to write to you concerning . . .
    B. I have been asked by Dr. Jones to write to you concerning . . .
    C. I am writing this letter on behalf of Dr. Jones concerning . . .
    D. On behalf of Dr. Jones, I am writing this letter concerning . . .
    E. On behalf of Dr. Jones, I am writing you concerning . . .

145. Which sentence contains correctly used words?
    A. The three medical assistants divided the laboratory work between them.
    B. The pharmaceutical company agreed to loan the films to the local chapter.
    C. Further testing will be necessary for the correct diagnosis.
    D. If you can return my call, I will be in the office after four o'clock.
    E. The medication does not appear to have an affect on the patient.

146. Using Elite type of 12 characters per inch and a left margin of 12, where would you place the right margin tab?
    A. 68
    B. 76
    C. 86
    D. 96
    E. 100

147. In preparing an announcement on WordPerfect, *justify* means to
    A. proofread the material for errors
    B. proofread the material for factual accuracy
    C. make typed information spread out evenly between right and left margins
    D. make typed information line up at the left margin
    E. footnote for calculation and reference purposes

148. Using a page width of 8.5 inches, 10 characters per inch, and left and right margin values of 10 and 68, how many characters of text can fit on one line?
    A. 58
    B. 65
    C. 68
    D. 78
    E. 85

149. Which of the following sentences needs the restrictive pronoun "that"?
     A. He felt that his big nose, which was crooked, needed surgical correction.
     B. He knew that he could not read the small print without his glasses.
     C. I am sure that she will return your call as soon as she is able.
     D. She found that she could not digest foods high in fat content.
     E. I discovered that I inadvertently omitted page 3.

150. Which of the following forms of inside address is proper when responding to a doctor who typed his signature:
     Harry M. Stone, Ph.D.
     Dean, Allied Health School of Medicine
     A. Dr. Harry M. Stone
     B. Dr. Harry M. Stone, Ph.D.
     C. Professor Harry M. Stone, Ph.D.
     D. Dr. Harry M. Stone, Dean
     E. Prof. Harry M. Stone, Ph.D.

151. Which sentence contains correctly used words or expressions?
     A. The patient felt nauseous shortly after each dose of the medication.
     B. The AMA meeting was chaired by Donna Mills.
     C. The topics included billing information, such as credit, debit, etc.
     D. Word processing is an alternative to photocopy production.
     E. The skin eruption in the second case appeared different than the first.

152. For attractive page placement of a short pica letter (100 words or less), the bottom margin can be set at
     A. 0.5 inch
     B. 1 inch
     C. 2 inch
     D. 5 spaces
     E. 10 spaces

153. True statements concerning Blue Shield reciprocity claim procedures include each of the following EXCEPT:
     A. The reciprocity plan letter and number are a part of the insured's group number.
     B. Reciprocity beneficiary claims are billed to the home Blue Shield.
     C. Nonreciprocity claims are billed to the home Blue Shield.
     D. Nonreciprocity claims should be filed on a HCFA 1500 form.
     E. A "N" plus three numbers in an arrow identifies a reciprocity policy.

154. An Explanation of Benefits (EOB) Form contains all of the following information EXCEPT:
     A. uncovered benefits
     B. deductibles
     C. copayment responsibilities
     D. payment-in-full advisories
     E. diagnosis codes

155. Each of the following statements about filing is true EXCEPT:
     A. Open-shelf filing takes 50% less space than vertical cabinet filing.
     B. Vertical files account for higher labor costs than open shelving.
     C. Vertical file cabinets require less floor space than open-shelf filing.
     D. Open-shelf files are ideal for a very active paper filing system.
     E. Open-shelf files are ideal for a large practice.

156. Which of the following possessive pronouns is correct?
     A. Her's
     B. It's
     C. Their's
     D. Your's
     E. one's

157. Each of the following is a correct form of address EXCEPT:
     A. John H. Howard Jr., MD
     B. Dr. John H. Howard, Jr.
     C. Dr. John H. Howard, III
     D. Dr. John H. Howard 3rd
     E. John H. Howard, Jr., FACP, MD

158. In the letter (Fig. 3–1), which of the following words is misspelled?
    A. boulevard
    B. absense
    C. acknowledging
    D. receipt
    E. sincerely

159. In the letter (Fig. 3–1), the punctuation pattern is
    A. open punctuation
    B. mixed punctuation
    C. closed punctuation
    D. modified punctuation
    E. incorrect

160. In the letter (Fig. 3–1), the style is
    A. modified block style
    B. semiblock style
    C. block style
    D. modified, semiblock style
    E. simplified style

161. In the letter (Fig. 3–1), all the following would be proper forms of address EXCEPT:
    A. Dear Doctor Pineda
    B. Dear Dr. Pineda
    C. Dear Doctor
    D. Dear Director Pineda
    E. My Dear Doctor Pineda

162. By using the diagram (Fig. 3–2), you know the patient is
    A. a single head of household
    B. the household breadwinner
    C. a wife
    D. a widow
    E. a blind person

163. By using the diagram (Fig. 3–2), you know the patient is entitled to
    A. hospital, office, and home visits
    B. prescription medical supplies
    C. inpatient and outpatient diagnostic services
    D. inpatient or outpatient surgical coverage
    E. room and board and special hospital services

164. By using the diagram (Fig. 3–2), you know the policyholder is a/an
    A. employee of the railroad
    B. retired railroad worker
    C. resident of the state of Washington
    D. state employee
    E. ward of the state

165. By using the diagram (Fig. 3–2), you know that claims should be mailed to
    A. a local fiscal agent of the Veterans Administration
    B. Social Security Administration
    C. Blue Cross/Blue Shield
    D. Department of Health and Human Services Health Care Financing Administration
    E. Travelers Insurance Company

166. By using the diagram (Fig. 3–2), you know that
    A. the beneficiary has had Medicare coverage since 1982
    B. the primary beneficiary died in 1982
    C. the beneficiary retired in 1982
    D. the card has expired
    E. the policy has expired

167. A patient with a history of hypertension makes a first appointment for a complete evaluation. Telephone instructions for this examination include
    A. NPO for 12 hours the day of the examination
    B. collecting a first voided specimen the morning of the examination
    C. a Fleet enema the morning of the examination
    D. bringing current medications to the appointment
    E. Hemoccult II screen

168. In computers with a two-drive floppy system, drive A is to drive B as
    A. source is to target
    B. original is to backup
    C. master is to blank
    D. first is to second
    E. hard drive is to floppy drive

169. In WordPerfect, the tab key can be used to move the cursor to each of the following EXCEPT
    A. to temporary margins (indents)
    B. to table tabulations
    C. to column tabulations
    D. into the left margin
    E. to a new line

Anna M. Robinson, MD
Letterhead Street Address
Letterhead City, ZP 32321-1234

May 23, 19--

Mariano Pineda, M.D.
Chief Medical Director
Sloane-Kettering Medical School
8900 Letterman Boulevard
Fort Johnson, ST 35567-4342

Dear Dr. Pineda

In the absense of Dr. Robinson, I am acknowledging receipt of your invitation for Dr. Robinson to speak at the State Medical Society's annual conference at the Fort Johnson Convention Center on August 10, 19--.

Dr. Robinson will return on June 10, 19--, after a trip to Canada. As soon as she returns, I will forward your letter to her promptly.

Sincerely yours

Joan Smith

Joan Smith, CMA-AC

Figure 3–1. Letter of acknowledgment.

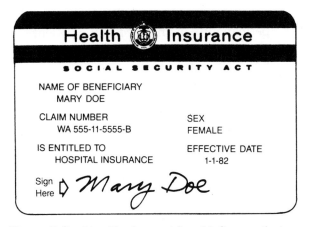

Figure 3–2. Identification card for a Medicare patient.

170. If you prematurely turn off a computer, each of the following may occur EXCEPT
    A. lost stored data on your hard disk files
    B. lost stored data on your floppy
    C. hard disk damage
    D. lost new data just entered into the system
    E. a power surge

171. To quickly move a cursor to the end of a WordPerfect document, press
    A. END
    B. HOME-END
    C. CTRL-PG DN
    D. END-END-END
    E. HOME-HOME-DOWNARROW

172. The physician is usually represented in small-claims court by
    A. the medical assistant
    B. an attorney
    C. either A or B
    D. himself
    E. either A or D

173. Patient checks that should be accepted include
    A. checks written for more than the amount due
    B. postdated checks
    C. third-party checks
    D. predated checks
    E. payroll checks

174. Materials necessary for business disbursements include:
    A. invoices
    B. chart of accounts
    C. both A and B
    D. aging analysis
    E. both A and D

175. In manual bookkeeping, proper NSF entries in the payment column of a ledger card include
    A. <$40.00>
    B. − $40.00
    C. both A and B
    D. $40.00
    E. both A and D

176. An adjustment entry will be necessary for which of the following?
    A. professional courtesy reductions
    B. when a patient has paid in advance
    C. both A and B
    D. write-off reductions
    E. both A and D

177. Each of the following patient benefits is true of an HMO EXCEPT:
    A. There is no need to pay money out-of-pocket for a visit.
    B. There is no need for approval before a member-specialist is seen.
    C. There is no need to file claims.
    D. Medical expenses are predictable.
    E. Routine physical examinations are often included.

178. CHAMPVA is an insurance program offering benefits and cost-sharing features to
    A. spouses and children of disabled or deceased veterans
    B. retired military personnel
    C. both A and B
    D. active-duty military personnel
    E. both A and D

179. Which of the following is required to be withheld from an employee's salary?
    A. disability insurance
    B. FICA
    C. workers' compensation insurance
    D. unemployment insurance
    E. health insurance

180. If the physician does not participate under the CHAMPUS program, true statements about the program include each of the following EXCEPT:
    A. The patient completes and submits the top half of Form 500/501.
    B. Forms must be received 1 year from the end of the year of service.
    C. The patient needs an itemized statement from the physician.
    D. Payment will go directly to the physician.
    E. The physician may bill the patient for charges above the CHAMPUS allowed.

181. The coding system that uses a maximum of three digits to code diagnoses is
    A. RBRVS
    B. DRG
    C. CPT
    D. ICD-9
    E. ICD-9-CM

182. Workers' compensation coverage includes each of the following EXCEPT
    A. temporary disability income
    B. death benefits
    C. permanent disability income
    D. rehabilitation benefits
    E. life insurance

183. True statements about records retention include
    A. Records of minors who are no longer patients are kept for three years.
    B. Patient records are kept indefinitely.
    C. Income tax records are kept for three years.
    D. Professional liability policies are kept until superseded by new ones.
    E. all of the above

184. In the letter (Fig. 3–3), which of the following patterns is correct?
    A. The date line is four lines below the letterhead.
    B. The inside address is five lines below the date line.
    C. The salutation is two lines below the inside address.
    D. The first paragraph is two lines below the salutation.
    E. all of the above

185. Telephone messages that should be permanently maintained in the patient's chart include each of the following EXCEPT
    A. a patient requesting a prescription renewal
    B. a patient requesting a change in appointment
    C. a patient reporting that a condition is improved
    D. a pharmacist requesting a prescription renewal
    E. a patient requesting a referral to a specialist

186. Postal OCR scanning directions include using each of the following EXCEPT
    A. room, apartment, or suite designation on a separate line
    B. capital letters for the entire address
    C. no punctuation
    D. fewer than 22 spaces on the last line
    E. one space between the state code and the zip code

187. Objective parts of the medical history include
    A. chief complaint
    B. present illness
    C. past history
    D. symptoms
    E. laboratory results

188. A patient refuses to follow medical advice, and the physician decides to terminate the physician-patient relationship. The letter to the patient should state each of the following EXCEPT
    A. the name(s) of referred physicians
    B. that the physician officially withdraws from the case
    C. that the patient needs further medical care
    D. a future date after which the physician is no longer available
    E. offering to make records available

189. On a balance sheet, assets include
    A. vendor payments due
    B. unpaid patient accounts
    C. real estate lease
    D. payroll
    E. payroll taxes

Anna M. Robinson, MD
Letterhead Street Address
Letterhead City, ZP 32321-1234

May 23, 19--

Mariano Pineda, M.D.
Chief Medical Director
Sloane-Kettering Medical School
8900 Letterman Boulevard
Fort Johnson, ST 35567-4342

Dear Dr. Pineda:

In the absence of Dr. Robinson, I am acknowledging
receipt of your May 18, 19-- consultation report on
our patient, James E. Johnson.

Dr. Robinson will return on June 10, 19--, after a
trip to Canada. Upon her return, I will make your
report immediately available to her.

Sincerely yours,

Joan Smith

Joan Smith, CMA-AC
Office Manager

Figure 3–3. Letter of acknowledgment.

190. Summaries identifying which patient accounts are 30, 60, 90, and over 90 days overdue include
    A. cash flow statements
    B. trial balance
    C. income and expense statements
    D. age analysis
    E. profit and loss analysis

191. The write-it-once check-writing system is capable of providing one-write entries of each of the following EXCEPT
    A. payee's address
    B. gross earnings
    C. withheld taxes
    D. health insurance deductions
    E. net earnings

192. Incoming patient calls that DO NOT require the immediate transfer to the physician include
    A. a 4-year-old child with a rectal temperature of 39.4°C (102.8°F)
    B. an adult patient on antibiotics who has developed a rash and ringing of the ears
    C. a nursing home charge nurse with an update on a resident
    D. an adult patient who reports recurrent low-grade fever over the past 2 weeks
    E. an adult patient who has passed out two times earlier in the day

193. Records that should be stored for up to 7 years include
    A. job applications
    B. time and attendance records
    C. letters of resignation
    D. performance reviews
    E. W-2 income transmittal forms

194. Manufacture sources for information on urinalysis supplies include
    A. Seimans Crop.
    B. Baxter Healthcare Corp.
    C. Ames Div. of Miles, Inc.
    D. MedicAlert
    E. Glaxo, Inc.

195. Manufacturers from which a pegboard system may be ordered include
    A. Safeguard Business Systems, Inc.
    B. AMA Council on Medical Service
    C. Healthcare Financing Administration
    D. Xerox Corporation
    E. St. Anthony's Publishing, Inc.

196. Figures used to calculate the RBRVS fee schedule include
    A. DRG dollar rates
    B. charges set by the physician
    C. customary charges within a specialty
    D. reasonable charges
    E. relative value units

197. The physician gives telephone orders to the pharmacist for the schedule V drug terpin hydrate with codeine. The medical assistant completes the necessary steps by
    A. using a DEA form
    B. handwriting the prescription for the physician to sign
    C. completing the prescription in multiple copies
    D. asking the physician to record the order on the medical record
    E. recording the order on the medical record

198. Third-party liability situations include
    A. Medicare
    B. a parent for a minor
    C. both A and B
    D. a husband for his wife
    E. both A and D

199. Procedures for which the patient can have only clear liquids the day of an examination include
    A. stool for culture and sensitivity
    B. sigmoidoscopy
    C. stool for occult blood
    D. barium enema
    E. pinworm test

200. A patient should void before each of the following examinations EXCEPT
    A. of the genitalia
    B. of the urinary tract
    C. of the abdomen
    D. of the rectum
    E. of the lower spine

Part 3—Clinical Procedures

Directions: *Each of the following questions or incomplete statements precedes five suggested answers or completions. Select the ONE answer or completion that is BEST in each case and fill in the circle containing the corresponding letter on the answer sheet.*

201. According to the Centers for Disease Control, what type of technique should be used for handling a patient when there is an increased risk of exposure to blood?
    A. protective isolation
    B. respiratory isolation
    C. enteric precautions
    D. wound and skin precautions
    E. universal blood and body-fluid precautions

202. After patient use of an oral thermometer, the medical assistant would *first*
    A. soak it in soap and cool water
    B. soak it in cool water
    C. wash it under the cool water faucet for a few seconds, then swab with alcohol
    D. swab with alcohol, then place it in a dry covered tray
    E. place it in a disinfecting solution for 1 hour

203. Infections in the medical office are most likely to be spread by
    A. soiled linens
    B. the hands of employees
    C. contaminated instruments and supplies
    D. drafts and currents caused by heating and air-conditioning units
    E. incomplete sterilization in the autoclave

204. One disease that is controlled by breaking the infection cycle of the insect (arthropod vector) populations is
    A. pinworm (*Enterobius vermicularis*)
    B. Lyme disease (*Borrelia burgdorferi*)
    C. ringworm (tinea)
    D. Legionnaires' disease (*Legionella pneumophila*)
    E. typhoid fever (*Salmonella* sp.)

205. Monilia is treated with a
    A. miconazole
    B. vinegar douche
    C. Flagyl
    D. estrogen
    E. Betadyne

206. An audiometer is used to examine
    A. disorders of equilibrium
    B. hearing acuity
    C. tympanic membrane trauma
    D. autistic children
    E. speech discrimination

207. A patient has a positive 6–7 mm induration tuberculin skin test. This screening suggests the patient
    A. has active tuberculosis
    B. has been exposed to tuberculosis in the past
    C. has had tuberculosis in the past
    D. has been infected with the tubercle bacilli
    E. is immune to tuberculosis

208. When one is obtaining a patient's blood pressure, the patient's arm should be
    A. slightly above heart level and resting
    B. at the level of the heart
    C. slightly below the level of the heart
    D. at waist level
    E. below waist level

209. In the male patient, which of the following early symptoms would confirm a diagnosis of gonorrhea rather than syphilis?
    A. skin rash
    B. painful urination
    C. blood in the urine
    D. an ulcer on the penis
    E. gumma

129

210. Before taking a patient's temperature, the medical assistant should shake the mercury column
   A. to below the lowest marking on the thermometer
   B. to the lowest marking on the thermometer
   C. to near 94°F (34°C)
   D. to near 97°F (36°C)
   E. to the arrow marking on the scale

211. The difference in a patient's apical and radial pulse is called the
   A. pulse pressure
   B. pulse deficit
   C. pulse differential
   D. basal blood pressure
   E. cardiac pressure

212. The medical assistant is asked to set up for a cerumen removal. Which of the following equipment will be required for the procedure?
   A. laryngeal mirror
   B. Reiner syringe
   C. biopsy pack
   D. cyst removal pack
   E. incision and drainage pack

213. In preparation for a physical examination, the medical assistant will have ready topical anesthesia if the physician wishes to
   A. test the patient's simple reflexes
   B. test the patient's nociceptive ("hot stove") reflexes
   C. perform a fundoscopic examination
   D. determine pressure within the patient's eye with a tonometer
   E. collect a specimen from the patient's cervix

214. A poorly secured stethoscope diaphragm may cause
   A. a blood pressure reading that is too high
   B. a blood pressure reading that is too low
   C. a distortion of the low-frequency blood pressure sounds
   D. tangling of the stethoscope tubing
   E. an inability to read the mercury column during the systolic phases

215. Before monilia infections are treated, it is important to obtain a
   A. Pap smear
   B. wet prep with normal saline
   C. potassium hydroxide (KOH) smear
   D. VDRL test
   E. rapid plasma reagen (RPR) test

216. The first sharp tapping sound that you hear when determining blood pressure is the
   A. arterial pressure
   B. venous pressure
   C. diastolic pressure
   D. systolic pressure
   E. pulse pressure

217. A child is brought into the office and the mother tells you he has been exposed to another child with rheumatic fever. One of the reported signs of rheumatic fever is
   A. cough
   B. sore throat 1 to 2 weeks previously
   C. runny nose
   D. nausea
   E. hyperactivity

218. The primary purpose for a drain is to
   A. hasten closure of the wound
   B. allow visual examination of the wound
   C. allow the exit of fluids or purulent material from a wound
   D. permit the introduction of antibiotics into the wound
   E. permit extravasation of blood from the wound

219. For which examination will the patient be placed in the knee-chest position?
   A. prostate
   B. rectum
   C. urinary bladder
   D. vaginal
   E. lumbar spine

220. A patient arrives for his appointment on a hot summer day and is drinking hot coffee in the waiting room. How long should you wait before measuring his body temperature orally?
   A. 1–2 minutes
   B. 3–4 minutes
   C. 5–10 minutes
   D. 15–30 minutes
   E. 45–60 minutes

221. A person's blood pressure is normally the lowest
   A. following exercise
   B. upon arising in the morning
   C. at mid-day
   D. after meals
   E. at bedtime

222. One of the first procedures performed for infertility couples is
   A. Rubin test
   B. hysterosalpingogram
   C. Huhner test
   D. basal temperature charting
   E. semen analysis

223. In preparation for palpation of the right breast for any masses, the medical assistant should position the patient by having her lie down and
   A. flex her neck
   B. turn her neck to the right
   C. extend her neck
   D. place a pillow under the right shoulder
   E. place a pillow under the left shoulder

224. A rectal thermometer should be inserted into the adult rectum to a depth of
   A. 0.5 inch
   B. 1.5 inches
   C. 3 inches
   D. 5 inches
   E. one-half the length of the thermometer

225. Each little square on the ECG paper is
   A. 1 mm square
   B. 5 mm square
   C. 10 mm square
   D. 1 cm square
   E. 5 cm square

226. To make an extremely small ECG complex larger, you would set the
   A. sensitivity switch to ½
   B. sensitivity switch to 1
   C. sensitivity switch to 2
   D. paper speed to 25 mm/sec
   E. paper speed to 50 mm/sec

227. The ECG device that touches the patient's skin is the
   A. amplifier
   B. galvanometer
   C. sensor
   D. stylus
   E. lead wire

228. When one is performing an ECG, the disadvantage of using electrolyte paste is
   A. sensors must be cleaned after each use
   B. it cannot be used on parts of the body with thick hair
   C. it cannot be used on the chest
   D. it is irritating to the patient's skin
   E. it stains clothing

229. The ECG reference electrode is the
   A. three-pronged plug
   B. right arm
   C. right leg
   D. left arm
   E. left leg

230. On an ECG, the QRS complex represents
   A. atrial contraction
   B. contraction conversing the A-V node
   C. ventricular contraction
   D. time interval between ventricular contraction and recovery
   E. ventricular relaxation

231. The portion of the ECG that relates to the time interval between the beginning of atrial contraction and the beginning of ventricular contraction is the
   A. P-R segment
   B. QRS complex
   C. S-T segment
   D. P-R interval
   E. Q-T interval

232. Because heat stroke is much more dangerous than heat exhaustion, it is important to distinguish between the two. The first symptom of heat stroke to differ sharply from heat exhaustion is
   A. headache
   B. dizziness
   C. weakness
   D. absence of sweating
   E. muscle cramping

233. If a patient appears to have a head injury, which of the following positions is contraindicated?
   A. supine
   B. Fowler's
   C. semi-Fowler's
   D. Sims
   E. Trendelenburg

234. During cardiopulmonary resuscitation, the medical assistant notices that the chest does not rise and fall with rescue breaths. The most probable cause for this is
    A. the patient's airway is not open
    B. breaths that are too shallow
    C. breaths that are administered too slowly
    D. cardiac pressure is too forceful
    E. the patient is beyond rescuing

235. After surveying the scene, the first action when finding a patient you suspect is not breathing is to
    A. open the patient's airway
    B. give two quick breaths to the patient
    C. call for help
    D. start cardiac compressions
    E. ask "Are you OK?"

236. When administering cardiopulmonary resuscitation to an adult, chest compression depth should be
    A. 0.5 to 1.0 inch
    B. 1.5 to 2.0 inches
    C. 2.5 to 3.0 inches
    D. 3.5 to 4.0 inches
    E. 4.5 to 5.0 inches

237. On a reagent pad, a urine positive for bacteriuria is
    A. yellow-orange
    B. pink
    C. red
    D. maroon
    E. green-blue

238. The urine in patients with uncontrolled diabetes smells of
    A. fruit
    B. garlic
    C. ammonia
    D. pine needles
    E. fish

239. A mammogram is useful for
    A. detecting breast tumors before symptoms appear
    B. detecting breast tumor locations prior to mastectomy
    C. differentiating types of breast tumors
    D. reducing the size of a tumor
    E. detecting whether or not breast tumors have metastasized

240. Controlling the quality of urine reagent testing includes the use of
    A. Attest
    B. Chek-stix
    C. Spore-O-Chex
    D. ethylene oxide indicators
    E. the Bowie and Dick Test

241. Of the following, which is the most commonly encountered parasite in urine testing?
    A. pinworm
    B. pinworm egg
    C. flagellates
    D. ameba
    E. blood fluke

242. Which of the following is an alkaline urine pH?
    A. 4.0
    B. 5.0
    C. 6.5
    D. 7.0
    E. 8.0

243. An antidote used to induce vomiting is
    A. activated charcoal
    B. Narcan
    C. syrup of ipecac
    D. Epsom salt
    E. milk

244. Salicylate (acetylsalicylic acid) drugs include
    A. Darvon-N
    B. Ecotrin
    C. Indocin
    D. Nuprin
    E. Tylenol

245. When treating an obese patient, the angle at which a 25-gauge 5/8-inch needle should be inserted for a subcutaneous injection is
    A. 10 degrees
    B. 20 degrees
    C. 45 degrees
    D. 60 degrees
    E. 180 degrees

246. Which of the following anesthetics is used as a local infiltration agent?
    A. lidocaine hydrochloride
    B. Isocaine
    C. Novocain
    D. Nupercainal
    E. tetracaine hydrochloride

247. The physician prescribes 120 mL of a liquid oral preparation. The pharmacist will dispense
A. 1 oz
B. 2 oz
C. 4 oz
D. 10 oz
E. 12 oz

248. Nitrates and nitrites are used as treatment for
A. angina
B. arthritis
C. cardiac arrhythmias
D. constipation
E. decubitis ulcers

249. How would the medical assistant instruct the patient to take the following medication:
Sig: ii tid 1h ac Refil prn
A. 1 hour before meals
B. whenever needed
C. 1 hour before meals, when needed
D. two times a day before meals
E. three times a day, 1 hour before meals

250. One brand name of local infiltration anesthesia used for minor surgery is
A. ethylene
B. Xylocaine
C. diethyl ether
D. benzocaine
E. ethyl chloride

251. One antidiarrheal agent that is still available by prescription only is
A. Kaopectolin
B. Imodium
C. Lactinex
D. Lomotil
E. Riopan

252. Translate the following order into household equivalents: "drams one quater in die."
A. ¼ tsp every day
B. ¼ dr every day
C. ¼ tsp four times a day
D. 1 tsp four times a day
E. 1 dr four times a day

253. One penicillin-based antimicrobial drug is
A. Ceclor
B. Amoxil
C. Cipro
D. E-mycin
E. Monistat

254. The physician orders 500 mg to be administered to a patient. The vial is labeled 500 mg/mL. What amount of medication would you draw up in the syringe?
A. 1 mg
B. 500 mg
C. 0.5 mL
D. 1 mL
E. 500 mL

255. Antacids are contraindicated in cases of
A. peptic ulcers
B. duodenal ulcers
C. tetracycline therapy
D. hyperacidity
E. management of phosphate urinary stone formation

256. After using disposable needle and syringe, the medical assistant would place it, uncapped and intact, in a rigid container to
A. avoid injury to self and other persons handling solid waste
B. discard equipment that cannot be sterilized
C. minimize space required for solid waste disposal
D. prevent reuse of the materials by unauthorized persons
E. minimize airborne infections

257. Lanoxin (digoxin) is a drug that
A. stimulates the heart muscle
B. relaxes the heart muscle
C. lowers blood pressure
D. increases respiration
E. decreases respiration

258. Theo-Dur (theophylline) is used to treat
A. migraine headache
B. bronchial asthma
C. gram positive bacteria
D. muscle spasm
E. gout

259. For preparing a medication, which of the following information is LEAST important?
    A. drug name
    B. drug indication
    C. usual dosage of the drug
    D. expected outcome
    E. manufacturer's name

260. To make Tincture of Zephiran (benzalkonium chloride) from a concentrated aqueous solution, which of the following ingredients are required?
    A. the concentrate, alcohol, and distilled water
    B. the concentrate and chemically deionized water
    C. the concentrate, soap, and alcohol
    D. the concentrate, soap, and water
    E. the concentrate and ether

261. Which of the following is a topical spray anesthetic?
    A. ethyl acetate
    B. ethyl alcohol
    C. ethyl chloride
    D. ethyl ether
    E. ether

262. In relation to the point of entry of an injection, where should the medical assistant begin cleansing the skin?
    A. above
    B. below
    C. to the left or right
    D. concentrically 1 to 2 inches away
    E. directly over the point

263. A diabetic patient should be taught to avoid which of the following foods?
    A. yogurt
    B. carrots
    C. pretzels
    D. popcorn
    E. mints

264. Cathartics (laxatives) are used for all of the following EXCEPT
    A. treatment of intestinal parasites
    B. chemical poisoning
    C. anorectal lesions
    D. appendicitis
    E. acute constipation

265. All of the following statements about antitussives are true EXCEPT
    A. Antitussives can be narcotic or nonnarcotic.
    B. Antitussives depress a cough either in the brain center or locally.
    C. Antitussives are contraindicated in pregnancy.
    D. Antitussives should be taken at least 15 minutes before eating or drinking.
    E. Antitussives are more effective in the treatment of the productive cough.

266. Specific human immune globulin products containing antibodies against specified diseases are now available for all of the following EXCEPT
    A. hepatitis B
    B. rabies
    C. measles
    D. botulism
    E. rubella

267. All of the following drugs are classified under schedule III EXCEPT
    A. Empirin compound with codeine
    B. Fiorinal with codeine
    C. Phenaphen with codeine
    D. Robitussin with codeine
    E. Tylenol with codeine

268. All of the following are used for the treatment of contact dermatitis EXCEPT
    A. hydrogen peroxide
    B. calamine
    C. cocoa butter
    D. collodion
    E. zinc oxide

269. Narcotic analgesics are used to treat all of the following EXCEPT
    A. head injuries following shock
    B. severe, dry coughs
    C. postoperative pain
    D. diarrhea
    E. severe pain following a heart attack

270. The type of fracture (Fig. 3–4) is
    A. complicated
    B. open
    C. comminuted
    D. compression
    E. green stick

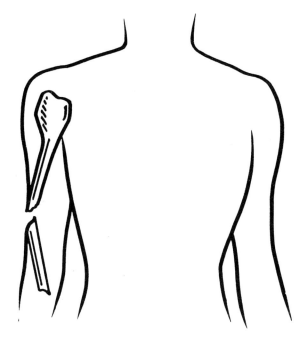

Figure 3–4. A patient enters the office with the injury above and falls to the floor. Another medical assistant calls for an ambulance to transport the patient to the hospital, while you help the physician attend to the patient. There is minimal wound bleeding. The patient is conscious and has also sprained her right knee. Using this case, answer questions 270–277.

271. Which of the following should the medical assistant do first?
    A. apply an ice bag to the right knee
    B. apply an Ace bandage to the right knee
    C. splint the arm without moving the patient
    D. move the patient to an examining table
    E. irrigate the wound with sterile saline

272. While waiting for the ambulance, cold application to the patient's right knee would be contraindicated if
    A. the knee is not swollen
    B. the knee is swollen
    C. a ligament injury is suspected
    D. another fracture is suspected
    E. the knee has an open wound

273. The physician asks the medical assistant to apply an Ace bandage to the patient's right leg. The medical assistant would begin bandaging
    A. above the knee
    B. at the knee
    C. below the knee
    D. at the ankle
    E. at the arch of the foot

274. While bandaging, how would the medical assistant position the patient's knee?
    A. slightly flexed
    B. slightly rotated
    C. extended
    D. abducted
    E. adducted

275. The patient's right toes begin to swell. The medical assistant most likely has applied the bandage
    A. unevenly
    B. too loosely
    C. too tightly
    D. over a pressure point
    E. correctly

276. The medical assistant takes the patient's vital signs. What would be the most likely vital sign?
    A. increased body temperature
    B. decreased pulse
    C. decreased respirations
    D. decreased blood pressure
    E. increased blood pressure

277. Until the patient is transported to the hospital, it is MOST important to
    A. keep the patient quiet to prevent further injury
    B. place the patient in a supine position to reduce shock
    C. reassure the patient to reduce fright
    D. administer oxygen to prevent tissue anoxia
    E. administer small sips of water to relieve thirst

278. In the diagram (Fig. 3–5), which of the following statements is true concerning the next step of the procedure?
    A. Strike the forceps against the inside rim to remove excess disinfectants.
    B. Wipe the forceps with sterile gauze to remove excess disinfectant.
    C. Lift the forceps up and away from the container with the grasping end downward.
    D. Turn the forceps end up to allow excess disinfectant to drip away from the tip.
    E. Place the forceps on a sterile field with the prongs in an open position.

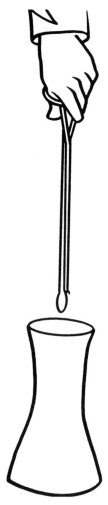

Figure 3–5. Using transfer forceps.

279. In the diagram (Fig. 3–5), the contained chemical is one that will destroy all living microorganisms, if the instrument is immersed for 10 hours. This chemical is
    A. 70% alcohol
    B. 10% formaldehyde
    C. sodium hypochlorite (bleach) 1:10
    D. quarternary ammonia
    E. 2% neutral glutaraldehyde

280. In the diagram (Fig.3–5), the contained chemical is
    A. inactivated in the presence of organic matter
    B. harmful to carbon steel or other plated materials
    C. harmful to rubber and plastic products
    D. both sporicidal and virucidal
    E. changed every day

281. Blood-borne pathogens will be present when collecting blood specimens from patients with
    A. infectious hepatitis B
    B. gonorrhea
    C. both A and B
    D. AIDS
    E. both A and D

282. A diabetic patient who has not eaten and taken insulin would exhibit first
    A. rapid, deep respirations
    B. +1 pulse
    C. hot, dry skin with deep red coloring
    D. fruity breath odor
    E. dizziness and faintness

283. During a fundoscopic examination, the physician will need
    A. a Snellen chart
    B. a tonometer
    C. anesthetic
    D. an ophthalmoscope
    E. miotic drops

284. One common infection of the vagina is caused by
    A. enteroviruses
    B. *Gardnerella* (*Haemophilus*)
    C. *Nocardia asteroides*
    D. helminths
    E. dermatophytes

285. Pain, by itself, will most likely affect the vital signs by increasing
    A. pulse
    B. blood pressure
    C. both A and B
    D. respirations
    E. both A and D

286. Abnormally colored urine can result from
    A. alcohol ingestion
    B. foods
    C. diuretic therapy
    D. uncontrolled diabetes mellitus
    E. diabetes insipidus

287. Elevated urine ketone levels occur as a by-product of
    A. the inflammatory process
    B. protein metabolism
    C. red blood cell destruction
    D. hemoglobin breakdown
    E. fat metabolism

288. A cloudy urine may be caused by
   A. sitting at room temperature
   B. refrigeration
   C. both A and B
   D. reagent strip testing
   E. both A and D

289. A urine specimen that is allowed to stand and cool will normally
   A. become alkaline
   B. have a sediment
   C. both A and B
   D. loose its odor
   E. both A and D

290. Infected urine may have which of the following odors?
   A. ammonia
   B. fruity
   C. both A and B
   D. putrid
   E. both A and D

291. Equipment for measuring urine specific gravity includes the
   A. urinometer
   B. reagent dipstick
   C. both A and B
   D. unimeter
   E. both A and D

292. Which of the following suture material properties would be appropriate for the skin closure of a superficial facial wound?
   A. nonabsorbable
   B. atraumatic
   C. both A and B
   D. 3–0
   E. both A and D

293. Because of the serum base of recombinant hepatitis B vaccines, immunization is contraindicated in patients with hypersensitivity to
   A. chickens
   B. ducks
   C. eggs
   D. yeast
   E. horse hair

294. Drugs that are administered using the transdermal patch include
   A. estrogen
   B. nicotine
   C. both A and B
   D. potassium chloride
   E. both A and D

295. Nonnarcotic analgesic and antipyretic drugs containing acetaminophen include
   A. Tylenol
   B. Empirin
   C. Bayer
   D. Advil
   E. Butazolidin

296. Vitamin K is used to
   A. prevent osteomalacia
   B. treat pernicious anemia
   C. treat sebaceous dermatosis
   D. prevent the danger of postoperative hemorrhage
   E. treat mental disturbances

297. When one is preparing a medication by injection, which of the following may NOT be touched?
   A. vial stopper
   B. plunger
   C. both A and B
   D. needle shaft
   E. both A and D

298. Tetracycline is safe to take
   A. in the last trimester of pregnancy
   B. during the neonatal period
   C. early childhood up to the age of 8
   D. after the onset of menopause
   E. during tooth development stages

299. Epinephrine (Adrenalin) produces each of the following EXCEPT
   A. raising blood pressure
   B. speeding up heart rate
   C. increasing cardiac output
   D. relaxing bronchial muscle
   E. dilating blood vessels

300. After examination, the physician asks you to record a diagnosis of "heart murmur, functional." Which is a true statement about this condition?
   A. A stress test will further confirm the diagnosis.
   B. The patient will be placed on a special diet.
   C. The condition is secondary to rheumatic fever.
   D. The physician will follow the case without surgical intervention.
   E. Chest x-ray examinations will be ordered.

1. **B.** Sebaceous glands produce sebum, an oily secretion that keeps the skin and hair from becoming brittle. Sebaceous cysts commonly occur on the scalp, back, and scrotum. There are no sebaceous glands on the palms of the hands and soles of the feet. *Gylys & Wedding, p. 66.*

2. **A.** The joints of the cranial bones are called sutures and are immovable. *Scanlon, p. 111.*

3. **C.** The autonomic nervous system regulates the activity of involuntary body functions, such as cardiac muscle, smooth muscle, and the glands; it exerts widespread influence over the entire body. *Gylys & Wedding, p. 319.*

4. **E.** The vertebrae become progressively larger down to the sacrum, and then become successively smaller. *Gylys & Wedding, p. 206.*

5. **A.** The occipital bone forms the base of the cranium. *Taber's, p. 1344.*

6. **E.** The proximal attachment of muscle to bone is called its origin. The opposite end is termed its insertion. *Scanlon, p. 132.*

7. **C.** Organs working together form a body system. *Gylys & Wedding, p. 45.*

8. **E.** Just as bone loses its mass with disease, muscle atrophies quickly if it is not used. The general term myopathy is applied to muscle disease. Contracture is commonly associated with bone injury or other disease. The muscular dystrophies are associated with structural changes, usually chemical in nature. Paralysis results from degeneration of a motor unit. *Sheldon, pp. 569–571.*

9. **B.** The sclera is the outermost, opaque layer of the eye. The front part of the sclera can be seen through the conjunctiva as "the white of the eye."*Gylys & Wedding, p. 344.*

10. **E.** The electrical currents of the brain are measured in the form of brain waves by electroencephalography. *Tamparo & Lewis, p. 400; Gylys & Wedding, p. 331.*

11. **A.** Voluntary muscular movement is controlled by the cerebral cortex portion of the cerebrum. *Gylys & Wedding, pp. 323.*

12. **B.** Myopia occurs when light entering the eye comes to a focus in front of the retina so that vision is better for nearby objects. This results from an eyeball that is too long from front to back. *Tamparo & Lewis, p. 336.*

13. **C.** Increased intraocular pressure is known as glaucoma. *Warden-Tamparo & Lewis, p. 339; Gylys & Wedding, p. 351.*

14. **D.** There are four curves, designed to give the spine strength to support the body and to give the body balance. The two concave curves are the cervical and lumbar curves; the two convex curves are the thoracic and sacral curves. *Gylys & Wedding, p. 206.*

15. **B.** The "shin bone" is a lay term for the tibia. *Taber's, p. 1996.*

16. **C.** The largest and strongest tendon in the body is the Achilles tendon, which connects the gastrocnemius to the heel bone. A tap on the Achilles tendon produces what is called the ankle jerk or Achilles reflex. *Taber's, p. 21.*

17. **B.** A pulse taken at the wrist is performed by trapping the radial artery against the radius. *Frew, Lane, Frew, p. 352.*

18. **A.** The action of flexion decreases the angle of a joint. *Gylys & Wedding, p. 211.*

19. **D.** There are 12 pairs of cranial nerves that, unlike the spinal nerves, have specific names. *Gylys & Wedding, p. 324.*

20. **D.** Synovial membrane is a vascular connective tissue that lines the inner surface of the joint capsule but does not cover articular cartilage. *Gylys & Wedding, p. 210.*

21. **D.** The distal end of the ulna forms the olecranon process. *Taber's, p. 1349.*

22. E. The folds in the cerebral cortex may be called convolutions or gyri. *Gyls & Wedding, p. 323.*

23. D. Vitamin D is necessary for bones to calcify and harden. *Frew, Lane, Frew, p. 522.*

24. E. The point of entrance of a nerve into a muscle is known as the motor point. *Taber's, p. 1240.*

25. D. The cells are bathed in fluids called interstitial (extracellular) fluids. *Sheldon, pp. 24–25.*

26. E. The small bones of the ear are called the ossicles or the auditory ossicles. *Gyls & Wedding, p. 347.*

27. D. The female pelvis has a wider subpubic angle, everted ischial tuberosities, and a shallower symphysis pubis. The female pelvis is tilted forward, and the bones are thinner and more delicate. *Gyls & Wedding, p. 208.*

28. D. The ventral or anterior aspect refers to the front of the body. *Gyls & Wedding, p. 46.*

29. B. Most new cells arise out of old cells by mitosis, which is the division of one cell into two. *Sheldon, p. 21.*

30. C. The chief function of red bone marrow is to manufacture erythrocytes, leukocytes, and platelets. Red bone marrow is responsible for the manufacture of most blood cells. *Sheldon, pp. 493–495.*

31. A. The knee joint is a condylar joint, which consists of two distinct articular surfaces, each called a condyle. *Scanlon, p. 558.*

32. A. The external intercostals elevate the ribs, and are therefore considered to be muscles of inspiration. *Gyls & Wedding, p. 123.*

33. A. The larynx is referred to as the voice box. *Gyls & Wedding, p. 122.*

34. B. Swimmer's ear, an inflammation of the external ear, is called otitis externa. *Tamparo & Lewis, p. 345.*

35. C. The average volume of air entering or leaving the respiratory passages with each breath (tidal volume) is 500 to 600 mL. *Sheldon, p. 359.*

36. D. The exchange of oxygen and carbon dioxide occurs in the alveoli, the microscopic air sacs of the lungs. *Sheldon, p. 359; Gyls & Wedding, p. 122.*

37. B. The posterior muscles of the thigh are often referred to as the hamstrings. *Taber's, p. 844.*

38. D. The heart's thickest walls are found in the left ventricle as it must pump oxygenated blood to the entire body. *Gyls & Wedding, p. 146.*

39. E. A lateral curvature of the spine (to the right or left) is termed scoliosis. *Gyls & Wedding, p. 219.*

40. D. The sternum forms the anterior portion of the bony wall of the thorax. It is composed of three parts: the manubrium, body, and xiphoid process. *Scanlon, p. 117.*

41. E. The basic functioning unit of the nervous system is the neuron, from the Greek *neuron,* meaning sinew-like structure. *Gyls & Wedding, p. 320.*

42. A. Nerves that carry impulses from the outside world to the brain and spinal cord are termed afferent (sensory) nerves. *Gyls & Wedding, p. 318.*

43. B. The hepatic vein carries blood from the liver to the inferior vena cava. *Sheldon, p. 387.*

44. B. The tympanic membrane, or ear drum, forms a partition between the external acoustic meatus and the tympanic cavity. *Gyls & Wedding, p. 347.*

45. C. Oxygen and carbon dioxide and nutrients and waste products exchange between the blood and the body cells in the capillaries. *Gyls & Wedding, pp. 123, 144.*

46. C. The shoulder joint has greater range of movement than any other joint, largely because of the scapular movement that generally accompanies movement at the shoulder joint. *Taber's, p. 1755.*

47. C. The 24 mobile, presacral vertebrae comprise 7 cervical, 12 thoracic, and 5 lumbar. The five vertebrae immediately below the lumbar are fused in the adult to form the sacrum. The lowermost four form the coccyx. *Gyls & Wedding, p. 208.*

48. **A.** The male urethra is about 20 cm long; the female urethra, 4 cm. This may explain why men are less subject to common urinary tract infections. Although the male urethra may be somewhat larger in lumen, the female urethra is quite distensible and can be dilated to about 1 cm without damage to it. *Tamparo & Lewis, pp. 91–92.*

49. **E.** The ventricles of the brain contain vascular choroid plexuses, from which an almost protein-free cerebrospinal fluid is formed. *Gylys & Wedding, p. 324.*

50. **E.** Three of the last five ribs (false ribs) join the cartilage immediately above. The last two are free from the sternum and are called floating ribs. *Gylys & Wedding, p. 207.*

51. **E.** The red blood cells carry oxygen combined with hemoglobin, called oxyhemoglobin, to all the cells of the body. *Gylys & Wedding, pp. 174–175.*

52. **B.** Another name for the bicuspid (two flaps) is the mitral valve. It separates the left atrium from the left ventricle and prevents reflux of blood into the atrium. *Gylys & Wedding, p. 148.*

53. **C.** The eustachian tube is connected to the nasopharynx. Infections may begin in the middle ear and transmit to the nasal cavity. *Gylys & Wedding, p. 347.*

54. **B.** There is no liability for mere negligent conduct, no matter what the intent. To have liability, there must be injury resulting from negligent conduct. *Lewis & Tamparo, pp. 60–61.*

55. **D.** The term litigation means lawsuit. *Lewis & Tamparo, p. 40.*

56. **D.** Negligence is the term for the failure to act in a reasonable and prudent manner resulting in damage to another person. *Lewis & Tamparo, pp. 60–61.*

57. **B.** Under the doctrine of respondeat superior, employers have a form of strict liability for the harm caused by agents or employees acting in the line and scope of authority. *Lewis & Tamparo, pp. 61–62.*

58. **E.** A patient's signature of informed consent should be obtained prior to the performance of a stress test or HIV antibody test. Facility policies vary, but rarely is a consent form necessary for the glucose tolerance test. *Lewis & Tamparo, pp 95–104.*

59. **E.** The medical assisting credential is limited to a period of 5 years. To maintain the credential, the medical assistant must complete a program of documented continuing education or retake the credentialling examination. *Frew, Lane, Frew, p. 9.*

60. **D.** Failure to bring about a promise, such as a cure, is a breach of contract. *Lewis & Tamparo, p. 63.*

61. **C.** It is most likely that the patient will sue the medical assistant under negligence and the physician under the law of agency's respondeat superior. *Lewis & Tamparo, pp. 61–62.*

62. **A.** Euphoria is a sense of well-being, or being without pain or distress. *Taber's, p. 683.*

63. **E.** The primary characteristic that differentiates psychosis from neurosis and other mental illnesses is that the patient is out of touch with reality. *Sheldon, pp. 517–518.*

64. **C.** To help persons best, it is best to encourage conversation and listen when the person is ready to talk about death. Never assume that you know what the patient is feeling. Instead ask, "Am I right that you are feeling . . . ?" or "Are you saying that . . . ?" *Davis, pp. 170–174.*

65. **D.** Allow the patient to express her feelings. Rationalizing or teaching is not helpful when a patient is too anxious to listen. Changing the subject will send a message either that it is not all right to talk about it or that the medical assistant does not care. *Davis, p. 102.*

66. **A.** The onset of schizophrenia is usually in adolescence or early adulthood. It may be found as early as the age of 2, but most often the onset is between 6 and 14 years of age. *Sheldon, p. 518.*

67. **D.** Viewing a human being as a whole rather than as body parts or systems is called holistic medicine. *Tamparo & Lewis, pp. 365–366.*

68. **C.** Although selections D and E are legally responsible on the part of the medical assistant, it is better to turn the question back to the patient, so the medical assistant can record the patient's feelings and relate them to the physician. The patient is obviously ready to talk about her progress, and it might be an opportunity that may not come up again. Always avoid giving medical opinion. *Davis, pp. 102, 104–105.*

69. **B.** Today, teaching in the health care field concentrates on helping people stay well by promoting good health. *Frew, Lane, Frew, pp. 74–75.*

70. **D.** Parathyroid. *Gylys & Wedding, p. 300.*

71. **D.** Myocardial infarction. *Taber's, p. 1262.*

72. **A.** Seborrheic dermatitis. *Gylys & Wedding, p. 79.*

73. **D.** Thyrotropin. *Taber's, p. 1996.*

74. **C.** Ophthalmology. *Taber's, p. 1361.*

75. **E.** Leukocyte. *Taber's, p. 1100.*

76. **C.** Urticaria. *Taber's, p. 2091.*

77. **D.** Pernicious anemia. *Taber's, p. 1479.*

78. **C.** Anesthesia. *Taber's, p. 100.*

79. **C.** The term for a discharge containing or producing pus is purulent. *Tamparo & Lewis, p. 391.*

80. **D.** Ascites. *Taber's, pp. 159.*

81. **D.** The prefix *dys* means painful or difficult; *uria* is the word element for urination. *Gylys & Wedding, pp. 37, 245.*

82. **C.** Articulation means joint; a place of union or junction between two or more bones of the skeleton. *Gylys & Wedding, p. 210.*

83. **D.** Abscess. *Taber's, p. 8.*

84. **B.** Orthopedic surgery. *Taber's, p. 1375.*

85. **C.** Current AMA Judicial Council opinions state that duties of the medical assistant include the collection of fees and that the completion of one routine, simplified insurance form should be performed without charge, as part of the service to the patient. If the patient has multiple insurance forms to be completed, the physician is justified in charging for the completion of insurance forms in excess of the first standard form. *Frew, Lane, Frew, p. 43.*

86. **E.** Mucus and the movement of cilia both help to trap and expel bacteria from the body, before it can cause disease. *Sheldon, p. 111.*

87. **D.** The chief function of the optic nerve is vision. Eye movement is controlled by the oculomotor, trochlear, and trigeminal nerves. The oculomotor nerve also controls miosis and accommodation. *Scanlon, p. 202.*

88. **D.** McBurney's point, about 2 inches from the right anterior superior spine of the ilium on a line to the umbilicus, corresponds with the normal position of the appendix. Pain from cholecystitis generally radiates to the URQ, epigastrium, or right scapula; from kidney stones, to the lumbar or hypogastric regions or the genitalia; and from gastric acid reflux (heartburn), to the sternum or epigastrium. *Tamparo & Lewis, pp. 148, 387.*

89. **E.** The functions of bone include providing a supporting framework for the body, providing a place of attachment for muscles, storing calcium, and producing blood cells. *Sheldon, pp. 550–551.*

90. **A.** Presbyopia is a refractive error that results from a loss of elasticity of the crystalline lens of the eye. This condition is a consequence of advancing age and is a form of far-sightedness (not to be confused with hyperopia). *Tamparo & Lewis, pp. 334–336.*

91. **E.** Epithelial tissues cover the body surfaces and line the body cavities, blood vessels, and glands. *Gylys & Wedding, p. 44.*

92. **B.** Leukemias are one of the malignant neoplasms of hematopoietic cells, such as lymphocytes, bone marrow, and plasma cells. Hodgkin's disease is the medical term for cancer of the lymph nodes. *Gylys & Wedding, p. 188.*

93. **C.** The sinuses develop as outgrowths of the nasal cavity; hence, they all drain, directly or indirectly, into the nasal cavity. *Taber's, p. 1802.*

94. **C.** The meninges is the collective term for the three layers of nonnervous tissue that protect the brain and spinal cord. The cerebral arteries (not the meninges) are involved in many types of headaches. *Sheldon, p. 549; Tamparo & Lewis, p. 387.*

95. **E.** Neural deafness may result from a lesion of the cochlea or cochlear nerve; conduction deafness may result from a disease of the middle ear. Although operable, otosclerosis of the walls of the inner ear may cause conductive deafness. Very rarely would an external ear infection or inflammation result in either neural or conduction deafness. *Gylys & Wedding, p. 352; Tamparo & Lewis, p. 347.*

96. **C.** Veins have valves that prevent blood backflow. They do not pulsate and do not spurt when bleeding occurs from them. Veins are more numerous than arteries and generally more variable. Their walls are thinner, and their diameters are usually larger than those of the corresponding arteries. Bleeding is controlled by applying pressure between the wound and the heart. *Gylys & Wedding, p. 146.*

97. **E.** A statute of limitation is extended past a patient's age of majority and in the case of a delay in the discovery of an injury due to negligence. *Lewis & Tamparo, p. 66.*

98. **C.** Communication may be verbal or nonverbal. Nonverbal communications include listening, facial expressions, gestures, touch, silence, and appearance. Verbal communication includes the spoken and written word. *Davis, pp. 147–148.*

99. **E.** Successful patient teaching depends on the patient being able to: understand the difference between disease and a state of wellness; adjust to and accept chronic illness as a condition other than a state of wellness that can be controlled; accept frustrations and failures without reacting with anxiety, depression, or anger; and remain a constructive participant in one's own treatment by setting personal goals and objectives of self-care and assessment. *Frew, Lane, Frew, pp. 68–73.*

100. **C.** The patient's response to illness is very dependent on family (cultural) attitudes, needs that motivate the individual, and a sense of self-esteem that develops from healthy physical and intellectual development, not level of education. *Frew, Lane, Frew, p. 69.*

101. **D.** The general journal is the daily ledger or daily log. The cash receipt book is used only when a patient pays in cash. Posting to accounts receivable (patient) ledger cards and disbursement journals (check registers) are accounting procedures that may not be completed every day. A fee schedule is revised when fees change, and it is distributed to patients when requested. *Lane, Keenon, Coleman (eds.), pp. 78–79.*

102. **D.** Saving a document under the same name stores the current version of the document for later use. *Walter, p. 126.*

103. **C.** F3 is used as a help screen function in WordPerfect. *Walter, p. 202.*

104. **D.** If you do not want new changes to an original document, escaping without saving the current work will automatically eliminate the material. Simply retrieve the original document under its saved name and start over with your work. Using the save command after changes will permanently alter the original document. *Walter, p. 188.*

105. **B.** RAM can be thought of as the "scratch pad" or working draft page. It contains the program instructions and the data that is currently being processed. ROM is the internal memory of the operating system itself and computer language. Before leaving newly entered material, it is necessary to "save" by whatever method the program uses. This gets the material to a disk, where it is permanently saved. It will not be lost when you exit the program or turn off the machine. *Walter, pp. 14, 188.*

106. **A.** The Disk Operating System is the DOS diskette. *Walter, p. 39.*

107. **B.** A review of the month's statements (patient billings) will give you a total of the expected income for the month. The ledger card totals represent the total accounts receivable [total amounts owed to the doctor(s)]; but not necessarily the expected income for one month. A chart of accounts is a listing of categories for posting income and expense transactions. Income expected within the next accounting cycle is considered current not fixed assets. Income is not a business liability. *Lane, Keenon, Coleman (eds.), p. 113.*

108. **D.** The payee may write in any of the omissions except for the signature. The lack of a signature makes the check nonnegotiable. *Lane, Keenon, Coleman (eds.), pp. 100–101.*

109. **E.** Principal ($2,000) × Rate (18% or 0.18) × Time (1 year) = Interest ($360). *Frew, Lane, Frew, p. 234.*

110. **A.** This invoice contains the following allowable discounts: take a 2% discount if you pay within 10 days; take a 1% discount if you pay within 20 days; you may wait 30 days and pay the full price. *Lane, Keenon, Coleman (eds.), p. 62.*

111. **D.** When you want to find a certain percentage of a number, you multiply the number by the equivalent decimal: 200 × 0.15 = 30. *Frew, Lane, Frew, p. 234.*

112. **B.** When reconciling an account, outstanding checks are those that have not yet cleared the bank. *Frew, Lane, Frew, p. 240.*

113. **B.** A successful trial balance means the total of the ledger cards equals the journal accounts receivable number (total of the charges, payments, and adjustments) for the month. The trial balance will not prove the accuracy of the accounts. For example, an incorrect charge may have been applied to both the journal and ledger card, or a charge or payment may have been applied to a wrong ledger card or omitted entirely. *Lane, Keenon, Coleman (eds.), p. 92.*

114. **B.** The petty cash fund is drawn from the business checking account and used to pay for incidental expenses. The amount of cash and the amounts of the petty cash receipts must always balance to the exact amount of the original starting draft. When the funds are low, the expenses are computed from the receipts and a new check is written for this amount, restoring the fund to its starting amount. The replenishing check will differ according to the expenses incurred during the period. *Frew, Lane, Frew, p. 280.*

115. **A.** Most physicians operate the business on a cash basis. *Lane, Keenon, Coleman (eds.), p. 124.*

116. **B.** Personal interviews with patients can be more effective than written agreements and correspondence. Face-to-face discussions beforehand can help you recognize special problems so that the proper plan can be designed for the patient. *Lane, Keenon, Coleman (eds.), p. 109.*

117. **E.** In any month, the deposit total must equal the total cash and checks received on account. The accounts receivable should equal the total of the patient ledger cards and should represent the total business for which money has not been received. The accounts payable for the month should equal the total of the business expenses paid out. The summary of practice-related business represents the total month's earnings, both paid and unpaid. It represents actual income and potential income. *Lane, Keenon, Coleman (eds.), p. 127.*

118. **D.** Forward the billing information to the collection agency and stop billing from the office. The physician does have a responsibility to continue treating the patient, unless he or she formally and properly withdraws from the case. Whenever possible, physicians should continue to treat these patients on a cash basis until their accounts are up-to-date. *Frew, Lane, Frew, p. 257; Lane, Keenon, Coleman (eds.), p. 119.*

119. **E.** An indemnity allowance (or schedule) is the fee amount to be paid by an insurance plan. Coverage differences must be paid by the patient. *Frew, Lane, Frew, p. 892.*

120. **A.** The new Medicare fee schedule, enacted in 1992, replaces the usual, customary, and reasonable (UCR) charge payment system and is based on the relative value of resources that physicians spend to provide services to Medicare patients. *Lane, Keenon, Coleman (eds.), p. 181.*

121. **E.** The assignment of benefits is executed by the patient to allow the insurance company to pay the doctor directly. *Frew, Lane, Frew, p. 316; Lane, Keenon, Coleman (eds.), pp. 170, 174.*

122. **B.** The use of either "no diagnosis established" or "for diagnostic purpose" is unacceptable. It is preferable to give a chief complaint if no diagnosis has been confirmed. If an insurance company covers annual physicals, a claim may be filed with "annual physical examination." *Lane, Keenon, Coleman (eds.), p. 194.*

123. **A.** Nonduplication of benefits is also called a coordination of benefits clause. *Frew, Lane, Frew, p. 290.*

124. **E.** In a fee-for-service, the patient sees the doctor and then gets a bill for the service. The insurance company then pays at least a portion of the bill. This is still the most common system. *Frew, Lane, Frew, pp. 301–302.*

125. **B.** When a physician signs a claim form, the physician agrees to participate only in that particular case. *Frew, Lane, Frew, p. 295.*

126. **A.** A pre-existing condition is one that is present before the effective date of the policy. *Frew, Lane, Frew, p. 892.*

127. **A.** Alphabetic filing best applies indexing rules to names of businesses, persons, and organizations. *Frew, Lane, Frew, pp. 105, 107.*

128. **C.** Allergies are closely related to the chemicals and preservatives used in drug therapy. *Lane, Medications, p. 102.*

129. **B.** In most states, when a patient requests a transfer of records, a physician is not legally bound to send a record in its entirety, whether original or photocopy. The physician is bound to send a written summary or photocopied excerpts. The doctrine of professional discretion allows the physician to protect the mentally or emotionally ill patient from viewing his record, unless the physician is ordered by the courts to do so. *Frew, Lane, Frew, pp. 38–39.*

130. **B.** SOAP is an acronym used in the problem-oriented medical records system. The initials stand for subjective data, objective data, assessment, and plan. *Frew, Lane, Frew, p. 85.*

131. **B.** Unless a case is closed or transferred to another physician, or the patient has not been in contact with the office for a number of years, the doctor-patient relationship is considered ongoing and the record remains in the inactive files. Inactive records should be transferred every 6 months to 1 year, depending on the size of the file space. *Lane, Keenon, Coleman (eds.), p. 24.*

132. **B.** In terminal-digit numeric filing, the active patients would be more evenly distributed with the inactive patients, and would require the most expansive area for active files retrieval. *Lane, Keenon, Coleman (eds.), p. 21.*

133. **C.** Problem-oriented medical records are organized and kept according to the patient's health problems and their resolutions. This is as opposed to arranging the record by date or incident and dividing the record into subsections. *Frew, Lane, Frew, p. 85.*

134. **E.** The numeric filing system is not designed to accommodate miscellaneous papers that do not warrant an individual folder or number. The other systems could be labeled as follows: alpha, "Misc." at the back or front of the filing system; subjective and descriptive "Miscellaneous"; and chronologic, "1989 Misc." *Frew, Lane, Frew, p. 106.*

135. **C.** Medical reports and progress notes are added chronologically with the newest notes on top. *Frew, Lane, Frew, p. 84; Lane, Keenon, Coleman (eds.), p. 26.*

136. **E.** Titles are considered in indexing if they indicate seniority. *Frew, Lane, Frew, p. 109.*

137. **C.** Gravida III = 3 pregnancies
UCD = usual childhood diseases
FH:HBP = family history of hypertension
PH:RHD = past history of rheumatic heart disease
PI:UTI = present illness includes urinary tract infection *Lane, Keenon, Coleman (eds.), pp. 696–698.*

138. **E.** A file of daily activities, kept on cards by month and day, is called a tickler file. *Frew, Lane, Frew, p. 113.*

139. **E.** The singular abbreviation for Esquire is Esq. If a courtesy title is used before the addressee's name, Esq. is omitted. *Fordney and Diehl, p. 15.*

140. **A.** Language should be concise and accurate. A sentence should not contain unnecessary words. Keep related words together. (Surely, Ms. Smith's biopsy was not enclosed!) *Strunk and White, pp. 23, 28.*

141. **B.** Close with the suggestion of action, but do not assume one's request will be honored. Wait until the service is rendered; then, make an appropriate acknowledgment of it or discuss further planning. "Irregardless" should be "regardless"; "anticipate" is an ambiguous word, and "contact" as a transitive verb is vague—use "phone you" or "get in touch with you." *Strunk and White, pp. 38–59.*

142. **A.** The proper order after the signature block is: identification initials, enclosure notations, carbon copy notations, and then the postscript, if used. *Lane, Keenon, Coleman (eds.), p. 39.*

143. **E.** The sentences in A, B, and C do not clarify whether it is the growth or the arm that is to the left of midline. In D, the interposed clause interrupts the flow of the main clause. *Strunk and White, pp. 28–31.*

144. **A.** Begin the letter using the active voice. Keep the composition direct and precise. *Strunk and White, p. 18.*

145. **C.** Further refers to time or quantity; farther, to distance. Between is used when referring to two people; among is used when more than two people are involved. Loan is a noun; the verb is lend. The future tense requires "shall" for the first person, "will" for the second and third persons. Affect means "influence"; as a noun, effect means "result." *Strunk and White, pp. 40, 45, 46, 58.*

146. **C.** A right margin tab of 86 would create a right margin slightly greater than one inch. *Frew, Lane, Frew, p. 127.*

147. **C.** Justification, or to justify, is an editing term for evenly spacing the words on each line to line up exactly with the left and right margins. *Walter, p. 129.*

148. **A.** With the left margin set at 10 and a right margin set at 68, 58 characters of text will fit on each line. *Frew, Lane, Frew, p. 127.*

149. **A.** Omit the "that" and you have "He felt his big nose . . ." The ear must decide when to retain the "that," when to omit it. Often "that" is omitted to make the thought simple and clear. *Strunk and White, p. 59.*

150. **A.** Either "Dr. Harry M. Stone" or "Harry M. Stone, Ph.D." is correct. Never use more than one of the following on one line with a surname: courtesy title, academic or medical degree, professional title. *Fordney and Diehl, p. 7.*

151. **D.** Alternative is correct when connoting a matter of choice; alternate means every other one in a series. Nauseous means "sickening to contemplate." Nauseated means the "unpleasant sensation preceding vomiting." Chaired is a noun incorrectly used as a verb. At the end of a list introduced by such as "etc." is incorrect. One thing differs "from" another. ***Strunk and White, pp. 40, 45–46, 54.***

152. **C.** For the short pica letter, bottom margins can be set at about 2″ (12 lines). ***Fordney and Diehl, p. 199.***

153. **B.** Reciprocity beneficiary claims are billed to the local Blue Shield; those claims that are not under reciprocity benefits are billed to the Blue Shield home office of the patient. When filing a claim outside the area, an HCFA 1500 form should be used. ***Lane, Keenon, Coleman (eds.), p. 161; Frew, Lane, Frew, pp. 301–302.***

154. **E.** The Explanation of Benefits will not list diagnosis codes. ***Lane, Keenon, Coleman (eds.), p. 182; Frew, Lane, Frew, pp. 312–313.***

155. **C.** Although the initial cost of open shelving may seem high, over time open shelving takes up 50% less space and costs less both in labor and in equipment. ***Lane, Keenon, Coleman (eds.), p. 123.***

156. **E.** The pronominal possessives have no apostrophe. Indefinite pronouns, however, use the apostrophe to show possession. ***Strunk and White, p. 1.***

157. **E.** In most medical correspondence and journals, MD takes precedence over other degrees and titles. Degrees and titles are usually listed in the order they are earned. Jr. and Sr. abbreviations may or may not be preceded by a comma. Second and third generation designations may be styled either as Roman numerals or as ordinals. ***Fordney and Diehl, pp. 15, 465.***

158. **B.** Absence is the correct spelling. ***Fordney and Diehl, p. 428.***

159. **A.** The punctuation pattern of this letter is called open punctuation, where the salutation and complimentary close are left unpunctuated. ***Frew, Lane, Frew, p. 125.***

160. **C.** All lines begin flush left; therefore, the style is block. ***Frew, Lane, Frew, p. 125.***

161. **C.** When "Doctor" appears in the salutation, it must be used with the addressee's surname. Doctor may be spelled out or abbreviated. Dean, or other professional titles, may be used rather than a courtesy title. Although rarely used, "My dear" is a very formal style of salutation. ***Fordney and Diehl, pp. 205–206.***

162. **C.** The code letter "B" at the end of the ID number means the patient is a spouse. ***Lane, Keenon, Coleman (eds.), p. 162.***

163. **E.** The patient is entitled to only hospital insurance. The card would contain the words "Medical Insurance" if the patient were entitled to medical insurance. ***Lane, Keenon, Coleman (eds.), p. 163.***

164. **B.** The initials "WA" before the ID indicates a retired railroad worker. ***Lane, Keenon, Coleman (eds.), pp. 163–164.***

165. **E.** Retired railroad workers claims are administered by Travelers Insurance Company. ***Lane, Keenon, Coleman (eds.), pp. 163–164.***

166. **A.** The patient has had coverage since 1982. ***Lane, Keenon, Coleman (eds.), pp. 163–164.***

167. **D.** Special study and test preparations are not typical for a first complete examination. It is always advisable to have the patients bring medications they are currently taking. ***Frew, Lane, Frew, p. 402.***

168. **D.** Drive A is the first drive; drive B, the second, and both refer to the system's hardware. Both source and target disks may be used in either drive. A backup is a second copy of an original program or file; it is created in case the original is damaged or destroyed. Either drive may run master or blank disks. ***Walter, pp. 22, 82–83; Gylys, p. 11.***

169. **E.** The tab key cannot move the cursor to a new line in WordPerfect. Only "Enter" can move the cursor to a new line. ***Walter, p. 121.***

170. **E.** If you turn off your computer without returning to a program main menu or without using a quit command, you may lose some or all of your data files, and you may even harm the hard disk system. *Gylys, p. 7.*

171. **E.** Pressing the Home key two times in succession, then the arrow down key will move the cursor to the end of a long document. *Walter, p. 122.*

172. **E.** A physician may represent himself or be represented by the medical assistant or other office employee. Parties to small claims may not be represented by an attorney or collection agencies. *Lane, Keenon, Coleman (eds.), pp. 119–122.*

173. **D.** A predated check is not a risk, unless of course, the check is predated more than 6 months. Checks that are written for more than the amount due will result in a cash or check refund, perhaps before you know whether or not the funds will clear the bank. Postdated checks are not negotiable. If you accept a third-party check, you will be accepting a check from someone unknown to you. *Lane, Keenon, Coleman (eds.), p. 101.*

174. **C.** Supplier invoices, the check register, checks, and a chart of accounts are necessary for accounts payable. Supplier statements may be used, but it is better to pay from invoice to avoid double payments. Aging analysis is a process of accounts receivable. *Lane, Keenon, Coleman (eds.), p. 93.*

175. **E.** An NSF entry is subtracted in the payment column and enclosed in brackets or with a circle drawn around it. *Lane, Keenon, Coleman (eds.), p. 91.*

176. **E.** Hand entries must be made for courtesy reductions and for write-offs. Prepayments will be later offset by transactions (refund and charge). *Lane, Keenon, Coleman (eds.), pp. 87–89.*

177. **B.** Approvals from a primary care provider may be needed before a specialist is seen, either within or outside the HMO plan. *Lane, Keenon, Coleman (eds.), p. 186.*

178. **A.** The spouse and child(ren) of a disabled or deceased veteran are eligible for benefits under CHAMPVA (Civilian Health and Medical Program of the Veterans Administration). *Frew, Lane, Frew, p. 294.*

179. **B.** State and federal disability insurance, unemployment, and workers' compensation are paid by the employer. FICA payments are divided equally by the employer and employee. Private disability insurance and health insurance deductions are at the election of the employee. *Lane, Keenon, Coleman (eds.), p. 239.*

180. **D.** Direct payment is made only to participating physicians. *Frew, Lane, Frew, p. 296.*

181. **B.** Diagnosis Related Groups (DRG's) use a three-digit numbering system from 1 to 471. *Lane, Keenon, Coleman (eds.), pp. 800–808.*

182. **E.** In addition to inpatient and outpatient medical treatment, workers' compensation may cover a weekly or monthly wage loss benefit for disability, burial allowance and cash benefits for dependents of those fatally injured, and rehabilitation/health education benefits. Life insurance benefits are not included. *Frew, Lane, Frew, p. 297.*

183. **B.** All patients' records, including the records of minors should be kept permanently or made available to another doctor of the patient's own choosing. Income tax records should be kept indefinitely. Even if an old professional liability policy is superseded by a new one, the old policy must be kept, in case there is a future claim of injury that took place while the old policy was in effect. *Frew, Lane, Frew, p. 102.*

184. **E.** On executive stationery, it is recommended that the date line appear three to five lines below the letterhead; the inside address may be three to eight lines below the date line, depending on the letter length; the salutation may be two to four lines below the inside address, depending on the letter length; and the first paragraph always begins two lines below the salutation. *Fordney and Diehl, p. 190.*

185. **B.** Notations of telephone calls should be made a part of the patient's medical record if the call is in reference to a change in condition during treatment, referral to another physician, a request for a prescription, and a new or refill order for a prescription. A change in appointment is recorded in the appointment book only, both by a line drawn through the original appointment, then the entry of the new date and time. Do not erase canceled appointments from the appointment book. *Frew, Lane, Frew, p. 171.*

186. **A.** OCR scanning directions include capital letters throughout; eliminating punctuation; using less than 22 spaces on the last line by abbreviating certain cities with longer than 13 spaces and using one space between city name and state code, two spaces for the state code, and one space between the state code and the zip code. A single delivery address line includes room, apartment, and suite numbers. *Lane, Keenon, Coleman (eds.), p. 39.*

187. **E.** Subjective information is supplied by the patient, and it includes chief complaint, details of present illness, symptoms and past history. Objective information is provided by the physician or in medical reports. *Frew, Lane, Frew, p. 322.*

188. **A.** A physician may withdraw from a case if a patient fails to follow instructions. To formally withdraw, a written notification—in the form of a letter—should be prepared for physician signature. It should include the reason for the dismissal and indicate a future date at which the physician is no longer responsible. The AMA, in *Medicolegal Forms with Legal Analysis,* also urges the physician to state in the letter that the patient still does require medical attention and urge the patient to see another physician. The letter should also state that the patient's records will be made available to a new physician once the patient signs the proper release form. *Lane, Keenon, Coleman (eds.), p. 281.*

189. **B.** Liabilities are the debts of the business and include real estate lease commitments and debts due in the form of vendor payments, payroll, and taxes. Patient accounts and equipment owned, whether it be used or new, are considered assets of a business. *Lane, Keenon, Coleman (eds.), p. 141.*

190. **D.** An age analysis breaks down the accounts receivable by which accounts are current and the length of time other accounts are overdue. This is used for billing and collections control. A cash flow statement is a breakdown of cash on hand and of cash expected within a period, less the expenses expected during that same period. A trial balance is necessary to determine that the books are accurate and in balance. An income and expense statement is the same as a profit and loss statement prepared after a designated period of business. *Frew, Lane, Frew, p. 256; Lane, Keenon, Coleman (eds.), pp. 121–122, 128.*

191. **A.** On one-write payroll systems, write-it-once features include entries for gross and net earnings, deductions, withheld taxes, and the payee's name. The payee's address is not included. *Lane, Keenon, Coleman (eds.), p. 132.*

192. **D.** Incoming calls that need immediate attention of the physician include young children with high fevers, possible or confirmed medication allergies, and other medical professionals who call the physician with updates on the conditions of patients. A patient who has had a low-grade fever, off and on, for more than a week should be given an appointment as soon as possible and the message of the call and the appointment should be placed on the physician's desk for approval. *Frew, Lane, Frew, pp. 165–168.*

193. **E.** In general, employee records should be kept active for three income tax return periods, then stored indefinitely in dead storage or destroyed. Copies of an employee's W-2 income transmittal forms should be saved for 7 years after an employee is discharged or voluntarily leaves the practice. *Lane, Keenon, Coleman (eds.), p. 257.*

194. **C.** Ames Co., Inc. manufactures urinalysis materials and equipment. *Lane, Keenon, Coleman (eds.), pp. 682–685.*

195. **A.** Safeguard Business Systems manufactures one type of pegboard system. *Lane, Keenon, Coleman (eds.), pp. 81–83.*

196. **E.** The Resource-Based Relative Value Scale is calculated based on three factors: relative value units, geographical cost indices, and a National Conversion factor. *Lane, Keenon, Coleman (eds.), p. 181.*

197. **E.** For Schedule IV and Schedule V drugs, a DEA prescription form (with the physician's DEA number) does not have to be used. The order may be issued orally by telephone to the pharmacist. *Lane, Medications, p. 41.*

198. **A.** Insurance carriers are considered third-party payers. A husband is legally responsible for debts incurred by his wife, and parents are legally responsible for services rendered to their minor children. *Frew, Lane, Frew, pp. 32, 248, 262.*

199. **D.** Before a barium enema, the patient may drink only clear liquids after the evening meal the day before. A special diet may be required prior to an occult blood test, and a light breakfast is allowed on the day of a sigmoidoscopy. No special diet is required before a pinworm test or a stool culture and sensitivity. *Frew, Lane, Frew, pp. 857–858.*

200. **E.** It is especially important that a patient void before any examination of the lower torso, unless the examination does not involve the palpation or examination of any of the organs involved. *Frew, Lane, Frew, p. 409; Lane, Keenon, Coleman (eds.), p. 323.*

201. **E.** The universal blood and body-fluid precaution system is designed to reduce the risk of cross-infection of any infective agent in any body substance in any patient. The CDC recommends this system be used solely and rather than any of the other, older systems of isolation. *Frew, Lane, Frew, pp. 344–345, 716–717, 898–900; Lane, Keenon, Coleman (eds.), pp. 770–777, 786–788, 815–820.*

202. **C.** Wash the thermometer in cool running water, then swab it with alcohol or soak it in a soap solution. Warm and hot water will damage the mercury column. A thermometer should not be soaked, sanitized, disinfected, or otherwise handled, without first rinsing off gross debris under the faucet. *Frew, Lane, Frew, p. 367.*

203. **B.** Many authorities believe that most infections in the medical facility are spread by the hands of health workers. Careful hand washing techniques are required for the decrease in the spread of infection. *Frew, Lane, Frew, pp. 343, 613.*

204. **B.** Lyme disease (Borrelia) is a spirochete transmitted by the tick (arthropod vector). *Lane, Keenon, Coleman (eds.), p. 436.*

205. **A.** Monilia are yeastlike (fungus) organisms treated with antifungal medications (miconazole or clotrimazole). *Lane, Keenon, Coleman (eds.), p. 446; Lane, Medications, p. 286.*

206. **B.** The audiometer is used to test hearing acuity. *Frew, Lane, Frew, p. 424.*

207. **D.** A 5–9 mm induration positive test means that the patient has not only been exposed to tuberculosis, but has also been infected with the tubercle bacilli. This does not mean that the patient has had or has active tuberculosis. *Repeat testing is indicated. Lane, Keenon, Coleman (eds.), p. 367.*

208. **B.** Blood pressure determination should always be done with the arm resting at cardiac level. *Frew, Lane, Frew, p. 318; Lane, Keenon, Coleman (eds.), p. 378.*

209. **B.** Early symptoms of gonorrhea include painful urination then later, urethral discharge. *Frew, Lane, Frew, p. 485; Lane, Keenon, Coleman (eds.), p. 628.*

210. **C.** The thermometer should be shaken so that the mercury column registers below 96°F (34C). *Frew, Lane, Frew, p. 367.*

211. **B.** The difference between the apical and radial pulse rate is called the pulse deficit. *Lane, Keenon, Coleman (eds.), pp. 312–313.*

212. **B.** Cerumen is the term for ear wax. An ear lavage setup includes a Reiner syringe, emesis basin, and otoscope. *Frew, Lane, Frew, pp. 449–551.*

213. **D.** Tetracaine, or other ophthalmic topical anesthesia, is required before placing a tonometer on the eyeball to measure ocular pressure. *Lane, Medications, pp. 244–245.*

214. **C.** A poorly secured stethoscope diaphragm will cause a distortion of low-frequency Korotkoff sounds. *Frew, Lane, Frew, pp. 357, 378.*

215. **C.** Monilia is a yeast infection. Before treatment, obtain potassium hydroxide (KOH) smears and/or cultures to confirm the diagnosis. *Lane, Keenon, Coleman (eds.), pp. 446–447; Lane, Medications, p. 286.*

216. **D.** The first sharp tapping sound you hear is the systolic pressure. *Frew, Lane, Frew, p. 359.*

217. **B.** Rheumatic fever is often preceded by a streptococcal sore throat. *Lane, Keenon, Coleman (eds.), p. 435.*

218. **C.** A drain is placed in a wound to keep the edges apart and allow a systematic drainage of fluids and discharges from a wound. All the other selections are not valid reasons for the use of a drain. *Frew, Lane, Frew, p. 640.*

219. **B.** The knee-chest position is one position used to examine the rectum. *Frew, Lane, Frew, p. 389; Lane, Keenon, Coleman (eds.), p. 322.*

220. **D.** The patient should not drink a hot beverage for at least 15 minutes prior to having his body temperature measured orally. *Frew, Lane, Frew, p. 364; Lane, Keenon, Coleman (eds.), p. 315.*

221. **B.** Blood pressure is usually lowest during sleep and is lowest upon arising from sleep. *Frew, Lane, Frew, p. 356.*

222. **D.** In order to check ovulation, one of the first procedures performed by the patient is keeping a basal temperature chart. Other early procedures include pelvic examination, culdoscopy, endometrial biopsy, and laparoscopy. *Lane, Keenon, Coleman (eds.), pp. 473–474.*

223. **D.** The patient should be positioned on her back with a pillow under her right shoulder and her right hand under her head. *Lane, Keenon, Coleman (eds.), p. 455.*

224. **B.** A thermometer should be inserted about 1.5 inches. Less will not render an accurate reading; more may damage the rectal mucosa. *Frew, Lane, Frew, p. 367.*

225. **A.** Each tiny square is 1 mm high and 1 mm wide. *Lane, Keenon, Coleman (eds.), p. 841.*

226. **C.** The sensitivity control regulates the output of the amplifier. Normal position is 1; the height of small complexes can be doubled by switching to 2. *Frew, Lane, Frew, p. 841.*

227. **C.** The human body acts as a transmitter, sending out electrical signals of the heart. These signals appear on the skin. The sensors serve as receiving antennas, detecting the voltage on the skin. *Frew, Lane, Frew, p. 842.*

228. **A.** While pastes and gels are adequate for accurate recordings, they can be messy for your instruments. Electrolyte pads maximize the "pickup" of electrical activity, and it may be used on any area of the body. It does not stain clothing or irritate the patient's skin or leave residue on electrodes. *Frew, Lane, Frew, p. 844.*

229. **C.** The right leg is called the "ground" or "reference electrode." *Frew, Lane, Frew, p. 842.*

230. **C.** The QRS complex represents ventricular depolarization or contraction. *Lane, Keenon, Coleman (eds.), p. 501.*

231. **D.** The P-R interval is the time interval between atrial depolarization and ventricular depolarization, when contraction traverses the A-V node. *Lane, Keenon, Coleman (eds.), p. 501.*

232. **D.** The early symptoms of headache, dizziness, weakness, and cramping of the muscles may occur in both heat stroke and heat exhaustion. In heat exhaustion the person turns pale and perspires profusely and the skin is cool and moist. In heat stroke, the body temperature becomes dangerously elevated and there is an absence of sweating. *Frew, Lane, Frew, p. 682.*

233. **E.** The Trendelenburg position should not be used with head injury patients. The Trendelenburg position increases blood flow to the head, which may already be edematous owing to injury. *Taber's, 2033; Frew, Lane, Frew, p. 672; Lane, Keenon, Coleman (eds.), p. 675.*

234. **A.** When the chest does not rise and fall with rescue breaths, it is most likely that there is an airway obstruction. *Lane, Keenon, Coleman (eds.), p. 667.*

235. **E.** Newer first aid guidelines specify that a rescuer first survey the scene (for things such as electrical wires or other dangers), next assess the victim for consciousness and breathing, then call for help. Then perform the ABC's: clear the airway, give rescue breaths, and if no pulse, begin cardiac compressions. *Frew, Lane, Frew, p. 671; Lane, Keenon, Coleman (eds.), p. 664.*

236. **B.** CPR guidelines require the rescuer to use 1.5- to 2.0-inch compressions. *Frew, Lane, Frew, p. 700; Lane, Keenon, Coleman (eds.), p. 666.*

237. **B.** The reagent turns pink when the urine is positive for nitrites. *Frew, Lane, Frew, p. 760; Lane, Keenon, Coleman (eds.), p. 569.*

238. **A.** Diabetic urine has a fruity odor because of the presence of ketones. *Wedding and Toenjes, p. 81.*

239. **A.** Mammography is useful in detecting tumors before symptoms appear. It is now recommended annually for women over 40. *Frew, Lane, Frew, p. 486.*

240. **B.** Chek-stix is a commercially prepared kit used to test and control the quality of macroscopic urine testing. *Frew, Lane, Frew, p. 764.*

241. **C.** The most commonly encountered parasite is the *Trichomonas vaginalis* organism, a flagellate which is found in the urine of men and as a vaginal contaminate in the urine of women. *Wedding and Toenjes, p. 117.*

242. **E.** 7.0 is neutral pH. Anything less than 7.0 is considered acid. Anything above 7.0 is considered alkaline (base). *Wedding and Toenjes, p. 98.*

243. **C.** Ipecac syrup is an emetic used to induce vomiting in case of acute poisoning. *Frew, Lane, Frew, p. 682.*

244. **B.** Only Ecotrin contains acetylsalicylic acid. Some others are Aspergum, Aspirin, A.S.A., and Decaprin. *Lane, Medications, p. 242.*

245. **C.** Subcutaneous injections should be angled 60–90 degrees in the obese patient. *Lane, Medications, p. 201.*

246. **A.** Lidocaine HC1 (Xylocaine) is particularly useful for peripheral nerveblock in amounts of 1 or more mm. *Lane, Medications, p. 252.*

247. **C.** 1 oz = 30 or 32 mL. *Lane, Medications, p. 12.*

248. **A.** Nitrites and nitrates (nitroglycerin) are peripheral vasodilators bringing relief to the pain of angina almost immediately. *Lane, Medications, pp. 247, 248.*

249. **E.** The directions to the patient are: take two, three times a day, one hour before meals. Refill when needed. *Lane, Medications, p. 40.*

250. **B.** Xylocaine (lidocaine HCl) is one anesthetic that is available in infiltration form. Ethylene and diethyl ether are general anesthetics. Benzocaine and ethyl chloride are topical anesthetics. *Lane, Medications, p. 252.*

251. **D.** Lomotil is diphenoxylate HCl with atropine. The drug remains by prescription to prevent is overuse, which might lead to dependence. *Lane, Keenon, Coleman (eds.), p. 338.*

252. **D.** The household equivalent of one dram is one teaspoon. Quater in die is translated four times in a day (four times a day). *Lane, Medications, p. 3, 12.*

253. **B.** Amoxil and Augmentin are examples of antimicrobials derived from penicillins. *Lane, Medications, pp. 272, 275–276.*

254. **D.** Milligram is the measurement of the drug's strength; milliliter is the unit of measurement for the amount to give. *Lane, Medications, pp 6–7.*

255. C. Aluminum hydroxide gels and magnesium salts reduce the ability of the intestine to absorb tetracyclines. Antacids are used for the treatment of gastric hyperacidity and ulcers. Aluminum-based antacids, in combination with a low phosphorus diet, help to prevent phosphate urinary stones by reducing urinary phosphate levels. *Lane, Medications, p. 191.*

256. A. Special care must be exercised to prevent injuries caused by contaminated needles. Not breaking down the syringe unit and not recapping minimizes handling and reduces risk. Special rigid containers are designed so that solid waste contents can be autoclaved before disposal. *Lane, Medications, pp. 98–99.*

257. A. Digitalis is a cardiotonic that stimulates the heart muscle to contract more forcefully and thus pump more blood to the body. *Lane, Medications, pp. 282–283.*

258. B. Theo-Dur (theophylline) is a bronchodilator that relaxes the smooth muscles of the bronchi and of the pulmonary blood vessels. *Lane, Medications, pp. 292–293.*

259. E. It is usually least important for the medical assistant to know the name of the manufacturer of the drug, unless one specific manufacturer's product is ordered by the physician. All the other selections are very important for the medical assistant to know before administering a medication to a patient. *Lane, Medications, p. 99.*

260. A. A tincture is an alcoholic preparation. Tincture of Zephiran (1:750) is 1 oz. Zephiran, 64 oz of alcohol, and distilled water q.s. ad 1 Gal. *Lane, Medications, p. 64.*

261. C. Ethyl chloride is a topical spray anesthetic used in some types of superficial skin surgery. *Frew, Lane, Frew, p. 630.*

262. E. Cleansing a site for injection begins directly over the point of entry and continues in widening concentric circles outward. *Lane, Medications, p. 208.*

263. E. Carbohydrates are high in candy and should be avoided. The other snacks are not necessarily contraindicated. *Frew, Lane, Frew, pp. 536–538.*

264. D. Cathartics should never be administered in suspected intestinal or abdominal rupture or hemorrhage. *Lane, Medications, p. 43.*

265. E. Antitussives are more effective in the treatment of nonproductive (dry) coughs. *Lane, Medications, p. 85.*

266. E. Although passive immunity may be administered in cases of rubella exposure, the serum used is the homologous immune serum globulin, a product obtained from the pooled plasma of human donors that contains antibodies against a variety of diseases including measles, rubella, poliomyelitis, and hepatitis B. There is yet no specific immune globulin for rubella as there are for the other selections. *Lane, Medications, p. 239.*

267. D. Although Robitussin A-C (schedule V) is subject to federal narcotic regulations, it is not classified under schedule III. *Lane, Keenon, Coleman (eds.), p. 338.*

268. A. Hydrogen peroxide prevents growth of surface organisms and does not reduce the reaction of the skin to irritation. *Lane, Medications, p. 84.*

269. A. Narcotic analgesics are contraindicated in head injuries because of their capacity to elevate intracranial pressure. They are contraindicated in shock because patients with reduced blood volume are susceptible to the hypotensive effects of narcotic analgesics. *Lane, Medications, pp. 239–242.*

270. B. An open fracture is a compound fracture. *Frew, Lane, Frew, p. 435; Lane, Keenon, Coleman (eds.), p. 674.*

271. C. The broken arm is the priority. Immobilize the arm where the patient is on the floor in order to prevent further injury to the bone or the surrounding tissues. *Lane, Keenon, Coleman (eds.), p. 664.*

272. B. Cold decreases circulation to a part. If the knee is already swollen, cold would not be applied. *Frew, Lane, Frew, pp. 454–455; Lane, Keenon, Coleman (eds.), pp. 400–401.*

273. E. A leg bandage is started at the arch of the foot. *Frew, Lane, Frew, p. 633; Lane, Keenon, Coleman (eds.), p. 395.*

274. **A.** For comfort and natural anatomic position, the knee should be slightly flexed. *Lane, Keenon, Coleman (eds.), p. 395.*

275. **C.** If the extremities become swollen, it is likely the bandage is too tight and interfering with circulation. *Lane, Keenon, Coleman (eds.), p. 396.*

276. **D.** Low-volume (hypovolemic) shock commonly occurs from blood loss due to fractures of large bones with hemorrhage into surrounding tissues. Neurogenic shock may be brought on by severe pain and fright. Most likely this patient is progressing into shock, which is marked by anxiety, hypotension, rapid breathing, and an increased pulse. *Frew, Lane, Frew, p. 676; Lane, Keenon, Coleman (eds.), p. 675.*

277. **B.** While first aid measures include reassuring the patient, keeping the patient quiet, warm, and comfortable, and perhaps administering a few small sips of water, it is most important to reduce and slow the process of shock of placing the patient in supine position. The patient should never to moved to another place until the paramedics arrive. *Lane, Keenon, Coleman (eds.), p. 674.*

278. **C.** Forceps should be removed from its container without touching the sides, without touching any item other than the instrument or material it is intended to grasp, with the grasping end downward to prevent disinfectant from flowing first to the contaminated ring-handle area then back down to the clean area, and with prongs together. Transfer forceps are never to be placed on a sterile field. *Frew, Lane, Frew, p. 620; Lane, Keenon, Coleman (eds.), pp. 378–379.*

279. **E.** Chemicals that destroy all living microorganisms are classified as sterilants. The glutaraldehydes are the only available EPA registered sterilants. *Frew, Lane, Frew, pp. 599–600.*

280. **D.** Neutral glutaraldehydes are effective in the presence of organic matter. They are not harmful to carbon steel, other plated materials, rubber, plastic, or rigid and flexible endoscopes. Neutral glutaraldehydes are effective sterilants against all microbial activity. The shelf life after activation is 14 to 28 days, depending on the brand and type used. *Frew, Lane, Frew, p. 600.*

281. **E.** Organisms are present in the blood in patients with AIDS and in those with hepatitis; therefore, handling blood specimens requires extreme care. *Wedding and Toenjes, p. 17.*

282. **E.** Diabetic insulin shock is a condition in which the patient has taken too much insulin, eaten too little, or exercised too much. The skin is pale and the patient feels dizzy and progresses to fainting. Vital signs are usually normal at this stage. *Lane, Keenon, Coleman (eds.), p. 672.*

283. **D.** The ophthalmoscope will be all that is needed to examine the retina. *Frew, Lane, Frew, p. 422; Lane, Keenon, Coleman (eds.), p. 327.*

284. **B.** Infection of the vagina is usually caused by three different kinds of organisms: trichomonas, a protozoan; *Candida*, a yeast; and *Gardnerella*, a bacterium. *Frew, Lane, Frew, pp. 722, 774–775.*

285. **E.** Pain, as a singular effect on vital signs, will most likely increase the pulse and respiration rates and decrease blood pressure with no effect on body temperature. *Frew, Lane, Frew, pp. 351, 356.*

286. **B.** Abnormally colored urine can result from pathologic conditions, bleeding, the presence of bilirubin, certain foods (such as beets), and many commonly used drugs (such as cathartics containing senna or cascara). *Lane, Keenon, Coleman (eds.), p. 565.*

287. **E.** Ketones are the end product of fat metabolism and are produced when carbohydrate intake or metabolism is deficient. *Wedding and Toenjes, p. 97.*

288. **C.** Cloudiness may be caused by cells, bacteria, contaminants, and certain foods with large amounts of fats and allowing urine to sit either at room temperature or refrigerated. *Wedding and Toenjes, p. 66; Lane, Keenon, Coleman (eds.), p. 565; Frew, Lane, Frew, p. 756.*

289. **C.** Urine allowed to cool will become cloudy as it becomes more alkaline and develops a sediment. Cooling does not cause urine to become less odorous. *Wedding and Toenjes, p. 66; Lane, Keenon, Coleman (eds.), p. 555.*

290. **E.** Infected urine has an unpleasant odor, and it may smell like ammonia from the breakdown of urea or putrid from the breakdown of bacteria and pus. ***Wedding and Toenjes, p. 81.***

291. **C.** Specific gravity can be measured using the urinometer float and cylinder, the Multistix 9 or 10 SG, or the refractometer. ***Wedding and Toenjes, pp. 82–85.***

292. **A.** Nonabsorbable sutures are used for superficial wounds where the sutures will be removed after healing has taken place. Although silk may be chosen, nylon is nonirritating to the tissue and is used mostly for skin suture. Atraumatic needles are used because they cause the least amount of tissue trauma. The 3–0 suture thread size would be too large a diameter for facial sutures. ***Frew, Lane, Frew, p. 609.***

293. **D.** Recombinant vaccines are derived from genetic recombinations of organisms. Recombinant hepatitis B vaccines are manufactured using yeast cells rather than human serum. Whenever a culture media or animal source immunization is ordered, the patient must be evaluated first for allergies related to the vaccine source. If a known allergy exists and the patient requires the vaccine, divided doses may be used, or a series of desensitizing injections may be given first. Emergency equipment should be readily available to manage any acute reaction. ***Lane, Medications, pp. 260–261.***

294. **C.** Drugs such as nitroglycerin, estrogen, motion sickness products, and nicotine are available as slow-release transdermal patches. ***Lane, Medications, pp. 65, 195.***

295. **A.** Datril, St. Joseph Fever Reducer, and Tylenol are all brand names for the para-aminophenol derivative acetaminophen. Advil is the nonsteroidal anti-inflammatory agent ibuprofen. ***Lane, Medications, pp. 242–244.***

296. **D.** Vitamin K is used to prevent postsurgical and postpartum hemorrhage from deficient prothrombin. Vitamin D is used to help prevent or treat osteomalacia; vitamin B2 (riboflavin) deficiency may result in sebaceous dermatosis; and vitamin B12 (cyanocobalamin) is used to treat pernicious anemia. ***Lane, Keenon, Coleman (eds.), p. 754.***

297. **A.** The plunger, barrel, and needle cap are the only parts that should be touched. The vial's rubber stopper should be cleaned with an antiseptic, then not touched. ***Lane, Medications, p. 217.***

298. **D.** Tetracycline may cause bone lesions and staining or deformity of teeth. It is to be avoided during tooth development stages, last trimester of pregnancy, neonatal period, and early childhood up to the age of 8. ***Taber's, p. 1972.***

299. **E.** Epinephrine is a vasopressor that increases blood pressure and increases heart rate and cardiac output; it is also an antispasmotic and is used to relive bronchial spasm. ***Lane, Medications, pp. 256–257.***

300. **D.** A heart murmur or any other condition classified as functional is one that occurs in the absence of structural changes. There is usually no treatment for this condition. ***Taber's, p. 767.***

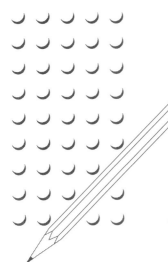

Sample Examination Simulation 4

- The following pages contain 300 test items.

- The examination is divided into:
    Part 1 - General Medical Knowledge
    Part 2 - Administrative Procedures
    Part 3 - Clinical Procedures.

- Answer sheets are provided for your use.

- The answer key immediately follows the test items and includes references with page numbers.

- References and suggested readings are at the end of the book.

Name _____ **Date** _____
　　　　　Last　　　　　　　First　　　　　　Middle

<table>
<tr><td colspan="2">

Directions for Marking Answers

- Use a black lead pencil (No. 2 or softer). Do NOT use pen or a pencil with hard lead.
- Make each mark heavy and black enough to completely obliterate the letter within the circle. Marks should fill the circles.
- Erase clearly any answer you wish to change.
- Make no stray marks on this answer sheet.
- Mark one and only one answer for each question. Multiple answers will be counted as wrong.

</td>
<td>

Example

WRONG   Ⓐ Ⓑ́ Ⓒ Ⓓ Ⓔ

WRONG   Ⓐ Ⓧ Ⓒ Ⓓ Ⓔ

WRONG   Ⓐ Ⓑ Ⓒ̊ Ⓓ Ⓔ

RIGHT   Ⓐ Ⓑ Ⓒ ● Ⓔ

</td></tr>
</table>

1 Ⓐ Ⓑ Ⓒ Ⓓ Ⓔ　　26 Ⓐ Ⓑ Ⓒ Ⓓ Ⓔ　　51 Ⓐ Ⓑ Ⓒ Ⓓ Ⓔ　　76 Ⓐ Ⓑ Ⓒ Ⓓ Ⓔ
2 Ⓐ Ⓑ Ⓒ Ⓓ Ⓔ　　27 Ⓐ Ⓑ Ⓒ Ⓓ Ⓔ　　52 Ⓐ Ⓑ Ⓒ Ⓓ Ⓔ　　77 Ⓐ Ⓑ Ⓒ Ⓓ Ⓔ
3 Ⓐ Ⓑ Ⓒ Ⓓ Ⓔ　　28 Ⓐ Ⓑ Ⓒ Ⓓ Ⓔ　　53 Ⓐ Ⓑ Ⓒ Ⓓ Ⓔ　　78 Ⓐ Ⓑ Ⓒ Ⓓ Ⓔ
4 Ⓐ Ⓑ Ⓒ Ⓓ Ⓔ　　29 Ⓐ Ⓑ Ⓒ Ⓓ Ⓔ　　54 Ⓐ Ⓑ Ⓒ Ⓓ Ⓔ　　79 Ⓐ Ⓑ Ⓒ Ⓓ Ⓔ
5 Ⓐ Ⓑ Ⓒ Ⓓ Ⓔ　　30 Ⓐ Ⓑ Ⓒ Ⓓ Ⓔ　　55 Ⓐ Ⓑ Ⓒ Ⓓ Ⓔ　　80 Ⓐ Ⓑ Ⓒ Ⓓ Ⓔ
6 Ⓐ Ⓑ Ⓒ Ⓓ Ⓔ　　31 Ⓐ Ⓑ Ⓒ Ⓓ Ⓔ　　56 Ⓐ Ⓑ Ⓒ Ⓓ Ⓔ　　81 Ⓐ Ⓑ Ⓒ Ⓓ Ⓔ
7 Ⓐ Ⓑ Ⓒ Ⓓ Ⓔ　　32 Ⓐ Ⓑ Ⓒ Ⓓ Ⓔ　　57 Ⓐ Ⓑ Ⓒ Ⓓ Ⓔ　　82 Ⓐ Ⓑ Ⓒ Ⓓ Ⓔ
8 Ⓐ Ⓑ Ⓒ Ⓓ Ⓔ　　33 Ⓐ Ⓑ Ⓒ Ⓓ Ⓔ　　58 Ⓐ Ⓑ Ⓒ Ⓓ Ⓔ　　83 Ⓐ Ⓑ Ⓒ Ⓓ Ⓔ
9 Ⓐ Ⓑ Ⓒ Ⓓ Ⓔ　　34 Ⓐ Ⓑ Ⓒ Ⓓ Ⓔ　　59 Ⓐ Ⓑ Ⓒ Ⓓ Ⓔ　　84 Ⓐ Ⓑ Ⓒ Ⓓ Ⓔ
10 Ⓐ Ⓑ Ⓒ Ⓓ Ⓔ　　35 Ⓐ Ⓑ Ⓒ Ⓓ Ⓔ　　60 Ⓐ Ⓑ Ⓒ Ⓓ Ⓔ　　85 Ⓐ Ⓑ Ⓒ Ⓓ Ⓔ
11 Ⓐ Ⓑ Ⓒ Ⓓ Ⓔ　　36 Ⓐ Ⓑ Ⓒ Ⓓ Ⓔ　　61 Ⓐ Ⓑ Ⓒ Ⓓ Ⓔ　　86 Ⓐ Ⓑ Ⓒ Ⓓ Ⓔ
12 Ⓐ Ⓑ Ⓒ Ⓓ Ⓔ　　37 Ⓐ Ⓑ Ⓒ Ⓓ Ⓔ　　62 Ⓐ Ⓑ Ⓒ Ⓓ Ⓔ　　87 Ⓐ Ⓑ Ⓒ Ⓓ Ⓔ
13 Ⓐ Ⓑ Ⓒ Ⓓ Ⓔ　　38 Ⓐ Ⓑ Ⓒ Ⓓ Ⓔ　　63 Ⓐ Ⓑ Ⓒ Ⓓ Ⓔ　　88 Ⓐ Ⓑ Ⓒ Ⓓ Ⓔ
14 Ⓐ Ⓑ Ⓒ Ⓓ Ⓔ　　39 Ⓐ Ⓑ Ⓒ Ⓓ Ⓔ　　64 Ⓐ Ⓑ Ⓒ Ⓓ Ⓔ　　89 Ⓐ Ⓑ Ⓒ Ⓓ Ⓔ
15 Ⓐ Ⓑ Ⓒ Ⓓ Ⓔ　　40 Ⓐ Ⓑ Ⓒ Ⓓ Ⓔ　　65 Ⓐ Ⓑ Ⓒ Ⓓ Ⓔ　　90 Ⓐ Ⓑ Ⓒ Ⓓ Ⓔ
16 Ⓐ Ⓑ Ⓒ Ⓓ Ⓔ　　41 Ⓐ Ⓑ Ⓒ Ⓓ Ⓔ　　66 Ⓐ Ⓑ Ⓒ Ⓓ Ⓔ　　91 Ⓐ Ⓑ Ⓒ Ⓓ Ⓔ
17 Ⓐ Ⓑ Ⓒ Ⓓ Ⓔ　　42 Ⓐ Ⓑ Ⓒ Ⓓ Ⓔ　　67 Ⓐ Ⓑ Ⓒ Ⓓ Ⓔ　　92 Ⓐ Ⓑ Ⓒ Ⓓ Ⓔ
18 Ⓐ Ⓑ Ⓒ Ⓓ Ⓔ　　43 Ⓐ Ⓑ Ⓒ Ⓓ Ⓔ　　68 Ⓐ Ⓑ Ⓒ Ⓓ Ⓔ　　93 Ⓐ Ⓑ Ⓒ Ⓓ Ⓔ
19 Ⓐ Ⓑ Ⓒ Ⓓ Ⓔ　　44 Ⓐ Ⓑ Ⓒ Ⓓ Ⓔ　　69 Ⓐ Ⓑ Ⓒ Ⓓ Ⓔ　　94 Ⓐ Ⓑ Ⓒ Ⓓ Ⓔ
20 Ⓐ Ⓑ Ⓒ Ⓓ Ⓔ　　45 Ⓐ Ⓑ Ⓒ Ⓓ Ⓔ　　70 Ⓐ Ⓑ Ⓒ Ⓓ Ⓔ　　95 Ⓐ Ⓑ Ⓒ Ⓓ Ⓔ
21 Ⓐ Ⓑ Ⓒ Ⓓ Ⓔ　　46 Ⓐ Ⓑ Ⓒ Ⓓ Ⓔ　　71 Ⓐ Ⓑ Ⓒ Ⓓ Ⓔ　　96 Ⓐ Ⓑ Ⓒ Ⓓ Ⓔ
22 Ⓐ Ⓑ Ⓒ Ⓓ Ⓔ　　47 Ⓐ Ⓑ Ⓒ Ⓓ Ⓔ　　72 Ⓐ Ⓑ Ⓒ Ⓓ Ⓔ　　97 Ⓐ Ⓑ Ⓒ Ⓓ Ⓔ
23 Ⓐ Ⓑ Ⓒ Ⓓ Ⓔ　　48 Ⓐ Ⓑ Ⓒ Ⓓ Ⓔ　　73 Ⓐ Ⓑ Ⓒ Ⓓ Ⓔ　　98 Ⓐ Ⓑ Ⓒ Ⓓ Ⓔ
24 Ⓐ Ⓑ Ⓒ Ⓓ Ⓔ　　49 Ⓐ Ⓑ Ⓒ Ⓓ Ⓔ　　74 Ⓐ Ⓑ Ⓒ Ⓓ Ⓔ　　99 Ⓐ Ⓑ Ⓒ Ⓓ Ⓔ
25 Ⓐ Ⓑ Ⓒ Ⓓ Ⓔ　　50 Ⓐ Ⓑ Ⓒ Ⓓ Ⓔ　　75 Ⓐ Ⓑ Ⓒ Ⓓ Ⓔ　　100 Ⓐ Ⓑ Ⓒ Ⓓ Ⓔ

Directions for Marking Answers

- Use a black lead pencil (No. 2 or softer). Do NOT use pen or a pencil with hard lead.
- Make each mark heavy and black enough to completely obliterate the letter within the circle. Marks should fill the circles.
- Erase clearly any answer you wish to change.
- Make no stray marks on this answer sheet.
- Mark one and only one answer for each question. Multiple answers will be counted as wrong.

Example

WRONG Ⓐ Ⓑ Ⓒ Ⓓ Ⓔ
WRONG Ⓐ Ⓑ Ⓒ Ⓓ Ⓔ
WRONG Ⓐ Ⓑ Ⓒ Ⓓ Ⓔ
RIGHT Ⓐ Ⓑ Ⓒ ● Ⓔ

101 Ⓐ Ⓑ Ⓒ Ⓓ Ⓔ	126 Ⓐ Ⓑ Ⓒ Ⓓ Ⓔ	151 Ⓐ Ⓑ Ⓒ Ⓓ Ⓔ	176 Ⓐ Ⓑ Ⓒ Ⓓ Ⓔ
102 Ⓐ Ⓑ Ⓒ Ⓓ Ⓔ	127 Ⓐ Ⓑ Ⓒ Ⓓ Ⓔ	152 Ⓐ Ⓑ Ⓒ Ⓓ Ⓔ	177 Ⓐ Ⓑ Ⓒ Ⓓ Ⓔ
103 Ⓐ Ⓑ Ⓒ Ⓓ Ⓔ	128 Ⓐ Ⓑ Ⓒ Ⓓ Ⓔ	153 Ⓐ Ⓑ Ⓒ Ⓓ Ⓔ	178 Ⓐ Ⓑ Ⓒ Ⓓ Ⓔ
104 Ⓐ Ⓑ Ⓒ Ⓓ Ⓔ	129 Ⓐ Ⓑ Ⓒ Ⓓ Ⓔ	154 Ⓐ Ⓑ Ⓒ Ⓓ Ⓔ	179 Ⓐ Ⓑ Ⓒ Ⓓ Ⓔ
105 Ⓐ Ⓑ Ⓒ Ⓓ Ⓔ	130 Ⓐ Ⓑ Ⓒ Ⓓ Ⓔ	155 Ⓐ Ⓑ Ⓒ Ⓓ Ⓔ	180 Ⓐ Ⓑ Ⓒ Ⓓ Ⓔ
106 Ⓐ Ⓑ Ⓒ Ⓓ Ⓔ	131 Ⓐ Ⓑ Ⓒ Ⓓ Ⓔ	156 Ⓐ Ⓑ Ⓒ Ⓓ Ⓔ	181 Ⓐ Ⓑ Ⓒ Ⓓ Ⓔ
107 Ⓐ Ⓑ Ⓒ Ⓓ Ⓔ	132 Ⓐ Ⓑ Ⓒ Ⓓ Ⓔ	157 Ⓐ Ⓑ Ⓒ Ⓓ Ⓔ	182 Ⓐ Ⓑ Ⓒ Ⓓ Ⓔ
108 Ⓐ Ⓑ Ⓒ Ⓓ Ⓔ	133 Ⓐ Ⓑ Ⓒ Ⓓ Ⓔ	158 Ⓐ Ⓑ Ⓒ Ⓓ Ⓔ	183 Ⓐ Ⓑ Ⓒ Ⓓ Ⓔ
109 Ⓐ Ⓑ Ⓒ Ⓓ Ⓔ	134 Ⓐ Ⓑ Ⓒ Ⓓ Ⓔ	159 Ⓐ Ⓑ Ⓒ Ⓓ Ⓔ	184 Ⓐ Ⓑ Ⓒ Ⓓ Ⓔ
110 Ⓐ Ⓑ Ⓒ Ⓓ Ⓔ	135 Ⓐ Ⓑ Ⓒ Ⓓ Ⓔ	160 Ⓐ Ⓑ Ⓒ Ⓓ Ⓔ	185 Ⓐ Ⓑ Ⓒ Ⓓ Ⓔ
111 Ⓐ Ⓑ Ⓒ Ⓓ Ⓔ	136 Ⓐ Ⓑ Ⓒ Ⓓ Ⓔ	161 Ⓐ Ⓑ Ⓒ Ⓓ Ⓔ	186 Ⓐ Ⓑ Ⓒ Ⓓ Ⓔ
112 Ⓐ Ⓑ Ⓒ Ⓓ Ⓔ	137 Ⓐ Ⓑ Ⓒ Ⓓ Ⓔ	162 Ⓐ Ⓑ Ⓒ Ⓓ Ⓔ	187 Ⓐ Ⓑ Ⓒ Ⓓ Ⓔ
113 Ⓐ Ⓑ Ⓒ Ⓓ Ⓔ	138 Ⓐ Ⓑ Ⓒ Ⓓ Ⓔ	163 Ⓐ Ⓑ Ⓒ Ⓓ Ⓔ	188 Ⓐ Ⓑ Ⓒ Ⓓ Ⓔ
114 Ⓐ Ⓑ Ⓒ Ⓓ Ⓔ	139 Ⓐ Ⓑ Ⓒ Ⓓ Ⓔ	164 Ⓐ Ⓑ Ⓒ Ⓓ Ⓔ	189 Ⓐ Ⓑ Ⓒ Ⓓ Ⓔ
115 Ⓐ Ⓑ Ⓒ Ⓓ Ⓔ	140 Ⓐ Ⓑ Ⓒ Ⓓ Ⓔ	165 Ⓐ Ⓑ Ⓒ Ⓓ Ⓔ	190 Ⓐ Ⓑ Ⓒ Ⓓ Ⓔ
116 Ⓐ Ⓑ Ⓒ Ⓓ Ⓔ	141 Ⓐ Ⓑ Ⓒ Ⓓ Ⓔ	166 Ⓐ Ⓑ Ⓒ Ⓓ Ⓔ	191 Ⓐ Ⓑ Ⓒ Ⓓ Ⓔ
117 Ⓐ Ⓑ Ⓒ Ⓓ Ⓔ	142 Ⓐ Ⓑ Ⓒ Ⓓ Ⓔ	167 Ⓐ Ⓑ Ⓒ Ⓓ Ⓔ	192 Ⓐ Ⓑ Ⓒ Ⓓ Ⓔ
118 Ⓐ Ⓑ Ⓒ Ⓓ Ⓔ	143 Ⓐ Ⓑ Ⓒ Ⓓ Ⓔ	168 Ⓐ Ⓑ Ⓒ Ⓓ Ⓔ	193 Ⓐ Ⓑ Ⓒ Ⓓ Ⓔ
119 Ⓐ Ⓑ Ⓒ Ⓓ Ⓔ	144 Ⓐ Ⓑ Ⓒ Ⓓ Ⓔ	169 Ⓐ Ⓑ Ⓒ Ⓓ Ⓔ	194 Ⓐ Ⓑ Ⓒ Ⓓ Ⓔ
120 Ⓐ Ⓑ Ⓒ Ⓓ Ⓔ	145 Ⓐ Ⓑ Ⓒ Ⓓ Ⓔ	170 Ⓐ Ⓑ Ⓒ Ⓓ Ⓔ	195 Ⓐ Ⓑ Ⓒ Ⓓ Ⓔ
121 Ⓐ Ⓑ Ⓒ Ⓓ Ⓔ	146 Ⓐ Ⓑ Ⓒ Ⓓ Ⓔ	171 Ⓐ Ⓑ Ⓒ Ⓓ Ⓔ	196 Ⓐ Ⓑ Ⓒ Ⓓ Ⓔ
122 Ⓐ Ⓑ Ⓒ Ⓓ Ⓔ	147 Ⓐ Ⓑ Ⓒ Ⓓ Ⓔ	172 Ⓐ Ⓑ Ⓒ Ⓓ Ⓔ	197 Ⓐ Ⓑ Ⓒ Ⓓ Ⓔ
123 Ⓐ Ⓑ Ⓒ Ⓓ Ⓔ	148 Ⓐ Ⓑ Ⓒ Ⓓ Ⓔ	173 Ⓐ Ⓑ Ⓒ Ⓓ Ⓔ	198 Ⓐ Ⓑ Ⓒ Ⓓ Ⓔ
124 Ⓐ Ⓑ Ⓒ Ⓓ Ⓔ	149 Ⓐ Ⓑ Ⓒ Ⓓ Ⓔ	174 Ⓐ Ⓑ Ⓒ Ⓓ Ⓔ	199 Ⓐ Ⓑ Ⓒ Ⓓ Ⓔ
125 Ⓐ Ⓑ Ⓒ Ⓓ Ⓔ	150 Ⓐ Ⓑ Ⓒ Ⓓ Ⓔ	175 Ⓐ Ⓑ Ⓒ Ⓓ Ⓔ	200 Ⓐ Ⓑ Ⓒ Ⓓ Ⓔ

Last   First   Middle

Directions for Marking Answers

- Use a black lead pencil (No. 2 or softer). Do NOT use pen or a pencil with hard lead.
- Make each mark heavy and black enough to completely obliterate the letter within the circle. Marks should fill the circles.
- Erase clearly any answer you wish to change.
- Make no stray marks on this answer sheet.
- Mark one and only one answer for each question. Multiple answers will be counted as wrong.

Example

WRONG (A) (B̸) (C) (D) (E)
WRONG (A) (B̸) (C) (D) (E)
WRONG (A) (B) (Ⓒ) (D) (E)
RIGHT (A) (B) (C) ● (E)

201 (A) (B) (C) (D) (E)	226 (A) (B) (C) (D) (E)	251 (A) (B) (C) (D) (E)	276 (A) (B) (C) (D) (E)
202 (A) (B) (C) (D) (E)	227 (A) (B) (C) (D) (E)	252 (A) (B) (C) (D) (E)	277 (A) (B) (C) (D) (E)
203 (A) (B) (C) (D) (E)	228 (A) (B) (C) (D) (E)	253 (A) (B) (C) (D) (E)	278 (A) (B) (C) (D) (E)
204 (A) (B) (C) (D) (E)	229 (A) (B) (C) (D) (E)	254 (A) (B) (C) (D) (E)	279 (A) (B) (C) (D) (E)
205 (A) (B) (C) (D) (E)	230 (A) (B) (C) (D) (E)	255 (A) (B) (C) (D) (E)	280 (A) (B) (C) (D) (E)
206 (A) (B) (C) (D) (E)	231 (A) (B) (C) (D) (E)	256 (A) (B) (C) (D) (E)	281 (A) (B) (C) (D) (E)
207 (A) (B) (C) (D) (E)	232 (A) (B) (C) (D) (E)	257 (A) (B) (C) (D) (E)	282 (A) (B) (C) (D) (E)
208 (A) (B) (C) (D) (E)	233 (A) (B) (C) (D) (E)	258 (A) (B) (C) (D) (E)	283 (A) (B) (C) (D) (E)
209 (A) (B) (C) (D) (E)	234 (A) (B) (C) (D) (E)	259 (A) (B) (C) (D) (E)	284 (A) (B) (C) (D) (E)
210 (A) (B) (C) (D) (E)	235 (A) (B) (C) (D) (E)	260 (A) (B) (C) (D) (E)	285 (A) (B) (C) (D) (E)
211 (A) (B) (C) (D) (E)	236 (A) (B) (C) (D) (E)	261 (A) (B) (C) (D) (E)	286 (A) (B) (C) (D) (E)
212 (A) (B) (C) (D) (E)	237 (A) (B) (C) (D) (E)	262 (A) (B) (C) (D) (E)	287 (A) (B) (C) (D) (E)
213 (A) (B) (C) (D) (E)	238 (A) (B) (C) (D) (E)	263 (A) (B) (C) (D) (E)	288 (A) (B) (C) (D) (E)
214 (A) (B) (C) (D) (E)	239 (A) (B) (C) (D) (E)	264 (A) (B) (C) (D) (E)	289 (A) (B) (C) (D) (E)
215 (A) (B) (C) (D) (E)	240 (A) (B) (C) (D) (E)	265 (A) (B) (C) (D) (E)	290 (A) (B) (C) (D) (E)
216 (A) (B) (C) (D) (E)	241 (A) (B) (C) (D) (E)	266 (A) (B) (C) (D) (E)	291 (A) (B) (C) (D) (E)
217 (A) (B) (C) (D) (E)	242 (A) (B) (C) (D) (E)	267 (A) (B) (C) (D) (E)	292 (A) (B) (C) (D) (E)
218 (A) (B) (C) (D) (E)	243 (A) (B) (C) (D) (E)	268 (A) (B) (C) (D) (E)	293 (A) (B) (C) (D) (E)
219 (A) (B) (C) (D) (E)	244 (A) (B) (C) (D) (E)	269 (A) (B) (C) (D) (E)	294 (A) (B) (C) (D) (E)
220 (A) (B) (C) (D) (E)	245 (A) (B) (C) (D) (E)	270 (A) (B) (C) (D) (E)	295 (A) (B) (C) (D) (E)
221 (A) (B) (C) (D) (E)	246 (A) (B) (C) (D) (E)	271 (A) (B) (C) (D) (E)	296 (A) (B) (C) (D) (E)
222 (A) (B) (C) (D) (E)	247 (A) (B) (C) (D) (E)	272 (A) (B) (C) (D) (E)	297 (A) (B) (C) (D) (E)
223 (A) (B) (C) (D) (E)	248 (A) (B) (C) (D) (E)	273 (A) (B) (C) (D) (E)	298 (A) (B) (C) (D) (E)
224 (A) (B) (C) (D) (E)	249 (A) (B) (C) (D) (E)	274 (A) (B) (C) (D) (E)	299 (A) (B) (C) (D) (E)
225 (A) (B) (C) (D) (E)	250 (A) (B) (C) (D) (E)	275 (A) (B) (C) (D) (E)	300 (A) (B) (C) (D) (E)

Directions for Marking Answers

Example

- Use a black lead pencil (No. 2 or softer). Do NOT use pen or a pencil with hard lead.
- Make each mark heavy and black enough to completely obliterate the letter within the circle. Marks should fill the circles.
- Erase clearly any answer you wish to change.
- Make no stray marks on this answer sheet.
- Mark one and only one answer for each question. Multiple answers will be counted as wrong.

WRONG (A) (B̸) (C) (D) (E)

WRONG (A) (B̶) (C) (D) (E)

WRONG (A) (B) (Ⓒ) (D) (E)

RIGHT (A) (B) (C) (●) (E)

1 (A)(B)(C)(D)(E)	26 (A)(B)(C)(D)(E)	51 (A)(B)(C)(D)(E)	76 (A)(B)(C)(D)(E)
2 (A)(B)(C)(D)(E)	27 (A)(B)(C)(D)(E)	52 (A)(B)(C)(D)(E)	77 (A)(B)(C)(D)(E)
3 (A)(B)(C)(D)(E)	28 (A)(B)(C)(D)(E)	53 (A)(B)(C)(D)(E)	78 (A)(B)(C)(D)(E)
4 (A)(B)(C)(D)(E)	29 (A)(B)(C)(D)(E)	54 (A)(B)(C)(D)(E)	79 (A)(B)(C)(D)(E)
5 (A)(B)(C)(D)(E)	30 (A)(B)(C)(D)(E)	55 (A)(B)(C)(D)(E)	80 (A)(B)(C)(D)(E)
6 (A)(B)(C)(D)(E)	31 (A)(B)(C)(D)(E)	56 (A)(B)(C)(D)(E)	81 (A)(B)(C)(D)(E)
7 (A)(B)(C)(D)(E)	32 (A)(B)(C)(D)(E)	57 (A)(B)(C)(D)(E)	82 (A)(B)(C)(D)(E)
8 (A)(B)(C)(D)(E)	33 (A)(B)(C)(D)(E)	58 (A)(B)(C)(D)(E)	83 (A)(B)(C)(D)(E)
9 (A)(B)(C)(D)(E)	34 (A)(B)(C)(D)(E)	59 (A)(B)(C)(D)(E)	84 (A)(B)(C)(D)(E)
10 (A)(B)(C)(D)(E)	35 (A)(B)(C)(D)(E)	60 (A)(B)(C)(D)(E)	85 (A)(B)(C)(D)(E)
11 (A)(B)(C)(D)(E)	36 (A)(B)(C)(D)(E)	61 (A)(B)(C)(D)(E)	86 (A)(B)(C)(D)(E)
12 (A)(B)(C)(D)(E)	37 (A)(B)(C)(D)(E)	62 (A)(B)(C)(D)(E)	87 (A)(B)(C)(D)(E)
13 (A)(B)(C)(D)(E)	38 (A)(B)(C)(D)(E)	63 (A)(B)(C)(D)(E)	88 (A)(B)(C)(D)(E)
14 (A)(B)(C)(D)(E)	39 (A)(B)(C)(D)(E)	64 (A)(B)(C)(D)(E)	89 (A)(B)(C)(D)(E)
15 (A)(B)(C)(D)(E)	40 (A)(B)(C)(D)(E)	65 (A)(B)(C)(D)(E)	90 (A)(B)(C)(D)(E)
16 (A)(B)(C)(D)(E)	41 (A)(B)(C)(D)(E)	66 (A)(B)(C)(D)(E)	91 (A)(B)(C)(D)(E)
17 (A)(B)(C)(D)(E)	42 (A)(B)(C)(D)(E)	67 (A)(B)(C)(D)(E)	92 (A)(B)(C)(D)(E)
18 (A)(B)(C)(D)(E)	43 (A)(B)(C)(D)(E)	68 (A)(B)(C)(D)(E)	93 (A)(B)(C)(D)(E)
19 (A)(B)(C)(D)(E)	44 (A)(B)(C)(D)(E)	69 (A)(B)(C)(D)(E)	94 (A)(B)(C)(D)(E)
20 (A)(B)(C)(D)(E)	45 (A)(B)(C)(D)(E)	70 (A)(B)(C)(D)(E)	95 (A)(B)(C)(D)(E)
21 (A)(B)(C)(D)(E)	46 (A)(B)(C)(D)(E)	71 (A)(B)(C)(D)(E)	96 (A)(B)(C)(D)(E)
22 (A)(B)(C)(D)(E)	47 (A)(B)(C)(D)(E)	72 (A)(B)(C)(D)(E)	97 (A)(B)(C)(D)(E)
23 (A)(B)(C)(D)(E)	48 (A)(B)(C)(D)(E)	73 (A)(B)(C)(D)(E)	98 (A)(B)(C)(D)(E)
24 (A)(B)(C)(D)(E)	49 (A)(B)(C)(D)(E)	74 (A)(B)(C)(D)(E)	99 (A)(B)(C)(D)(E)
25 (A)(B)(C)(D)(E)	50 (A)(B)(C)(D)(E)	75 (A)(B)(C)(D)(E)	100 (A)(B)(C)(D)(E)

Directions for Marking Answers

- Use a black lead pencil (No. 2 or softer). Do NOT use pen or a pencil with hard lead.
- Make each mark heavy and black enough to completely obliterate the letter within the circle. Marks should fill the circles.
- Erase clearly any answer you wish to change.
- Make no stray marks on this answer sheet.
- Mark one and only one answer for each question. Multiple answers will be counted as wrong.

Example

WRONG   Ⓐ Ⓑ Ⓒ Ⓓ Ⓔ

WRONG   Ⓐ Ⓧ Ⓒ Ⓓ Ⓔ

WRONG   Ⓐ Ⓑ Ⓒ Ⓓ Ⓔ

RIGHT   Ⓐ Ⓑ Ⓒ ● Ⓔ

101 Ⓐ Ⓑ Ⓒ Ⓓ Ⓔ	126 Ⓐ Ⓑ Ⓒ Ⓓ Ⓔ	151 Ⓐ Ⓑ Ⓒ Ⓓ Ⓔ	176 Ⓐ Ⓑ Ⓒ Ⓓ Ⓔ
102 Ⓐ Ⓑ Ⓒ Ⓓ Ⓔ	127 Ⓐ Ⓑ Ⓒ Ⓓ Ⓔ	152 Ⓐ Ⓑ Ⓒ Ⓓ Ⓔ	177 Ⓐ Ⓑ Ⓒ Ⓓ Ⓔ
103 Ⓐ Ⓑ Ⓒ Ⓓ Ⓔ	128 Ⓐ Ⓑ Ⓒ Ⓓ Ⓔ	153 Ⓐ Ⓑ Ⓒ Ⓓ Ⓔ	178 Ⓐ Ⓑ Ⓒ Ⓓ Ⓔ
104 Ⓐ Ⓑ Ⓒ Ⓓ Ⓔ	129 Ⓐ Ⓑ Ⓒ Ⓓ Ⓔ	154 Ⓐ Ⓑ Ⓒ Ⓓ Ⓔ	179 Ⓐ Ⓑ Ⓒ Ⓓ Ⓔ
105 Ⓐ Ⓑ Ⓒ Ⓓ Ⓔ	130 Ⓐ Ⓑ Ⓒ Ⓓ Ⓔ	155 Ⓐ Ⓑ Ⓒ Ⓓ Ⓔ	180 Ⓐ Ⓑ Ⓒ Ⓓ Ⓔ
106 Ⓐ Ⓑ Ⓒ Ⓓ Ⓔ	131 Ⓐ Ⓑ Ⓒ Ⓓ Ⓔ	156 Ⓐ Ⓑ Ⓒ Ⓓ Ⓔ	181 Ⓐ Ⓑ Ⓒ Ⓓ Ⓔ
107 Ⓐ Ⓑ Ⓒ Ⓓ Ⓔ	132 Ⓐ Ⓑ Ⓒ Ⓓ Ⓔ	157 Ⓐ Ⓑ Ⓒ Ⓓ Ⓔ	182 Ⓐ Ⓑ Ⓒ Ⓓ Ⓔ
108 Ⓐ Ⓑ Ⓒ Ⓓ Ⓔ	133 Ⓐ Ⓑ Ⓒ Ⓓ Ⓔ	158 Ⓐ Ⓑ Ⓒ Ⓓ Ⓔ	183 Ⓐ Ⓑ Ⓒ Ⓓ Ⓔ
109 Ⓐ Ⓑ Ⓒ Ⓓ Ⓔ	134 Ⓐ Ⓑ Ⓒ Ⓓ Ⓔ	159 Ⓐ Ⓑ Ⓒ Ⓓ Ⓔ	184 Ⓐ Ⓑ Ⓒ Ⓓ Ⓔ
110 Ⓐ Ⓑ Ⓒ Ⓓ Ⓔ	135 Ⓐ Ⓑ Ⓒ Ⓓ Ⓔ	160 Ⓐ Ⓑ Ⓒ Ⓓ Ⓔ	185 Ⓐ Ⓑ Ⓒ Ⓓ Ⓔ
111 Ⓐ Ⓑ Ⓒ Ⓓ Ⓔ	136 Ⓐ Ⓑ Ⓒ Ⓓ Ⓔ	161 Ⓐ Ⓑ Ⓒ Ⓓ Ⓔ	186 Ⓐ Ⓑ Ⓒ Ⓓ Ⓔ
112 Ⓐ Ⓑ Ⓒ Ⓓ Ⓔ	137 Ⓐ Ⓑ Ⓒ Ⓓ Ⓔ	162 Ⓐ Ⓑ Ⓒ Ⓓ Ⓔ	187 Ⓐ Ⓑ Ⓒ Ⓓ Ⓔ
113 Ⓐ Ⓑ Ⓒ Ⓓ Ⓔ	138 Ⓐ Ⓑ Ⓒ Ⓓ Ⓔ	163 Ⓐ Ⓑ Ⓒ Ⓓ Ⓔ	188 Ⓐ Ⓑ Ⓒ Ⓓ Ⓔ
114 Ⓐ Ⓑ Ⓒ Ⓓ Ⓔ	139 Ⓐ Ⓑ Ⓒ Ⓓ Ⓔ	164 Ⓐ Ⓑ Ⓒ Ⓓ Ⓔ	189 Ⓐ Ⓑ Ⓒ Ⓓ Ⓔ
115 Ⓐ Ⓑ Ⓒ Ⓓ Ⓔ	140 Ⓐ Ⓑ Ⓒ Ⓓ Ⓔ	165 Ⓐ Ⓑ Ⓒ Ⓓ Ⓔ	190 Ⓐ Ⓑ Ⓒ Ⓓ Ⓔ
116 Ⓐ Ⓑ Ⓒ Ⓓ Ⓔ	141 Ⓐ Ⓑ Ⓒ Ⓓ Ⓔ	166 Ⓐ Ⓑ Ⓒ Ⓓ Ⓔ	191 Ⓐ Ⓑ Ⓒ Ⓓ Ⓔ
117 Ⓐ Ⓑ Ⓒ Ⓓ Ⓔ	142 Ⓐ Ⓑ Ⓒ Ⓓ Ⓔ	167 Ⓐ Ⓑ Ⓒ Ⓓ Ⓔ	192 Ⓐ Ⓑ Ⓒ Ⓓ Ⓔ
118 Ⓐ Ⓑ Ⓒ Ⓓ Ⓔ	143 Ⓐ Ⓑ Ⓒ Ⓓ Ⓔ	168 Ⓐ Ⓑ Ⓒ Ⓓ Ⓔ	193 Ⓐ Ⓑ Ⓒ Ⓓ Ⓔ
119 Ⓐ Ⓑ Ⓒ Ⓓ Ⓔ	144 Ⓐ Ⓑ Ⓒ Ⓓ Ⓔ	169 Ⓐ Ⓑ Ⓒ Ⓓ Ⓔ	194 Ⓐ Ⓑ Ⓒ Ⓓ Ⓔ
120 Ⓐ Ⓑ Ⓒ Ⓓ Ⓔ	145 Ⓐ Ⓑ Ⓒ Ⓓ Ⓔ	170 Ⓐ Ⓑ Ⓒ Ⓓ Ⓔ	195 Ⓐ Ⓑ Ⓒ Ⓓ Ⓔ
121 Ⓐ Ⓑ Ⓒ Ⓓ Ⓔ	146 Ⓐ Ⓑ Ⓒ Ⓓ Ⓔ	171 Ⓐ Ⓑ Ⓒ Ⓓ Ⓔ	196 Ⓐ Ⓑ Ⓒ Ⓓ Ⓔ
122 Ⓐ Ⓑ Ⓒ Ⓓ Ⓔ	147 Ⓐ Ⓑ Ⓒ Ⓓ Ⓔ	172 Ⓐ Ⓑ Ⓒ Ⓓ Ⓔ	197 Ⓐ Ⓑ Ⓒ Ⓓ Ⓔ
123 Ⓐ Ⓑ Ⓒ Ⓓ Ⓔ	148 Ⓐ Ⓑ Ⓒ Ⓓ Ⓔ	173 Ⓐ Ⓑ Ⓒ Ⓓ Ⓔ	198 Ⓐ Ⓑ Ⓒ Ⓓ Ⓔ
124 Ⓐ Ⓑ Ⓒ Ⓓ Ⓔ	149 Ⓐ Ⓑ Ⓒ Ⓓ Ⓔ	174 Ⓐ Ⓑ Ⓒ Ⓓ Ⓔ	199 Ⓐ Ⓑ Ⓒ Ⓓ Ⓔ
125 Ⓐ Ⓑ Ⓒ Ⓓ Ⓔ	150 Ⓐ Ⓑ Ⓒ Ⓓ Ⓔ	175 Ⓐ Ⓑ Ⓒ Ⓓ Ⓔ	200 Ⓐ Ⓑ Ⓒ Ⓓ Ⓔ

Name _____ **Date** _____

Last   First   Middle

201 Ⓐ Ⓑ Ⓒ Ⓓ Ⓔ	226 Ⓐ Ⓑ Ⓒ Ⓓ Ⓔ	251 Ⓐ Ⓑ Ⓒ Ⓓ Ⓔ	276 Ⓐ Ⓑ Ⓒ Ⓓ Ⓔ
202 Ⓐ Ⓑ Ⓒ Ⓓ Ⓔ	227 Ⓐ Ⓑ Ⓒ Ⓓ Ⓔ	252 Ⓐ Ⓑ Ⓒ Ⓓ Ⓔ	277 Ⓐ Ⓑ Ⓒ Ⓓ Ⓔ
203 Ⓐ Ⓑ Ⓒ Ⓓ Ⓔ	228 Ⓐ Ⓑ Ⓒ Ⓓ Ⓔ	253 Ⓐ Ⓑ Ⓒ Ⓓ Ⓔ	278 Ⓐ Ⓑ Ⓒ Ⓓ Ⓔ
204 Ⓐ Ⓑ Ⓒ Ⓓ Ⓔ	229 Ⓐ Ⓑ Ⓒ Ⓓ Ⓔ	254 Ⓐ Ⓑ Ⓒ Ⓓ Ⓔ	279 Ⓐ Ⓑ Ⓒ Ⓓ Ⓔ
205 Ⓐ Ⓑ Ⓒ Ⓓ Ⓔ	230 Ⓐ Ⓑ Ⓒ Ⓓ Ⓔ	255 Ⓐ Ⓑ Ⓒ Ⓓ Ⓔ	280 Ⓐ Ⓑ Ⓒ Ⓓ Ⓔ
206 Ⓐ Ⓑ Ⓒ Ⓓ Ⓔ	231 Ⓐ Ⓑ Ⓒ Ⓓ Ⓔ	256 Ⓐ Ⓑ Ⓒ Ⓓ Ⓔ	281 Ⓐ Ⓑ Ⓒ Ⓓ Ⓔ
207 Ⓐ Ⓑ Ⓒ Ⓓ Ⓔ	232 Ⓐ Ⓑ Ⓒ Ⓓ Ⓔ	257 Ⓐ Ⓑ Ⓒ Ⓓ Ⓔ	282 Ⓐ Ⓑ Ⓒ Ⓓ Ⓔ
208 Ⓐ Ⓑ Ⓒ Ⓓ Ⓔ	233 Ⓐ Ⓑ Ⓒ Ⓓ Ⓔ	258 Ⓐ Ⓑ Ⓒ Ⓓ Ⓔ	283 Ⓐ Ⓑ Ⓒ Ⓓ Ⓔ
209 Ⓐ Ⓑ Ⓒ Ⓓ Ⓔ	234 Ⓐ Ⓑ Ⓒ Ⓓ Ⓔ	259 Ⓐ Ⓑ Ⓒ Ⓓ Ⓔ	284 Ⓐ Ⓑ Ⓒ Ⓓ Ⓔ
210 Ⓐ Ⓑ Ⓒ Ⓓ Ⓔ	235 Ⓐ Ⓑ Ⓒ Ⓓ Ⓔ	260 Ⓐ Ⓑ Ⓒ Ⓓ Ⓔ	285 Ⓐ Ⓑ Ⓒ Ⓓ Ⓔ
211 Ⓐ Ⓑ Ⓒ Ⓓ Ⓔ	236 Ⓐ Ⓑ Ⓒ Ⓓ Ⓔ	261 Ⓐ Ⓑ Ⓒ Ⓓ Ⓔ	286 Ⓐ Ⓑ Ⓒ Ⓓ Ⓔ
212 Ⓐ Ⓑ Ⓒ Ⓓ Ⓔ	237 Ⓐ Ⓑ Ⓒ Ⓓ Ⓔ	262 Ⓐ Ⓑ Ⓒ Ⓓ Ⓔ	287 Ⓐ Ⓑ Ⓒ Ⓓ Ⓔ
213 Ⓐ Ⓑ Ⓒ Ⓓ Ⓔ	238 Ⓐ Ⓑ Ⓒ Ⓓ Ⓔ	263 Ⓐ Ⓑ Ⓒ Ⓓ Ⓔ	288 Ⓐ Ⓑ Ⓒ Ⓓ Ⓔ
214 Ⓐ Ⓑ Ⓒ Ⓓ Ⓔ	239 Ⓐ Ⓑ Ⓒ Ⓓ Ⓔ	264 Ⓐ Ⓑ Ⓒ Ⓓ Ⓔ	289 Ⓐ Ⓑ Ⓒ Ⓓ Ⓔ
215 Ⓐ Ⓑ Ⓒ Ⓓ Ⓔ	240 Ⓐ Ⓑ Ⓒ Ⓓ Ⓔ	265 Ⓐ Ⓑ Ⓒ Ⓓ Ⓔ	290 Ⓐ Ⓑ Ⓒ Ⓓ Ⓔ
216 Ⓐ Ⓑ Ⓒ Ⓓ Ⓔ	241 Ⓐ Ⓑ Ⓒ Ⓓ Ⓔ	266 Ⓐ Ⓑ Ⓒ Ⓓ Ⓔ	291 Ⓐ Ⓑ Ⓒ Ⓓ Ⓔ
217 Ⓐ Ⓑ Ⓒ Ⓓ Ⓔ	242 Ⓐ Ⓑ Ⓒ Ⓓ Ⓔ	267 Ⓐ Ⓑ Ⓒ Ⓓ Ⓔ	292 Ⓐ Ⓑ Ⓒ Ⓓ Ⓔ
218 Ⓐ Ⓑ Ⓒ Ⓓ Ⓔ	243 Ⓐ Ⓑ Ⓒ Ⓓ Ⓔ	268 Ⓐ Ⓑ Ⓒ Ⓓ Ⓔ	293 Ⓐ Ⓑ Ⓒ Ⓓ Ⓔ
219 Ⓐ Ⓑ Ⓒ Ⓓ Ⓔ	244 Ⓐ Ⓑ Ⓒ Ⓓ Ⓔ	269 Ⓐ Ⓑ Ⓒ Ⓓ Ⓔ	294 Ⓐ Ⓑ Ⓒ Ⓓ Ⓔ
220 Ⓐ Ⓑ Ⓒ Ⓓ Ⓔ	245 Ⓐ Ⓑ Ⓒ Ⓓ Ⓔ	270 Ⓐ Ⓑ Ⓒ Ⓓ Ⓔ	295 Ⓐ Ⓑ Ⓒ Ⓓ Ⓔ
221 Ⓐ Ⓑ Ⓒ Ⓓ Ⓔ	246 Ⓐ Ⓑ Ⓒ Ⓓ Ⓔ	271 Ⓐ Ⓑ Ⓒ Ⓓ Ⓔ	296 Ⓐ Ⓑ Ⓒ Ⓓ Ⓔ
222 Ⓐ Ⓑ Ⓒ Ⓓ Ⓔ	247 Ⓐ Ⓑ Ⓒ Ⓓ Ⓔ	272 Ⓐ Ⓑ Ⓒ Ⓓ Ⓔ	297 Ⓐ Ⓑ Ⓒ Ⓓ Ⓔ
223 Ⓐ Ⓑ Ⓒ Ⓓ Ⓔ	248 Ⓐ Ⓑ Ⓒ Ⓓ Ⓔ	273 Ⓐ Ⓑ Ⓒ Ⓓ Ⓔ	298 Ⓐ Ⓑ Ⓒ Ⓓ Ⓔ
224 Ⓐ Ⓑ Ⓒ Ⓓ Ⓔ	249 Ⓐ Ⓑ Ⓒ Ⓓ Ⓔ	274 Ⓐ Ⓑ Ⓒ Ⓓ Ⓔ	299 Ⓐ Ⓑ Ⓒ Ⓓ Ⓔ
225 Ⓐ Ⓑ Ⓒ Ⓓ Ⓔ	250 Ⓐ Ⓑ Ⓒ Ⓓ Ⓔ	275 Ⓐ Ⓑ Ⓒ Ⓓ Ⓔ	300 Ⓐ Ⓑ Ⓒ Ⓓ Ⓔ

Name _____ **Date** _____

Last   First   Middle

Directions for Marking Answers

Example

- Use a black lead pencil (No. 2 or softer). Do NOT use pen or a pencil with hard lead.

WRONG   Ⓐ Ⓑ̷ Ⓒ Ⓓ Ⓔ

- Make each mark heavy and black enough to completely obliterate the letter within the circle. Marks should fill the circles.

WRONG   Ⓐ Ⓧ Ⓒ Ⓓ Ⓔ

- Erase clearly any answer you wish to change.

WRONG   Ⓐ Ⓑ Ⓒ̊ Ⓓ Ⓔ

- Make no stray marks on this answer sheet.

RIGHT   Ⓐ Ⓑ Ⓒ ● Ⓔ

- Mark one and only one answer for each question. Multiple answers will be counted as wrong.

1 Ⓐ Ⓑ Ⓒ Ⓓ Ⓔ	26 Ⓐ Ⓑ Ⓒ Ⓓ Ⓔ	51 Ⓐ Ⓑ Ⓒ Ⓓ Ⓔ	76 Ⓐ Ⓑ Ⓒ Ⓓ Ⓔ
2 Ⓐ Ⓑ Ⓒ Ⓓ Ⓔ	27 Ⓐ Ⓑ Ⓒ Ⓓ Ⓔ	52 Ⓐ Ⓑ Ⓒ Ⓓ Ⓔ	77 Ⓐ Ⓑ Ⓒ Ⓓ Ⓔ
3 Ⓐ Ⓑ Ⓒ Ⓓ Ⓔ	28 Ⓐ Ⓑ Ⓒ Ⓓ Ⓔ	53 Ⓐ Ⓑ Ⓒ Ⓓ Ⓔ	78 Ⓐ Ⓑ Ⓒ Ⓓ Ⓔ
4 Ⓐ Ⓑ Ⓒ Ⓓ Ⓔ	29 Ⓐ Ⓑ Ⓒ Ⓓ Ⓔ	54 Ⓐ Ⓑ Ⓒ Ⓓ Ⓔ	79 Ⓐ Ⓑ Ⓒ Ⓓ Ⓔ
5 Ⓐ Ⓑ Ⓒ Ⓓ Ⓔ	30 Ⓐ Ⓑ Ⓒ Ⓓ Ⓔ	55 Ⓐ Ⓑ Ⓒ Ⓓ Ⓔ	80 Ⓐ Ⓑ Ⓒ Ⓓ Ⓔ
6 Ⓐ Ⓑ Ⓒ Ⓓ Ⓔ	31 Ⓐ Ⓑ Ⓒ Ⓓ Ⓔ	56 Ⓐ Ⓑ Ⓒ Ⓓ Ⓔ	81 Ⓐ Ⓑ Ⓒ Ⓓ Ⓔ
7 Ⓐ Ⓑ Ⓒ Ⓓ Ⓔ	32 Ⓐ Ⓑ Ⓒ Ⓓ Ⓔ	57 Ⓐ Ⓑ Ⓒ Ⓓ Ⓔ	82 Ⓐ Ⓑ Ⓒ Ⓓ Ⓔ
8 Ⓐ Ⓑ Ⓒ Ⓓ Ⓔ	33 Ⓐ Ⓑ Ⓒ Ⓓ Ⓔ	58 Ⓐ Ⓑ Ⓒ Ⓓ Ⓔ	83 Ⓐ Ⓑ Ⓒ Ⓓ Ⓔ
9 Ⓐ Ⓑ Ⓒ Ⓓ Ⓔ	34 Ⓐ Ⓑ Ⓒ Ⓓ Ⓔ	59 Ⓐ Ⓑ Ⓒ Ⓓ Ⓔ	84 Ⓐ Ⓑ Ⓒ Ⓓ Ⓔ
10 Ⓐ Ⓑ Ⓒ Ⓓ Ⓔ	35 Ⓐ Ⓑ Ⓒ Ⓓ Ⓔ	60 Ⓐ Ⓑ Ⓒ Ⓓ Ⓔ	85 Ⓐ Ⓑ Ⓒ Ⓓ Ⓔ
11 Ⓐ Ⓑ Ⓒ Ⓓ Ⓔ	36 Ⓐ Ⓑ Ⓒ Ⓓ Ⓔ	61 Ⓐ Ⓑ Ⓒ Ⓓ Ⓔ	86 Ⓐ Ⓑ Ⓒ Ⓓ Ⓔ
12 Ⓐ Ⓑ Ⓒ Ⓓ Ⓔ	37 Ⓐ Ⓑ Ⓒ Ⓓ Ⓔ	62 Ⓐ Ⓑ Ⓒ Ⓓ Ⓔ	87 Ⓐ Ⓑ Ⓒ Ⓓ Ⓔ
13 Ⓐ Ⓑ Ⓒ Ⓓ Ⓔ	38 Ⓐ Ⓑ Ⓒ Ⓓ Ⓔ	63 Ⓐ Ⓑ Ⓒ Ⓓ Ⓔ	88 Ⓐ Ⓑ Ⓒ Ⓓ Ⓔ
14 Ⓐ Ⓑ Ⓒ Ⓓ Ⓔ	39 Ⓐ Ⓑ Ⓒ Ⓓ Ⓔ	64 Ⓐ Ⓑ Ⓒ Ⓓ Ⓔ	89 Ⓐ Ⓑ Ⓒ Ⓓ Ⓔ
15 Ⓐ Ⓑ Ⓒ Ⓓ Ⓔ	40 Ⓐ Ⓑ Ⓒ Ⓓ Ⓔ	65 Ⓐ Ⓑ Ⓒ Ⓓ Ⓔ	90 Ⓐ Ⓑ Ⓒ Ⓓ Ⓔ
16 Ⓐ Ⓑ Ⓒ Ⓓ Ⓔ	41 Ⓐ Ⓑ Ⓒ Ⓓ Ⓔ	66 Ⓐ Ⓑ Ⓒ Ⓓ Ⓔ	91 Ⓐ Ⓑ Ⓒ Ⓓ Ⓔ
17 Ⓐ Ⓑ Ⓒ Ⓓ Ⓔ	42 Ⓐ Ⓑ Ⓒ Ⓓ Ⓔ	67 Ⓐ Ⓑ Ⓒ Ⓓ Ⓔ	92 Ⓐ Ⓑ Ⓒ Ⓓ Ⓔ
18 Ⓐ Ⓑ Ⓒ Ⓓ Ⓔ	43 Ⓐ Ⓑ Ⓒ Ⓓ Ⓔ	68 Ⓐ Ⓑ Ⓒ Ⓓ Ⓔ	93 Ⓐ Ⓑ Ⓒ Ⓓ Ⓔ
19 Ⓐ Ⓑ Ⓒ Ⓓ Ⓔ	44 Ⓐ Ⓑ Ⓒ Ⓓ Ⓔ	69 Ⓐ Ⓑ Ⓒ Ⓓ Ⓔ	94 Ⓐ Ⓑ Ⓒ Ⓓ Ⓔ
20 Ⓐ Ⓑ Ⓒ Ⓓ Ⓔ	45 Ⓐ Ⓑ Ⓒ Ⓓ Ⓔ	70 Ⓐ Ⓑ Ⓒ Ⓓ Ⓔ	95 Ⓐ Ⓑ Ⓒ Ⓓ Ⓔ
21 Ⓐ Ⓑ Ⓒ Ⓓ Ⓔ	46 Ⓐ Ⓑ Ⓒ Ⓓ Ⓔ	71 Ⓐ Ⓑ Ⓒ Ⓓ Ⓔ	96 Ⓐ Ⓑ Ⓒ Ⓓ Ⓔ
22 Ⓐ Ⓑ Ⓒ Ⓓ Ⓔ	47 Ⓐ Ⓑ Ⓒ Ⓓ Ⓔ	72 Ⓐ Ⓑ Ⓒ Ⓓ Ⓔ	97 Ⓐ Ⓑ Ⓒ Ⓓ Ⓔ
23 Ⓐ Ⓑ Ⓒ Ⓓ Ⓔ	48 Ⓐ Ⓑ Ⓒ Ⓓ Ⓔ	73 Ⓐ Ⓑ Ⓒ Ⓓ Ⓔ	98 Ⓐ Ⓑ Ⓒ Ⓓ Ⓔ
24 Ⓐ Ⓑ Ⓒ Ⓓ Ⓔ	49 Ⓐ Ⓑ Ⓒ Ⓓ Ⓔ	74 Ⓐ Ⓑ Ⓒ Ⓓ Ⓔ	99 Ⓐ Ⓑ Ⓒ Ⓓ Ⓔ
25 Ⓐ Ⓑ Ⓒ Ⓓ Ⓔ	50 Ⓐ Ⓑ Ⓒ Ⓓ Ⓔ	75 Ⓐ Ⓑ Ⓒ Ⓓ Ⓔ	100 Ⓐ Ⓑ Ⓒ Ⓓ Ⓔ

Name _____ **Date** _____
  Last   First   Middle

101 Ⓐ Ⓑ Ⓒ Ⓓ Ⓔ   126 Ⓐ Ⓑ Ⓒ Ⓓ Ⓔ   151 Ⓐ Ⓑ Ⓒ Ⓓ Ⓔ   176 Ⓐ Ⓑ Ⓒ Ⓓ Ⓔ
102 Ⓐ Ⓑ Ⓒ Ⓓ Ⓔ   127 Ⓐ Ⓑ Ⓒ Ⓓ Ⓔ   152 Ⓐ Ⓑ Ⓒ Ⓓ Ⓔ   177 Ⓐ Ⓑ Ⓒ Ⓓ Ⓔ
103 Ⓐ Ⓑ Ⓒ Ⓓ Ⓔ   128 Ⓐ Ⓑ Ⓒ Ⓓ Ⓔ   153 Ⓐ Ⓑ Ⓒ Ⓓ Ⓔ   178 Ⓐ Ⓑ Ⓒ Ⓓ Ⓔ
104 Ⓐ Ⓑ Ⓒ Ⓓ Ⓔ   129 Ⓐ Ⓑ Ⓒ Ⓓ Ⓔ   154 Ⓐ Ⓑ Ⓒ Ⓓ Ⓔ   179 Ⓐ Ⓑ Ⓒ Ⓓ Ⓔ
105 Ⓐ Ⓑ Ⓒ Ⓓ Ⓔ   130 Ⓐ Ⓑ Ⓒ Ⓓ Ⓔ   155 Ⓐ Ⓑ Ⓒ Ⓓ Ⓔ   180 Ⓐ Ⓑ Ⓒ Ⓓ Ⓔ
106 Ⓐ Ⓑ Ⓒ Ⓓ Ⓔ   131 Ⓐ Ⓑ Ⓒ Ⓓ Ⓔ   156 Ⓐ Ⓑ Ⓒ Ⓓ Ⓔ   181 Ⓐ Ⓑ Ⓒ Ⓓ Ⓔ
107 Ⓐ Ⓑ Ⓒ Ⓓ Ⓔ   132 Ⓐ Ⓑ Ⓒ Ⓓ Ⓔ   157 Ⓐ Ⓑ Ⓒ Ⓓ Ⓔ   182 Ⓐ Ⓑ Ⓒ Ⓓ Ⓔ
108 Ⓐ Ⓑ Ⓒ Ⓓ Ⓔ   133 Ⓐ Ⓑ Ⓒ Ⓓ Ⓔ   158 Ⓐ Ⓑ Ⓒ Ⓓ Ⓔ   183 Ⓐ Ⓑ Ⓒ Ⓓ Ⓔ
109 Ⓐ Ⓑ Ⓒ Ⓓ Ⓔ   134 Ⓐ Ⓑ Ⓒ Ⓓ Ⓔ   159 Ⓐ Ⓑ Ⓒ Ⓓ Ⓔ   184 Ⓐ Ⓑ Ⓒ Ⓓ Ⓔ
110 Ⓐ Ⓑ Ⓒ Ⓓ Ⓔ   135 Ⓐ Ⓑ Ⓒ Ⓓ Ⓔ   160 Ⓐ Ⓑ Ⓒ Ⓓ Ⓔ   185 Ⓐ Ⓑ Ⓒ Ⓓ Ⓔ
111 Ⓐ Ⓑ Ⓒ Ⓓ Ⓔ   136 Ⓐ Ⓑ Ⓒ Ⓓ Ⓔ   161 Ⓐ Ⓑ Ⓒ Ⓓ Ⓔ   186 Ⓐ Ⓑ Ⓒ Ⓓ Ⓔ
112 Ⓐ Ⓑ Ⓒ Ⓓ Ⓔ   137 Ⓐ Ⓑ Ⓒ Ⓓ Ⓔ   162 Ⓐ Ⓑ Ⓒ Ⓓ Ⓔ   187 Ⓐ Ⓑ Ⓒ Ⓓ Ⓔ
113 Ⓐ Ⓑ Ⓒ Ⓓ Ⓔ   138 Ⓐ Ⓑ Ⓒ Ⓓ Ⓔ   163 Ⓐ Ⓑ Ⓒ Ⓓ Ⓔ   188 Ⓐ Ⓑ Ⓒ Ⓓ Ⓔ
114 Ⓐ Ⓑ Ⓒ Ⓓ Ⓔ   139 Ⓐ Ⓑ Ⓒ Ⓓ Ⓔ   164 Ⓐ Ⓑ Ⓒ Ⓓ Ⓔ   189 Ⓐ Ⓑ Ⓒ Ⓓ Ⓔ
115 Ⓐ Ⓑ Ⓒ Ⓓ Ⓔ   140 Ⓐ Ⓑ Ⓒ Ⓓ Ⓔ   165 Ⓐ Ⓑ Ⓒ Ⓓ Ⓔ   190 Ⓐ Ⓑ Ⓒ Ⓓ Ⓔ
116 Ⓐ Ⓑ Ⓒ Ⓓ Ⓔ   141 Ⓐ Ⓑ Ⓒ Ⓓ Ⓔ   166 Ⓐ Ⓑ Ⓒ Ⓓ Ⓔ   191 Ⓐ Ⓑ Ⓒ Ⓓ Ⓔ
117 Ⓐ Ⓑ Ⓒ Ⓓ Ⓔ   142 Ⓐ Ⓑ Ⓒ Ⓓ Ⓔ   167 Ⓐ Ⓑ Ⓒ Ⓓ Ⓔ   192 Ⓐ Ⓑ Ⓒ Ⓓ Ⓔ
118 Ⓐ Ⓑ Ⓒ Ⓓ Ⓔ   143 Ⓐ Ⓑ Ⓒ Ⓓ Ⓔ   168 Ⓐ Ⓑ Ⓒ Ⓓ Ⓔ   193 Ⓐ Ⓑ Ⓒ Ⓓ Ⓔ
119 Ⓐ Ⓑ Ⓒ Ⓓ Ⓔ   144 Ⓐ Ⓑ Ⓒ Ⓓ Ⓔ   169 Ⓐ Ⓑ Ⓒ Ⓓ Ⓔ   194 Ⓐ Ⓑ Ⓒ Ⓓ Ⓔ
120 Ⓐ Ⓑ Ⓒ Ⓓ Ⓔ   145 Ⓐ Ⓑ Ⓒ Ⓓ Ⓔ   170 Ⓐ Ⓑ Ⓒ Ⓓ Ⓔ   195 Ⓐ Ⓑ Ⓒ Ⓓ Ⓔ
121 Ⓐ Ⓑ Ⓒ Ⓓ Ⓔ   146 Ⓐ Ⓑ Ⓒ Ⓓ Ⓔ   171 Ⓐ Ⓑ Ⓒ Ⓓ Ⓔ   196 Ⓐ Ⓑ Ⓒ Ⓓ Ⓔ
122 Ⓐ Ⓑ Ⓒ Ⓓ Ⓔ   147 Ⓐ Ⓑ Ⓒ Ⓓ Ⓔ   172 Ⓐ Ⓑ Ⓒ Ⓓ Ⓔ   197 Ⓐ Ⓑ Ⓒ Ⓓ Ⓔ
123 Ⓐ Ⓑ Ⓒ Ⓓ Ⓔ   148 Ⓐ Ⓑ Ⓒ Ⓓ Ⓔ   173 Ⓐ Ⓑ Ⓒ Ⓓ Ⓔ   198 Ⓐ Ⓑ Ⓒ Ⓓ Ⓔ
124 Ⓐ Ⓑ Ⓒ Ⓓ Ⓔ   149 Ⓐ Ⓑ Ⓒ Ⓓ Ⓔ   174 Ⓐ Ⓑ Ⓒ Ⓓ Ⓔ   199 Ⓐ Ⓑ Ⓒ Ⓓ Ⓔ
125 Ⓐ Ⓑ Ⓒ Ⓓ Ⓔ   150 Ⓐ Ⓑ Ⓒ Ⓓ Ⓔ   175 Ⓐ Ⓑ Ⓒ Ⓓ Ⓔ   200 Ⓐ Ⓑ Ⓒ Ⓓ Ⓔ

Name _____ **Date** _____

Last   First   Middle

Directions for Marking Answers

- Use a black lead pencil (No. 2 or softer). Do NOT use pen or a pencil with hard lead.
- Make each mark heavy and black enough to completely obliterate the letter within the circle. Marks should fill the circles.
- Erase clearly any answer you wish to change.
- Make no stray marks on this answer sheet.
- Mark one and only one answer for each question. Multiple answers will be counted as wrong.

Example

WRONG   Ⓐ Ⓑ̸ Ⓒ Ⓓ Ⓔ

WRONG   Ⓐ Ⓧ Ⓒ Ⓓ Ⓔ

WRONG   Ⓐ Ⓑ Ⓒ̲ Ⓓ Ⓔ

RIGHT   Ⓐ Ⓑ Ⓒ ● Ⓔ

201 Ⓐ Ⓑ Ⓒ Ⓓ Ⓔ	226 Ⓐ Ⓑ Ⓒ Ⓓ Ⓔ	251 Ⓐ Ⓑ Ⓒ Ⓓ Ⓔ	276 Ⓐ Ⓑ Ⓒ Ⓓ Ⓔ
202 Ⓐ Ⓑ Ⓒ Ⓓ Ⓔ	227 Ⓐ Ⓑ Ⓒ Ⓓ Ⓔ	252 Ⓐ Ⓑ Ⓒ Ⓓ Ⓔ	277 Ⓐ Ⓑ Ⓒ Ⓓ Ⓔ
203 Ⓐ Ⓑ Ⓒ Ⓓ Ⓔ	228 Ⓐ Ⓑ Ⓒ Ⓓ Ⓔ	253 Ⓐ Ⓑ Ⓒ Ⓓ Ⓔ	278 Ⓐ Ⓑ Ⓒ Ⓓ Ⓔ
204 Ⓐ Ⓑ Ⓒ Ⓓ Ⓔ	229 Ⓐ Ⓑ Ⓒ Ⓓ Ⓔ	254 Ⓐ Ⓑ Ⓒ Ⓓ Ⓔ	279 Ⓐ Ⓑ Ⓒ Ⓓ Ⓔ
205 Ⓐ Ⓑ Ⓒ Ⓓ Ⓔ	230 Ⓐ Ⓑ Ⓒ Ⓓ Ⓔ	255 Ⓐ Ⓑ Ⓒ Ⓓ Ⓔ	280 Ⓐ Ⓑ Ⓒ Ⓓ Ⓔ
206 Ⓐ Ⓑ Ⓒ Ⓓ Ⓔ	231 Ⓐ Ⓑ Ⓒ Ⓓ Ⓔ	256 Ⓐ Ⓑ Ⓒ Ⓓ Ⓔ	281 Ⓐ Ⓑ Ⓒ Ⓓ Ⓔ
207 Ⓐ Ⓑ Ⓒ Ⓓ Ⓔ	232 Ⓐ Ⓑ Ⓒ Ⓓ Ⓔ	257 Ⓐ Ⓑ Ⓒ Ⓓ Ⓔ	282 Ⓐ Ⓑ Ⓒ Ⓓ Ⓔ
208 Ⓐ Ⓑ Ⓒ Ⓓ Ⓔ	233 Ⓐ Ⓑ Ⓒ Ⓓ Ⓔ	258 Ⓐ Ⓑ Ⓒ Ⓓ Ⓔ	283 Ⓐ Ⓑ Ⓒ Ⓓ Ⓔ
209 Ⓐ Ⓑ Ⓒ Ⓓ Ⓔ	234 Ⓐ Ⓑ Ⓒ Ⓓ Ⓔ	259 Ⓐ Ⓑ Ⓒ Ⓓ Ⓔ	284 Ⓐ Ⓑ Ⓒ Ⓓ Ⓔ
210 Ⓐ Ⓑ Ⓒ Ⓓ Ⓔ	235 Ⓐ Ⓑ Ⓒ Ⓓ Ⓔ	260 Ⓐ Ⓑ Ⓒ Ⓓ Ⓔ	285 Ⓐ Ⓑ Ⓒ Ⓓ Ⓔ
211 Ⓐ Ⓑ Ⓒ Ⓓ Ⓔ	236 Ⓐ Ⓑ Ⓒ Ⓓ Ⓔ	261 Ⓐ Ⓑ Ⓒ Ⓓ Ⓔ	286 Ⓐ Ⓑ Ⓒ Ⓓ Ⓔ
212 Ⓐ Ⓑ Ⓒ Ⓓ Ⓔ	237 Ⓐ Ⓑ Ⓒ Ⓓ Ⓔ	262 Ⓐ Ⓑ Ⓒ Ⓓ Ⓔ	287 Ⓐ Ⓑ Ⓒ Ⓓ Ⓔ
213 Ⓐ Ⓑ Ⓒ Ⓓ Ⓔ	238 Ⓐ Ⓑ Ⓒ Ⓓ Ⓔ	263 Ⓐ Ⓑ Ⓒ Ⓓ Ⓔ	288 Ⓐ Ⓑ Ⓒ Ⓓ Ⓔ
214 Ⓐ Ⓑ Ⓒ Ⓓ Ⓔ	239 Ⓐ Ⓑ Ⓒ Ⓓ Ⓔ	264 Ⓐ Ⓑ Ⓒ Ⓓ Ⓔ	289 Ⓐ Ⓑ Ⓒ Ⓓ Ⓔ
215 Ⓐ Ⓑ Ⓒ Ⓓ Ⓔ	240 Ⓐ Ⓑ Ⓒ Ⓓ Ⓔ	265 Ⓐ Ⓑ Ⓒ Ⓓ Ⓔ	290 Ⓐ Ⓑ Ⓒ Ⓓ Ⓔ
216 Ⓐ Ⓑ Ⓒ Ⓓ Ⓔ	241 Ⓐ Ⓑ Ⓒ Ⓓ Ⓔ	266 Ⓐ Ⓑ Ⓒ Ⓓ Ⓔ	291 Ⓐ Ⓑ Ⓒ Ⓓ Ⓔ
217 Ⓐ Ⓑ Ⓒ Ⓓ Ⓔ	242 Ⓐ Ⓑ Ⓒ Ⓓ Ⓔ	267 Ⓐ Ⓑ Ⓒ Ⓓ Ⓔ	292 Ⓐ Ⓑ Ⓒ Ⓓ Ⓔ
218 Ⓐ Ⓑ Ⓒ Ⓓ Ⓔ	243 Ⓐ Ⓑ Ⓒ Ⓓ Ⓔ	268 Ⓐ Ⓑ Ⓒ Ⓓ Ⓔ	293 Ⓐ Ⓑ Ⓒ Ⓓ Ⓔ
219 Ⓐ Ⓑ Ⓒ Ⓓ Ⓔ	244 Ⓐ Ⓑ Ⓒ Ⓓ Ⓔ	269 Ⓐ Ⓑ Ⓒ Ⓓ Ⓔ	294 Ⓐ Ⓑ Ⓒ Ⓓ Ⓔ
220 Ⓐ Ⓑ Ⓒ Ⓓ Ⓔ	245 Ⓐ Ⓑ Ⓒ Ⓓ Ⓔ	270 Ⓐ Ⓑ Ⓒ Ⓓ Ⓔ	295 Ⓐ Ⓑ Ⓒ Ⓓ Ⓔ
221 Ⓐ Ⓑ Ⓒ Ⓓ Ⓔ	246 Ⓐ Ⓑ Ⓒ Ⓓ Ⓔ	271 Ⓐ Ⓑ Ⓒ Ⓓ Ⓔ	296 Ⓐ Ⓑ Ⓒ Ⓓ Ⓔ
222 Ⓐ Ⓑ Ⓒ Ⓓ Ⓔ	247 Ⓐ Ⓑ Ⓒ Ⓓ Ⓔ	272 Ⓐ Ⓑ Ⓒ Ⓓ Ⓔ	297 Ⓐ Ⓑ Ⓒ Ⓓ Ⓔ
223 Ⓐ Ⓑ Ⓒ Ⓓ Ⓔ	248 Ⓐ Ⓑ Ⓒ Ⓓ Ⓔ	273 Ⓐ Ⓑ Ⓒ Ⓓ Ⓔ	298 Ⓐ Ⓑ Ⓒ Ⓓ Ⓔ
224 Ⓐ Ⓑ Ⓒ Ⓓ Ⓔ	249 Ⓐ Ⓑ Ⓒ Ⓓ Ⓔ	274 Ⓐ Ⓑ Ⓒ Ⓓ Ⓔ	299 Ⓐ Ⓑ Ⓒ Ⓓ Ⓔ
225 Ⓐ Ⓑ Ⓒ Ⓓ Ⓔ	250 Ⓐ Ⓑ Ⓒ Ⓓ Ⓔ	275 Ⓐ Ⓑ Ⓒ Ⓓ Ⓔ	300 Ⓐ Ⓑ Ⓒ Ⓓ Ⓔ

SIMULATION TEST 4

Part 1—General Medical Knowledge

Directions: *Each of the following questions or incomplete statements precedes five suggested answers or completions. Select the ONE answer or completion that is BEST in each case and fill in the circle containing the corresponding letter on the answer sheet.*

1. Joints that are freely movable are called
   A. synarthrotic
   B. amphiarthrotic
   C. diarthrotic
   D. manubriotic
   E. acromial

2. Inoculations of specific antibodies to provide temporary immunity against a disease are manufactured using human or animal
   A. plasma
   B. serum
   C. thymus gland
   D. bone marrow
   E. lymph

3. On examination, the area of mucous membrane that lines the nose and throat would be referred to as the
   A. nasal septum
   B. nasal cavity oropharynx
   C. nasopharynx
   D. laryngopharynx
   E. urula

4. One treatment for a hyperventilating patient is to have the patient breathe into a paper bag. This procedure is based on which of the following principles?
   A. Hyperventilation results in carbon dioxide depletion.
   B. Hyperventilation results in carbon dioxide saturation.
   C. Carbon dioxide depresses the respiratory center of the brain.
   D. Carbon dioxide dilates the bronchi.
   E. Oxygen stimulates the respiratory center of the brain.

5. The membrane lining the digestive tract is
   A. mucous membrane
   B. serous membrane
   C. synovial membrane
   D. fibrous membrane
   E. cutaneous membrane

6. Adipose tissue is one type of
   A. epithelial tissue
   B. muscle tissue
   C. nerve tissue
   D. connective tissue
   E. osseous connective tissue

7. A protozoan present in most normal individuals but causing severe opportunistic infections in AIDS patients is
   A. Kaposi's sarcoma
   B. *Pneumocystis carinii*
   C. cytomegalovirus
   D. *Candida albicans*
   E. herpes simplex

8. A fat-soluble vitamin essential to the coagulation process is vitamin
   A. A
   B. B
   C. E
   D. K
   E. B_{12}

9. Fingernails are formed from the
   A. epidermis
   B. dermis
   C. bone
   D. osseous connective tissue
   E. dense fibrous connective tissue

10. The skin acts as a protective barrier against bacteria by
    A. secreting sebum
    B. producing hair
    C. remaining intact
    D. the evaporation of perspiration
    E. transporting body wastes with perspiration

11. Of the following, which is the simplest structure in the body?
    A. cells
    B. tissues
    C. membranes
    D. organs
    E. systems

12. A nerve impulse continuing from one nerve to another in a chain event is a
    A. reflex
    B. reflex arc
    C. impulse
    D. circumduction
    E. synapse

13. A component of blood that aids in blood clotting is
    A. hemoglobin
    B. phagocytes
    C. platelets
    D. erythrocytes
    E. leukocytes

14. The term for the adjustment of the lens for near and far vision is
    A. coloboma
    B. accommodation
    C. miosis
    D. mydriasis
    E. dilation

15. The innermost coat of the eyeball is the
    A. fornix
    B. vitreous body
    C. sclera
    D. choroid
    E. retina

16. The cranial nerve affecting the functions of coughing, sneezing, heart rate, and hunger sensations is the
    A. trochlear
    B. abducens
    C. vagus
    D. vestibulocochlear
    E. hypoglossal

17. The healthy tympanic membrane has which appearance?
    A. pink and shiny
    B. pearl-gray and shiny
    C. pink and dull
    D. pearl-gray and dull
    E. white and translucent

18. The part of the inner ear that is concerned with equilibrium is the
    A. malleus
    B. incus
    C. stapes
    D. vestibule
    E. cochlea

19. The inner lining of the heart is most likely to be involved in which the following diseases?
    A. subacute bacterial endocarditis
    B. pericardial infusion
    C. myocardial infarction
    D. ischemic heart disease
    E. congestive heart failure

20. In men, the normal red blood cell count per cubic millimeter of blood is
    A. 4500 to 5000
    B. 5000 to 10,000
    C. 4.5 million to 6.0 million
    D. 5.0 million to 10 million
    E. 12 to 15 million

21. The functions of respiration, heart rate, and constriction of the blood vessels are controlled by the
    A. cerebrum
    B. cerebellum
    C. medulla oblongata
    D. pons
    E. brain stem

22. To ensure the daily requirement for "high-quality protein" that contains all the essential amino acids, which of the following diets must be carefully planned?
    A. fish, poultry, vegetables; no milk, red meats or eggs
    B. eggs, vegetables, fruits, legumes; no animal meats or milk
    C. milk, vegetables, fruits, legumes; no animal meats or eggs
    D. vegetables, fruits, grains; no animal meats or animal products
    E. meats, milk, eggs, grains; little vegetables, fruits, fish or poultry

23. Melanin gives the skin
    A. elasticity
    B. moisture
    C. color
    D. fingerprints
    E. oil

24. The skull turns by pivoting around which vertebra?
    A. atlas
    B. axis
    C. arch
    D. pedicle
    E. hyoid vertebral prominence

25. Which of the following describes the adult sacral spine?
    A. four mobile vertebrae
    B. four fused vertebrae
    C. five mobile vertebrae
    D. five fused vertebrae
    E. seven mobile vertebrae

26. Cardiac muscle is referred to as
    A. striated, voluntary
    B. striated, involuntary
    C. smooth, voluntary
    D. smooth, involuntary
    E. smooth, striated

27. The anterior fontanel normally closes by what age?
    A. 1 month
    B. 3 months
    C. 4 months
    D. 6 months
    E. 15 months

28. The average, healthy adult requires how many glasses of water daily?
    A. One per meal
    B. 2–3
    C. 4–5
    D. 6–8
    E. 10–12

29. Ovulation occurs approximately how long before menstruation?
    A. 5 days
    B. 10 to 12 days
    C. 12 to 14 days
    D. 2 weeks
    E. 3 weeks

30. A pathologic or accentuated posterior, convex curvature of the spine, also known as "hunchback," is referred to as
    A. kyphosis
    B. lordosis
    C. functional scoliosis
    D. structural socliosis
    E. spondylolisthesis

31. The two organisms that most frequently cause subacute bacterial endocarditis are *Staphylococcus aureus* and
    A. *Haemophilus influenzae*
    B. *Mycobacterium tuberculosis*
    C. *Streptococcus viridans*
    D. *Chlamydia trachomatis*
    E. *Histoplasma capsulatum*

32. The distal portion of the sternum is termed the
    A. manubrium
    B. body
    C. xiphoid process
    D. acromion process
    E. coracoid process

33. The heart's pacemaker is located in the
    A. sinoatrial node
    B. atrioventricular node
    C. bundle of His
    D. chordae tendineae
    E. papillary muscles

34. A temperature that is fluctuating between normal and 102°F in a 24-hour period is called
    A. remittent
    B. constant
    C. intermittent
    D. relapsing
    E. lysis

35. Tonometry measures the intraocular pressure of the
    A. cornea
    B. lens
    C. aqueous humor
    D. retina
    E. sclera

36. The muscle that abducts the upper arm is the
    A. biceps brachii
    B. triceps brachii
    C. coracobrachialis
    D. brachialis
    E. deltoid

37. The connective tissue that connects muscle to bone is
    A. bursa
    B. tendon
    C. fascia
    D. aponeurosis
    E. ligament

38. If a nerve to a muscle is given a brief electrical shock, the muscle responds by a brief contraction called
    A. treppe
    B. tetany
    C. tone
    D. twitch
    E. tension

39. When we inhale, the diaphragm
    A. flattens
    B. rises
    C. decreases the thorax vertically
    D. contracts and lowers
    E. does not change

40. A legal order to present records, correspondence, and documents as evidence is a(n)
    A. interrogatory
    B. deposition
    C. subpoena
    D. citation
    E. warrant

41. The term for the patient agreeing to a procedure with reasonable knowledge of and a capacity to understand the procedure is
    A. burden of proof
    B. informed consent
    C. implied consent
    D. expressed consent
    E. written consent

42. In a negligence case, the most crucial element in determining whether or not a medical assistant used due care is
    A. the medical assistant's length of experience
    B. the medical assistant's training and background
    C. the professional credentials of the medical assistant
    D. the reasonable, prudent conduct of others in the same circumstance
    E. contributory negligence on the part of the patient

43. A living will is written to ensure which of the following patient rights?
    A. refuse treatment while mentally competent
    B. choose a physician
    C. make certain arrangements concerning disposition of a body after death
    D. name a power of attorney
    E. choose types of treatments to be allowed when death is imminent

44. Ethical practices for the medical assistant include which of the following?
    A. Turning over a patient account to a collection agency without the doctor's review.
    B. Using sample nonprescription drugs without the physician's knowledge.
    C. Charging for a cancellation, if the policy is known beforehand by the patients.
    D. Saying to a patient "I'm sure the doctor will make you feel better."
    E. Saying to a patient "We don't use that type of treatment here."

45. Which of the following could involve a statute of limitations?
    A. real estate deed
    B. power of attorney
    C. promissory note
    D. uncashed check
    E. returned check

46. An elderly patient in good health states she wishes her life would end. The medical assistant would regard this patient as a person who is
    A. feeling sorry for herself
    B. dissatisfied with her medical care
    C. lonely
    D. out of touch with reality
    E. a potential suicide

47. During the pediatric appointment, infants need to be close to their mothers during the examination. This is related to Erikson's first stage of development, which is
    A. dependence
    B. trust
    C. autonomy
    D. stranger anxiety
    E. object permanence

48. A hypochondriac is one who is
    A. clinically depressed over an illness
    B. fearful of injury to one's body
    C. abnormally concerned with one's health
    D. abnormally concerned with one's environment
    E. abnormally concerned with one's body

49. Which of the following is an illustration of verbal communication?
    A. a baby's cry
    B. a stranger's frown
    C. a friend's smile
    D. shaking the head from side to side to say "no"
    E. the patient's medical record

50. An incident in which the patient refuses to go into the bathroom because he believes there are spiders in all bathrooms would be recorded as the patient having
    A. delusions
    B. illusions
    C. fantasies
    D. hallucinations
    E. phobias

51. When dealing with a mentally ill patient, it is appropriate for the medical assistant to
    A. talk about the patient's mental problem
    B. keep conversation to a minimum to avoid extremes of mood in the patient
    C. relax the atmosphere by making light of a patient's fears, if they are silly
    D. get the patient to laugh at his or her own fears
    E. talk with the patient at a lesser level of reasoning

52. A patient having an examination prior to being admitted for a biopsy and possible mastectomy is upset. A primary reason women are afraid to have a mastectomy is that they fear
    A. a permanent loss of being femininely attractive
    B. that the physician may have made an incorrect diagnosis
    C. loss of use of the arm on the affected side
    D. a loss of control in decision making
    E. a loss of control in fighting the spread of the disease

53. A patient confides in you that he is afraid of what might happen if his test results are positive. How would the medical assistant best respond to this patient?
    A. "What type of thoughts concern you?"
    B. "Don't be afraid when you have made so much progress."
    C. "The doctor says you are doing just fine."
    D. "Why are you afraid? We are here to take care of you."
    E. "What you need to do now is work at getting better."

54. A patient says to the medical assistant, "I don't want you to tell the doctor, but I don't like the way he treats me or talks to me." The medical assistant should explain to the patient
    A. that he should not say such things
    B. that he should not feel that way
    C. why the patient feels that way
    D. why the doctor acts in a certain way
    E. why you want to let the physician know of his complaint

55. Which of the following is correct?
    A. contusion
    B. contussion
    C. contution
    D. contutian
    E. contuscion

56. A food exchange list is a
    A. guide to monounsaturated, saturated, and polyunsaturated fats
    B. guide to the recommended dietary allowances of vitamins and minerals
    C. computation formula for determining specific caloric needs (energy intake)
    D. table of daily caloric requirements, by age, of the four basic food groups
    E. standard caloric diet model for measuring daily food intake

57. Which of the following is correct?
    A. assymptomatic
    B. assymptamatic
    C. assymtomatic
    D. asymtomatic
    E. asymptomatic

58. An invasive procedure is
    A. surgical entry into tissues, where bleeding occurs or may occur
    B. infection control for limiting the transmission of disease
    C. one performed without the patient's knowledge
    D. the entry and spread of microorganisms in the human tissues
    E. the use of interferon as treatment for viral diseases

59. A fungal condition of the foot, called athlete's foot, is also termed
    A. pediculosis
    B. phthiriasis
    C. pityriasis
    D. tinea pedis
    E. tinea versicolor

60. Which of the following is the correct spelling in the NOUN form?
    A. mucous
    B. mucus
    C. moucous
    D. moucus
    E. mucosal

61. The term for menstruating less frequently than normal is
    A. amenorrhea
    B. menorrhagia
    C. metrorrhagia
    D. menometrorrhagia
    E. oligomenorrhea

62. Which of the following is correct?
    A. parithyroid
    B. parethyroid
    C. parothyroid
    D. parathyroid
    E. perithyroid

63. One condition in which the patient has a strong tendency to bleed is
    A. von Willebrand's disease
    B. thalassemia
    C. thrombophlebitis
    D. leukemia
    E. sickle cell disease

64. Bulimia is
    A. an eating disorder characterized by binge eating followed by purging
    B. excessive appetite
    C. a mass of food
    D. a condition of lesions larger than 1 cm
    E. inflammation of the bulb of the urethra

65. Small, purplish, hemorrhagic spots on the skin are called
    A. petechiae
    B. chloasma
    C. ecchymosis
    D. onychia
    E. nevi

66. The medical term for a stroke is
    A. aneurysm
    B. cerebral vascular accident
    C. cerebral contusion
    D. cerebroma
    E. angina

67. Which of the following is correct?
    A. arythmia
    B. arythmea
    C. arhythmia
    D. arrythmia
    E. arrhythmia

68. A microorganism that lives in the presence of free oxygen is said to be aero-
    A. bic
    B. genic
    C. pathic
    D. pnagic
    E. philic

69. Desquamation is a term meaning
    A. tanning of the skin
    B. sloughing of skin cells
    C. the formation of a scab
    D. the healing of wound edges
    E. the production of new skin

70. Which of the following is correct?
    A. diabetes melitus
    B. diabetes mellitus
    C. diabetis melitus
    D. diabetis mellitus
    E. diabetis mellitis

71. The medical term for tissue forcibly torn from the body is
    A. laceration
    B. puncture
    C. abrasion
    D. avulsion
    E. adhesion

72. The presence of increased protein in the urine is called
    A. albuminuria
    B. ketonuria
    C. urobilinogenuria
    D. urobilinuria
    E. pyuria

73. Drugs used to dilate the pupils of the eyes are called
    A. mycterics
    B. mydriatics
    C. myectopics
    D. myopics
    E. myotonics

74. Which of the following is correct?
    A. nucular isotoap
    B. nuclear isotoap
    C. nuculer isotope
    D. nuclear isotope
    E. nucular isotope

75. The most common nonmedical term for a myocardial infarction is
    A. stroke
    B. heart failure
    C. heart attack
    D. angina
    E. rheumatic fever

76. Which of the following is correct?
    A. decubitis ulcer
    B. decubites ulcer
    C. decubitus ulcer
    D. decubites ulser
    E. decubitis ulser

77. Which of the following is correct?
    A. optician
    B. optition
    C. optitian
    D. optisian
    E. optishian

78. Characteristics of white blood cells include each of the following EXCEPT
    A. They filter out foreign bacteria.
    B. They aid in combating foreign bacteria.
    C. They are part of the formation of pus.
    D. They help to repair tissue.
    E. They regulate metabolism.

79. Which of the following neoplasms is a malignant tumor of nerve tissue?
    A. nevus
    B. multiple myeloma
    C. meningioma
    D. glioma
    E. neuroma

80. Each of the following patients has an established, implied contract with the physician EXCEPT
    A. emergency victims
    B. incompetent adults
    C. minors
    D. pro bono patients
    E. patients covered in full by insurance carriers

81. Each of the following is true concerning the patient-physician relationship EXCEPT
    A. A contract is usually implied.
    B. A contract must be expressed.
    C. Services must be provided.
    D. The relationship begins when the patient arrives for the first appointment.
    E. The patient must understand the relationship.

82. Drainage of congested paranasal sinuses may be by
    A. suction set up during blowing of the nose
    B. lymphatic osmosis
    C. both A and B
    D. ciliary action
    E. both A and D

83. The air spaces that make up the paranasal sinuses include the
    A. frontal sinuses
    B. maxillary sinuses
    C. both A and B
    D. mastoid sinuses
    E. both A and D

84. Ear wax is made up of secretions from
    A. apocrine glands
    B. auricular glands
    C. both A and B
    D. ceruminous glands
    E. both A and D

85. Examples of nociceptive reflexes include
    A. winking
    B. coughing
    C. both A and B
    D. Babinski reflex
    E. both A and D

86. On normal examination, cerebrospinal fluid contains
    A. white blood cells
    B. red blood cells
    C. both A and B
    D. protein
    E. both A and D

87. The gluteus maximus muscle is important in
    A. walking
    B. rising from a sitting position
    C. both A and B
    D. erect standing posture
    E. both A and D

88. The skin helps to regulate
    A. body temperature
    B. electrolyte balance
    C. both A and B
    D. waste elimination
    E. both A and D

89. The dorsal cavity includes the
    A. lungs and heart
    B. stomach
    C. both A and B
    D. spinal cord and spinal cord nerve roots
    E. both A and D

90. The posterior nasal cavity may be examined through the
    A. nostril
    B. pharynx
    C. both A and B
    D. auditory tube
    E. both A and D

91. The sternoclavicular joint is formed by the sternum, the clavicle, and the
    A. vertebrae
    B. first costal cartilage
    C. humerus
    D. scapula
    E. xiphoid process

92. The central nervous system is composed of the brain and the
    A. cranial nerves
    B. peripheral nerves
    C. spinal cord
    D. sympathetic and parasympathetic systems
    E. motor nerves

93. Minerals important to bone formation include calcium and
    A. phosphorus
    B. iron
    C. magnesium
    D. sodium
    E. potassium

94. In the patient-physician contract, the implied consent of the patient includes a willingness to
    A. follow the physician's advice
    B. pay for services rendered
    C. both A and B
    D. release records to third-party providers
    E. both A and D

95. Persons licensed to prescribe a drug include the
    A. physician
    B. pharmacy assistant
    C. both A and B
    D. pharmacist
    E. both A and D

96. In cases of negligence, defenses include which of the following?
    A. informed consent
    B. contributory negligence
    C. both A and B
    D. res ipsa loquitur
    E. both A and D

97. A tort is an injury or wrong committed
    A. by one person to another person or property of another
    B. either by omission or wrongful act
    C. both A and B
    D. for which the wrongdoer is subject to punishment by the state
    E. both A and D

98. Prothrombin and fibrinogen, which aid in the clotting of blood, are produced in the
    A. liver
    B. spleen
    C. bone marrow
    D. pancreas
    E. lymph nodes

99. Diets that control disorders of carbohydrate metabolism are used to treat
    A. anorexia nervosa
    B. obesity
    C. bulimia
    D. diabetes mellitus
    E. starvation

100. Terms for headache include
    A. cephalodynia
    B. cephalalgia
    C. both A and B
    D. neuralgia
    E. both A and D

Part 2—Administrative Procedures

Directions: *Each of the following questions or incomplete statements precedes five suggested answers or completions. Select the ONE answer or completion that is BEST in each case and fill in the circle containing the corresponding letter on the answer sheet.*

101. When setting an appointment for a pelvic examination, the patient should be instructed
    A. not to douche for 2 weeks
    B. not to douche for 1 week
    C. not to douche for 1 to 2 days
    D. to douche the evening before the examination
    E. to douche the morning of the examination

102. The time scheduled for a first visit of a patient with a history of hypertension should be
    A. 15 minutes
    B. 20 minutes
    C. 30 minutes
    D. 45 minutes
    E. 1.5 hours

103. A collection of forms that have the same design and are stored together on a disk under one particular file name is a
    A. database
    B. data file
    C. document file
    D. field
    E. working copy

104. A dot followed by three letters added to the end of a file name is called an
    A. alternate field name
    B. enhancement
    C. extension
    D. identifier spec
    E. ordering number

105. A path indicating a particular disk, directory, and file name may be entered on the computer as
    A. C:/Directory/File
    B. C:Directory/File
    C. C:Directory:File
    D. C\Directory\File
    E. C:\Directory\File

106. After retrieving a manuscript, you accidentally delete a major portion of the work on the screen. You would
    A. rekey the deleted material
    B. rename the document, then retrieve the stored version again
    C. exit your work without saving and retrieve the stored version again
    D. save the current work, then retrieve the stored version again
    E. delete the current file, then retrieve the stored version again

107. If you are not on-line, which of the following computer equipment can be eliminated?
    A. CPU
    B. monitor
    C. disk drive
    D. printer
    E. modem

108. The proofreader mark "stet" means
    A. take out
    B. let stand as originally set
    C. straighten alignment
    D. query to author: has this been set as intended?
    E. character of a wrong size or cap style

109. The proofreader mark "#" tells the typesetter to
   A. add a number
   B. begin a new paragraph
   C. insert a space
   D. indent
   E. enclose in brackets

110. The Index Medicus is published by
   A. Medical Economics, Inc.
   B. Slack, Inc.
   C. American Medical Association
   D. National Library of Medicine
   E. American Hospital Association

111. The computer equivalent to Index Medicus is
   A. MEDALERT
   B. MEDLINE
   C. MEDLINE/Health File
   D. EMBASE
   E. EMPIRES

112. On the calculator, if the CE key is depressed before striking the arithmetic function key, it will
   A. clear an incorrectly depressed number key
   B. erase the keyboard register
   C. erase the operating register
   D. erase the keyboard register and the operating register
   E. erase the keyboard register, the operating register, and storage memory

113. Funds can be automatically transferred from one account to the other by
   A. a one-write check-writing system
   B. using a software program to print checks
   C. opening up a special checking account
   D. electronic fund transfer systems at the bank
   E. going on-line with a bank

114. When you are purchasing supplies, a manufacturer offers an item at $20 each less 5% each if you purchase six or more. You buy six and will pay the invoice price of
   A. $6
   B. $84
   C. $90
   D. $114
   E. $120

115. In double-entry bookkeeping, the book of original entry is the
   A. patient ledger card
   B. daily log
   C. appointment book
   D. general ledger
   E. chart of accounts

116. The business-related accounts receivable is considered a business
   A. current asset
   B. fixed asset
   C. current liability
   D. long-term liability
   E. owner's equity

117. If a pegboard system is not used, patient receipts should be issued if the patient
   A. requests one
   B. pays in cash
   C. pays by check
   D. makes no payment
   E. has insurance coverage

118. Which of the following must be completed with the patient if a payment plan is set up for more than four payments?
   A. promissory note
   B. truth-in-lending statement
   C. fee schedule
   D. medical insurance record
   E. surgical cost estimate

119. A $40.00 invoice offers a 3% discount if paid within 10 days. Within that time period, you would make the check for
   A. $28.00
   B. $37.00
   C. $38.00
   D. $38.80
   E. $39.88

120. Calculate the amount of simple interest you would have to pay if you borrowed $500 at 12% for 6 months.
   A. $12
   B. $30
   C. $60
   D. $72
   E. $120

121. The fee for service may be reduced if a patient
    A. refuses to pay the bill
    B. has received a bill for the full amount and says she cannot afford to pay it
    C. complains that the fee is excessive
    D. has died
    E. has had a poor result from treatment

122. Banking fees will appear on a monthly statement in the form of a
    A. credit
    B. voucher check
    C. service charge
    D. withdrawal
    E. draft

123. A plan for both basic medical insurance and services beyond those covered in the basic medical portion is
    A. major medical plan
    B. reciprocity program
    C. indemnity plan
    D. service benefit plan
    E. usual, customary, and reasonable fee plan

124. The spouse of an active-duty marine is being treated for a difficult pregnancy. The patient has a Blue Shield plan, as well as CHAMPUS. The medical assistant would bill first
    A. CHAMPVA
    B. CHAMPUS
    C. Blue Shield and CHAMPVA
    D. Blue Shield and CHAMPUS
    E. Blue Shield

125. If a physician's fee is to be paid through coinsurance, the medical assistant will bill
    A. the patient and the patient's employer
    B. the patient's employer only
    C. a primary and secondary insurer
    D. the insurance carrier and workers' compensation
    E. the patient and the insurance carrier

126. Workers' compensation payments are made
    A. directly to the physician
    B. by the patient who is reimbursed
    C. after the patient meets a deductible
    D. on an 80%–20% copayment plan with the patient
    E. by the patient's employer

127. CHAMPUS dependents are issued an identification card at
    A. birth
    B. age 10
    C. age 16
    D. age 18
    E. age 21

128. Which of the following is an insurance claim processing error?
    A. stating the substance, amount, and route for injections
    B. itemizing surgical trays and supplies as separate fees
    C. itemizing multiple visits occurring on the same date
    D. entering referred consultations, but not referred laboratory or x-ray work-ups
    E. stating presurgical care is for a medical diagnosis rather than surgery

129. Under Medicare, a retired couple has to pay an annual deductible
    A. per illness
    B. per admission
    C. per person
    D. per family unit
    E. every 15 months

130. Nonduplication of benefits means that
    A. benefits will not cover the same condition twice
    B. benefits will not cover pre-existing conditions
    C. the physician may not bill more than one insurance company
    D. benefits will not cover conditions covered by a previous insurance policy
    E. benefits will be coordinated between two separate insurance companies

131. The correct transcription of the underlined dictation "the wound was closed with *four oh* black silk" is
    A. 4–0
    B. four-0
    C. either 4–0 or four-0
    D. 0000
    E. either 4–0 or 0000

132. For an ICD-9 diagnostic code to be valid, the maximum number of code digits is
    A. two
    B. three
    C. four
    D. five
    E. six

133. For ambulatory surgery, which of the following is ICD-9 CM coded first?
    A. previous conditions that require patient care
    B. coexisting conditions that require patient care
    C. coexisting conditions that affect patient treatment
    D. preoperative diagnosis
    E. postoperative diagnosis

134. A patient with acute chest pain is examined by the doctor. An ECG and enzyme studies are ordered. The diagnosis reads: "rule out acute myocardial infarction." The medical assistant would code the case
    A. "acute myocardial infarction"
    B. "rule out acute myocardial infarction"
    C. "probable myocardial infarction"
    D. "acute and chronic coronary artery disease"
    E. "chest pain"

135. Capital equipment purchases must be recorded and documented separately because they are
    A. under warranty
    B. expendable
    C. taken as a tax credit within the year
    D. depreciated over a period of years
    E. appreciated over a period of years

136. Filing of medical records should be completed
    A. once a week
    B. daily
    C. twice a day
    D. when the file box is full
    E. after the use of each record

137. Which filing system will provide the greatest amount of confidentiality?
    A. alphabetic
    B. numeric
    C. subject by disease
    D. geographic
    E. descriptive

138. When collecting patient data, which of the following questions should you avoid?
    A. "What brings you here?"
    B. "How would you describe your general health?"
    C. "Do you have any brothers or sisters?"
    D. "Is there anything else you would like to tell me?"
    E. "What do you think is the matter with you?"

139. Records may be released without further signature
    A. after the patient has transferred his care to a new doctor
    B. after the patient has died
    C. to insurance companies
    D. as long as there is a blanket release signed and on file
    E. if the release signature is for the current request

140. An example of a subjective note in a patient's medical record is the
    A. medical history
    B. examination finding
    C. laboratory report
    D. diagnosis
    E. treatment

141. A patient who had a testicular mass discovered during a routine physical examination is being referred to a surgeon. Which of the following is the correct way to handle this referral before the patient leaves the office?
    A. Write the name and number of the referral on office stationery.
    B. Give the patient the business card of the referral physician.
    C. Call and notify the referral office that the patient will be calling.
    D. Set the appointment for the patient before he leaves.
    E. Tell the patient you will set the appointment later and call him with the date.

142. In keeping patient medical records, records for patients who have allergies should be
   A. kept in a separate filing system
   B. kept in folders of a specific color
   C. labeled with their specific allergies on the front of the record
   D. labeled with their specific allergies on every page of the medical record
   E. labeled with the word allergy on the filing folder

143. The abbreviation for the system of medical record-keeping that is based on the patient's health problems is
   A. MICR
   B. POMR
   C. CPT
   D. ICD-9
   E. CRVS

144. Which of the following processes would be the same for all filing systems?
   A. inspecting
   B. indexing
   C. coding
   D. sorting
   E. storing

145. Which of the following statements is true concerning current trends in the use of the patient's medical record?
   A. Patients are being allowed to see their records.
   B. Patients are participating by making their own entries on their records.
   C. Health facilities are being discouraged from automating medical records.
   D. Medical assistants have less access to patient confidential information.
   E. Health facility use of premanufactured history forms is decreasing.

146. The best filing system for medical and scientified reports is
   A. alphabetic
   B. numeric
   C. subject
   D. chronologic
   E. by publisher

147. The patient's name is Mary Louise Hoffman-Jones. She is married to Alan Richard Jones. Which is her third indexing unit?
   A. Mary
   B. Louise
   C. Hoffman
   D. Mrs.
   E. Alan

148. In terminal-digit filing, which number would come after 88 34 23?
   A. 88 34 24
   B. 88 34 33
   C. 88 35 23
   D. 89 34 23
   E. 89 34 24

149. The abbreviations RUQ, LUQ, RLQ, LLQ describe an examination of the patient's
   A. electric impulses of the brain
   B. electric currents generated by the heart
   C. chest
   D. abdomen
   E. retina

150. When you receive a call placed by a referring physician, you should
   A. make the appointment
   B. put the call through to the physician
   C. take a message and have the physician return the call
   D. take the patient's information and call the patient to set the appointment
   E. take the patient's information and give it to your physician to call

151. In the terminal-digit filing system, a folder is numbered 88 34 23. This number would be filed in
   A. section 23, guide 34, 88th in sequence
   B. section 88, guide 34, 23rd in sequence
   C. section 23, guide 88, 34th in sequence
   D. section 88, guide 23, 34th in sequence
   E. section 34, guide 23, 88th in sequence

152. Under which guide should an equipment inventory based on useful life be filed?
   A. Equipment-Receipts
   B. Equipment-Master List
   C. Equipment-Budget
   D. Equipment-Maintenance and Repairs
   E. Equipment-Purchases

153. The name of the filing system used to call patients to set appointments or confirm appointments is the
   A. follow-up file
   B. tickler file
   C. both A and B
   D. appointment file
   E. both A and D

154. The group is considering the purchase of a computer system for all business functions. A discount mail-order supply house has a special discount for bulk ordering of typewriter ribbons. Which is the cost effective consideration?
   A. Will the quantity be used in reasonable time to justify the current cash output?
   B. Will deterioration take place before the ribbons can be used?
   C. Will there be space to conveniently store the ribbons?
   D. Will you discontinue using the product before the supply is used?
   E. Will the manufacturer accept return of the product if there are defects?

155. Which of the following is permissible to abbreviate in the inside address of a letter?
   A. Mister
   B. William
   C. Road
   D. Street
   E. Kansas City

156. Which of the following is considered a friendly and informal close when the writer and reader are on a first-name basis and a comma is used after the salutation?
   A. Very truly yours
   B. Yours very truly
   C. Sincerely yours
   D. Best wishes
   E. Sincerely

157. "*Tapping* of the *achilles* tendon produced a normal reflex. There appears to be no injury to the spinal cord or leg muscles, which *supersedes* my *preliminary* diagnosis." Which of the italicized words is an error in transcription?
   A. Tapping
   B. achilles
   C. ,
   D. supersedes
   E. preliminary

158. How would you transcribe the dictation: "auscultation revealed a grade four reflux on the right"?
   A. grade four
   B. Grade four
   C. Grade 4
   D. grade iv
   E. grade IV

159. In the following correspondence, which part can be omitted?
   Mabel Smith, M.D.
   Department of Radiography
   Building 4 - Room 301
   P.O. Box 225
   2345 Meeting Street
   Atlanta, GA 00101
   A. Department of Radiography
   B. Building 4
   C. Room 301
   D. P.O. Box 225
   E. 2345 Meeting Street

160. A letter prepared with mixed punctuation will use which punctuation after the salutation?
   A. none
   B. comma
   C. semicolon
   D. colon
   E. period

161. If the writer wishes copies of a letter distributed to a list of people without the list shown on the original,
   A. type "cc:" but no names on all copies
   B. type "bcc:" and the recipient names on each of the carbon copies
   C. make no notation either on the original or on the carbon copies
   D. stamp "blind carbon copies sent" on the original only
   E. recommend the writer not use blind carbon copies

162. In professional correspondence to a woman holding a doctorate degree and her husband, one proper inside address and salutation would be
   A. Mr. and Mrs. Alan E. Jones
      Dear Mr. and Mrs. Jones:
   B. Mr. and Dr. Alan E. Jones
      Dear Mr. Jones and Dr. Jones:
   C. Mr. Alan E. Jones and Jane L. Jones, MD
      Dear Dr. and Mr. Jones:
   D. Dr. Jane L. Jones and Mr. Alan E. Jones
      Dear Dr. Jones and Mr. Jones
   E. Jane L. Jones, MD and Mr. Alan E. Jones
      Dear Dr. and Mr. Jones

163. Each of the following would receive copies of workers' compensation reports EXCEPT
   A. the employer
   B. the employee
   C. the insurance carrier
   D. the physician
   E. the state compensation board

164. On the HCFA 1500 claim form, each of the following is true EXCEPT which?
   A. For Medicaid, one diagnosis will be allowed.
   B. For Medicaid, only two diagnoses will be allowed.
   C. Past diagnoses are not submitted if they have no impact on the current diagnosis.
   D. The principal diagnosis submitted by the doctor and the hospital must be the same.
   E. Separate records are sent with claims only if requested.

165. Each of the following business documents should be kept permanently EXCEPT
   A. tax records older than the last three returns
   B. receipts for depreciated business equipment
   C. cancelled checks older than 3 years
   D. professional liability policies no longer in effect
   E. case histories of patients moved to another physician

166. Concerning patient medical records, each of the following statements is true EXCEPT which?
   A. They are used for research purposes.
   B. They are inadmissable in a court of law.
   C. They are used by review committees for evaluating the quality of care.
   D. They are used for exchanging information among medical assisting staff.
   E. They are used to teach medical and allied health students.

167. Each of the following statements about numeric filing is true EXCEPT which?
   A. Numeric filing allows unlimited expansion without folder shifting.
   B. Shelving or drawers are filled evenly.
   C. Filing activity is greatest at the end of the numeric series.
   D. The system is recommended for offices with greater than 15,000 files
   E. The system requires less training.

168. Each of the following statements concerning filing is true EXCEPT which?
   A. Microfiche is a transparent rectangle of film.
   B. Roll microfilm storage is ideal for records that need frequent updating.
   C. Microfiche is a small half-sheet document that is filed horizontally.
   D. A visible label is placed on microfiche to serve as a "drawer label."
   E. Computer output microfilm eliminates the paper printout.

169. Each of the following medical record notations is appropriate following the examination of a woman suspected to be a victim of spouse abuse EXCEPT
   A. recorder's initials
   B. time of the examination
   C. date of the examination
   D. the position of the patient during the examination
   E. the types of specimens collected

170. Each of the following should be noted in the patient's medical record EXCEPT
    A. collections telephone conversation
    B. telephone conversation about an insurance claim
    C. letter from the patient stating thank you for a particular treatment
    D. pharmacist's phone request for a prescription renewal
    E. a no-show appointment

171. After loading DOS into RAM, the operating disk is necessary for which of the following commands?
    A. Type
    B. Dir
    C. Save
    D. Format
    E. Retrieve

172. Which of the following records must be permanently kept?
    A. a patient's note of appreciation
    B. a patient's request to transfer records to another physician
    C. both A and B
    D. a patient's request for an annual itemized statement
    E. both A and D

173. Which of the following provides the sender with a record of delivery?
    A. registered mail
    B. certificate of mailing
    C. certified mail
    D. special delivery
    E. return receipt requested

174. Which of the following would be found on a balance sheet?
    A. assets
    B. liabilities
    C. both A and B
    D. income and expenses
    E. both A and D

175. Medicare, Part B covers
    A. elective cosmetic surgery
    B. routine physical examinations
    C. eyeglasses and hearing aid examinations
    D. prescription drugs
    E. immunizations for travel

176. When a physician agrees to participate in CHAMPUS, the medical assistant must
    A. accept the insurance payment as payment in full
    B. write off the difference between what was billed and what was paid
    C. bill the patient for the full amount and collect from the patient
    D. directly bill the CHAMPUS fiscal intermediary
    E. provide the patient a statement to submit for direct reimbursement

177. For which of the following must a patient be 65 years of age or older to receive Medicare coverage?
    A. renal dialysis
    B. heart bypass
    C. permanent disability
    D. kidney transplant donor
    E. blind

178. The International Classification of Diseases is used to code
    A. operations
    B. laboratory tests
    C. imaging studies
    D. psychologic testing
    E. diagnoses

179. Medicare patients who are treated by nonparticipating physicians must
    A. participate in the plan for 3 months
    B. pay for their charges than apply for reimbursement
    C. pay a higher deductible
    D. complete their forms themselves
    E. pay for services not covered by Medicare provided they are informed in advance that the service is not covered.

180. A patient is diagnosed with a chronic duodenal ulcer that is now perforated and bleeding. The medical assistant should properly code the case with which of the following ICD-9 specifics?
    A. acute condition; hemorrhage involved
    B. acute condition; hemorrhage involved; perforation involved
    C. acute condition; perforation involved
    D. acute condition; chronic history involved; perforation involved
    E. acute condition; hemorrhage involved; perforation involved; chronic history involved

181. X-ray examination findings must accompany radiology charges when submitting
    A. Medicare claims
    B. CHAMPUS claims
    C. CHAMPVA claims
    D. Medicaid claims
    E. workers' compensation claims

182. Persons who qualify for Medicare Part A benefits without charge include
    A. dependent widows or widowers between ages 50 and 65
    B. the blind and disabled of any age
    C. both A and B
    D. those who have not worked enough quarters to qualify for SS
    E. both A and D

183. When a shipment of medical supplies is received, the medical assistant should record in an inventory log
    A. catalog prices
    B. order request date
    C. amounts received
    D. freight/delivery charges
    E. volume discounts

184. The following responses represent on-arrival notations typed on envelopes. Upon arrival, which incoming mail pieces may NOT be opened by the medical assistant?
    A. "HOLD FOR ARRIVAL"
    B. "Attention: John Poroski, M.D."
    C. "PLEASE FORWARD"
    D. "CONFIDENTIAL"
    E. "Special Delivery"

185. For a letter requiring quick delivery service, which is the most economical way to get it there?
    A. Federal Express Priority Mail
    B. Federal Express Second Day
    C. Federal Express Standard Overnight
    D. U.S. Post Office Priority Mail
    E. UPS Overnight Delivery

186. If a patient cancels an appointment, the medical assistant should
    A. draw a line through the appointment
    B. write "canceled" above the patient's name
    C. write in the date the patient canceled
    D. write in the reason the patient cancelled
    E. erase the appointment

187. A written release of records is required when sending information to
    A. Medicare
    B. referral physician
    C. spouse
    D. a police department investigating an abuse case
    E. a health department communicable disease division

188. A referral letter should contain
    A. the condition for which the patient is being referred
    B. the entire past history of the patient
    C. both A and B
    D. a description of the treatment (if any) given so far
    E. both A and D

189. True statements about the medical record include which of the following?
    A. The patient owns the information.
    B. The physician owns the record.
    C. Legally, if it is not recorded, it was not done.
    D. A signed release is waived for subpoenaed records.
    E. all of the above

190. Color-coded files enable
    A. unlimited expansion without periodic shifting of folders
    B. filing without indexing
    C. better confidentiality of records
    D. better visualization of misfiles
    E. easier grouping of miscellaneous records

191. An address in which the abbreviated form of "esquire" is correctly used is
    A. Simpson, Tyler, and MacDonald, Esqs.
    B. Hon. Mary Barnes, Esq.
    C. Ms. Carolyn B. West, Esq. Attorney-at-Law
    D. Mr. Clyde Simpson, Esq.
    E. Honorable Wilson, Esq.

192. The correct style for enclosure notations is
    A. Enclosure
    B. enclosure
    C. encl:
    D. enc
    E. encl

193. When finalizing transcribed dictation for signature, the physician has the responsibility to
    A. correct improper sentence structure
    B. make sure material makes grammatical sense
    C. correct punctuation
    D. spell each word correctly
    E. correct meaning and content

194. "A prescription for flagyl was written by the referring physician to treat a recurrent infection of trichomonas vaginalis." From this dictation, words that need a capitalized first letter include:
    A. flagyl
    B. trichomonas
    C. both A and B
    D. vaginalis
    E. both A and D

195. In the letter (Fig. 4–1), the letter style is
    A. block
    B. modified block
    C. semiblock
    D. modfied semiblock
    E. official

196. In the letter style (Fig. 4–1), each of the following may be positioned flush left EXCEPT
    A. special mailing notation
    B. on-arrival notation
    C. Attention line
    D. carbon copy notation
    E. postscript

197. In the letter style (Fig. 4–1), an attention line would be positioned
    A. single-spaced and directly below the date line
    B. two lines above the inside address
    C. two lines below the inside address
    D. two lines below the salutation
    E. two lines above the first paragraph

198. In the letter (Fig. 4–1), each of the following designations is correct EXCEPT
    A. the addressee's full name and academic degree
    B. the addressee's professional title
    C. the salutation
    D. the courtesy titles in the message
    E. the signature block

199. If you were to include a reference line in the letter (Fig. 4–1), it would be positioned
    A. flush left above the date line
    B. one line above the date line and blocked with the date line
    C. one line above the salutation and flush left
    D. blocked with the date line, one line above the salutation
    E. flush left one line below the salutation

200. Which of the following sources would have the most comprehensive information concerning the control of infection?
    A. a state health department
    B. U.S. Public Health Service
    C. American Medical Association
    D. Federal Food and Drug Administration
    E. The World Health Organization

Anna M. Robinson, MD
Letterhead Street Address
Letterhead City, ST 32321-1234
Tele: (101) 555-1212

May 23, 19--

Reginald Graves, Ph.D.
Vice President of Academic Affairs
Sloane-Kettering Medical School
8900 Letterman Boulevard
Fort Johnson, ST 35567-4342

Dear Dr. Graves:

In the absence of Dr. Robinson, I am acknowledging receipt of your invitation for Dr. Robinson to speak at the Society's Annual Conference on August 10, 19-- at the Fort Johnson Convention Center.

Dr. Robinson will return on June 10, 19--, after a trip to Canada. As soon as she returns, I will make your letter available to her promptly.

Sincerely yours,

Joan Smith

Joan Smith, CMA
Certified Medical Assistant

Figure 4–1. Letter of acknowledgment.

SIMULATION TEST 4

Part 3—Clinical Procedures

Directions: *Each of the following questions or incomplete statements precedes five suggested answers or completions. Select the ONE answer or completion that is BEST in each case and fill in the circle containing the corresponding letter on the answer sheet.*

201. The quickest method of sterilization for instruments with sharp, cutting edges is
    A. steam under pressure autoclave
    B. dry oven autoclave
    C. chemical sterilant
    D. boiling water
    E. cold chemical disinfection

202. Which of the following is the acceptable practice with a contaminated syringe needle?
    A. recapping the needle after use
    B. if a needle must be preserved, recapping with one hand against a countertop
    C. bending and breaking the needle using a gauze 4×4, then double bagging the needle
    D. with the needle cap, bending and breaking the needle inside the cap
    E. breaking the needle using a destructclip or similar device

203. During minor surgery, the circulating assistant is requested to place sterile dressings from a covered, sterile Bard-Parker tray onto the sterile field. Which of the following is the correct procedure for the tray lid while the dressings are being transferred?
    A. placing the lid inside up on a counter
    B. placing the lid inside down on a counter
    C. placing the lid inside down on the sterile field
    D. holding the lid over the sterile field inside up
    E. holding the lid above and to the side of the tray, inside down

204. On a Celsius scale, a Fahrenheit temperature of 103.8° would be
    A. 38°
    B. 29°
    C. 39.9°
    D. 40.5°
    E. 41.1°

205. During an irrigation of the eye, the patient's head should be
    A. tilted with the eye to be treated uppermost, the patient gazing downward
    B. tilted with the eye to be treated uppermost, the patient gazing upward
    C. tilted with the eye to be treated downward, the patient gazing downward
    D. tilted with the eye to be treated downward, the patient gazing upward
    E. positioned in straight alignment with the body, the patient gazing upward

206. When one is clamping a suture needle with the needle holder, it is important to clamp the needle
    A. just above the atraumatic point
    B. at the lower one third of the curve
    C. at midpoint
    D. at the upper one third of the curve
    E. just below the point of attachment with the thread

207. On the ordinary radiograph, which part of the musculoskeletal system is not visible?
    A. periosteum
    B. compact bone
    C. spongy bone
    D. epiphysial line
    E. muscle

208. The medical assistant is asked to remove cerumen from a patient. What instrument would be used?
    A. Lucae bayonet forceps
    B. Larry probe
    C. Hartmann alligator ear forceps
    D. Buck ear curette
    E. Reiner ear syringe

209. The physician performs a breast examination. The method of examination used is
    A. mensuration
    B. palpation
    C. inspection
    D. percussion
    E. tapotement

210. During ophthalmoscopy, the physician examines the
    A. conjunctiva
    B. sclera
    C. choroid
    D. retina
    E. lacrimal gland

211. If a "fading sound" heard from 84 mm to 72 mm is to be included in the recording of a patient's blood pressure, you would chart it as
    A. 13/84-72/72
    B. 130/84-72
    C. 130/84/72
    D. 130/72/84
    E. 130/72

212. A physician reports on the medical record that the patient has carotid stenosis. This condition is detected by auscultation of the
    A. coronary artery system
    B. aorta
    C. arteries supplying the arms and legs
    D. valves of the heart
    E. arteries of the neck and head

213. A patient's blood pressure is 160/95. Her pulse pressure is
    A. 1.7
    B. 65
    C. 95
    D. 160
    E. 255

214. During determination of a patient's blood pressure, an auscultatory gap (loss of Korotkoff sound) occurs in
    A. phase I
    B. phase II
    C. phase III
    D. phase IV
    E. phase V

215. The medical assistant obtains the following vital signs on a patient with hypertension and a history of myocardial infarction: T - 99.7F (37.6C); P-.60; R-20; BP-140/96/70 (lying); BP-152/98/80 (standing). Which one should the assistant report promptly?
    A. temperature
    B. pulse
    C. respiration
    D. blood pressure lying to standing
    E. fading sound changes

216. An oral thermometer should not be used in the rectum because it
    A. may injure the rectal mucosa
    B. may fall out
    C. will become contaminated with intestinal microorganisms
    D. is designed to register 1° less than rectal thermometers
    E. is designed to register 1° higher than rectal thermometers

217. The early diagnosis of prostatic conditions is most often made after which of the following examinations?
    A. urine
    B. blood
    C. rectal
    D. proctoscopic
    E. cystoscopic

218. The frontal and paranasal sinuses are initially examined with
    A. palpation
    B. illuminated tongue depressor
    C. Vienna nasal speculum
    D. otoscope
    E. ophthalmoscope

219. When reviewing a patient's past history, which of the following conditions would likely predispose a patient to breast cancer?
    A. breast-feeding four children
    B. having a first child at age 17
    C. having a last child at age 42
    D. having fibrocystic disease
    E. having an abscess of the breast that occurred during lactation

220. When obtaining a blood pressure reading, before placing the stethoscope over the brachial artery the medical assistant would FIRST
    A. palpate the radial artery and inflate cuff 30 mm above pulse disappearance
    B. palpate the brachial artery and inflate 30 mm above pulse disappearance
    C. complete an entire inflation and deflation palpating the radial artery
    D. complete an entire inflation and deflation palpating the brachial artery
    E. palpate the brachial artery

221. If the pulse is irregular, it is recommended that the medical assistant count the pulse rate for a minimum of
    A. 10 seconds
    B. 15 seconds
    C. 30 seconds
    D. 1 minute
    E. 2 minutes

222. One of the typical problems examining a menopausal patient is
    A. urinary incontenance
    B. pain on digital examination
    C. flatulence
    D. bowel incontenance
    E. increased vaginal discharges

223. If a patient develops an allergic reaction to oral penicillin, which is the most likely early reaction?
    A. rash and itching
    B. dizziness and fainting
    C. both A and B
    D. sudden elevation of body temperature
    E. both A and D

224. Too much sensor paste between the patient and the electrode will cause
    A. wandering baseline
    B. AC interference
    C. somatic tremor
    D. recording breaks along the complexes
    E. overdamped stylus

225. In recording lead I of an ECG, you notice a negative R wave. You would
    A. ignore it and continue recording
    B. immediately stop the recording and notify the physician
    C. stop recording and check that the lead wires are connected properly
    D. stop recording and check to see if the patient's limbs are comfortable
    E. stop the recording and reprep the patient's skin

226. You have a large amount of AC interference on leads I and III. The source of the interference is in the direction of the
    A. right arm
    B. left arm
    C. right arm and left arm
    D. left leg
    E. left arm and left leg

227. For which of the following leads must sensors be placed at a specific area for accuracy of the ECG recording?
    A. lead I
    B. inspiration lead
    C. rhythm strip
    D. AVR
    E. V3

228. The P wave represents
    A. atrial depolarization
    B. atrial repolarization
    C. ventricular depolarization
    D. ventricular repolarization
    E. depolarization transversing the A-V node

229. In ECG, leads I, II, and III are the
    A. standard leads
    B. augmented leads
    C. unipolar leads
    D. chest leads
    E. precordial leads

230. Until help arrives the relation of cardiac compressions to rescue breaths during cardiopulmonary resuscitation is
    A. one to five
    B. one to ten
    C. one to fifteen
    D. two to five
    E. two to fifteen

231. Which artery is most often used to check an adult patient's condition in an emergency?
    A. apical
    B. radial
    C. carotid
    D. temporal
    E. femoral

232. Which is the preferred position for administering the Heimlich maneuver?
    A. prone
    B. Sims'
    C. recumbent
    D. sitting
    E. standing

233. A physician orders confirmatory urine testing for albuminuria. The medical assistant would use
    A. sulfosalicylic acid test
    B. Acetest reagent tablets
    C. Ictotest reagent tablets
    D. Clinitest reagent tablets
    E. Benedict's test

234. One selective culture media used for urine cultures is
    A. blood agar
    B. eosin-methylene blue agar
    C. Thayer-Martin agar
    D. chocolate agar
    E. Mueller-Hinton agar

235. One characteristic of the organism that causes gonorrhea is that it is
    A. acid-fast
    B. spore-producing
    C. gram-positive
    D. gram-negative
    E. aerobic

236. For which procedure should a patient's fat intake be limited for at least 12 hours prior to the procedure?
    A. cystogram
    B. IVP
    C. cholecystogram
    D. upper GI
    E. barium enema

237. Which of the following urine constituents evaporate at room temperature and therefore should be tested immediately?
    A. nitrites
    B. phenylketones
    C. protein
    D. glucose
    E. ketones

238. The instrument used to measure urine specific gravity by passing light through solids in a liquid is the
    A. centrifuge
    B. microscope
    C. refractometer
    D. urinometer
    E. unimeter

239. An alternative to reagent strip testing for ketones is
    A. Clinitest
    B. Acetest
    C. Ictotest
    D. sulfosalicyclic acid precipitation test
    E. Phenistix

240. Which of the following urinalysis values is most likely to vary with the specific gravity?
    A. pH
    B. Odor
    C. Appearance
    D. Color
    E. Ketones

241. A green urine may indicate the presence of
    A. urobilinogen
    B. diruetics
    C. high fluid intake
    D. carotine
    E. *Pseudomonas* organisms

242. Protective eyewear should be worn when
    A. handling soiled linens
    B. performing venipuncture
    C. centrifuging specimens
    D. packaging specimens
    E. cleaning work surfaces

243. Screening newborns for phenylketonuria (PKU) with Phenistix is
    A. not necessary for breast-fed babies
    B. performed at 6 months of age
    C. performed on three separate occasions
    D. performed on three filter paper circles
    E. performed with urine collected in a pediatric urine bag or on a diaper

244. For which procedure is a test meal ordered for the patient?
    A. barium swallow
    B. barium enema
    C. occult blood
    D. glucose tolerance test
    E. gastroscopy

245. To perform a nonspecific glucose test, you would use
    A. Ictotest
    B. Clinitest
    C. Chemstrip GP
    D. Multistix 8 SG
    E. Chek-stix

246. Which of the following medications should be taken 1 hour before meals or 2 to 3 hours after meals?
    A. oral penicillin G
    B. erythromycin
    C. ibuprofen
    D. potassium chloride
    E. naproxen

247. The label has fallen off a 3-ounce bottle of medication. There is approximately 1 ounce left and the expiration date is still 1 year away. The medical assistant would
    A. discard the medication down a drain connected to a sanitary sewer
    B. glue the label back onto the bottle
    C. scotch tape the label back onto the bottle
    D. write another label and attach it by covering it entirely with clear tape
    E. return the bottle to the manufacture as defective

248. To prepare 1 gallon of an aqueous solution of Zephiran chloride 1:750 from a stock solution of 17% Zephiran chloride concentrate, you would add:
    A. 1 ounce of water and 750 parts Zephiran
    B. 1 ounce of Zephiran and 127 ounces of water
    C. 1 ounce of Zephiran and 128 ounces of water
    D. 1 ounce of Zephiran and 750 ounces of water
    E. 1 ounce of Zephiran and 63 ounces of water

249. The correct site for the intramuscular injection of an infant is the
    A. deltoid
    B. gluteus maximus
    C. gluteus medius
    D. gluteus minimus
    E. vastus lateralis

250. The physician orders 500 mg to be administered to a patient. The vial is labeled 1 g/mL. How much medication would you administer?
    A. 250 mg
    B. 1/2 mL
    C. 1 mL
    D. 2 mL
    E. 250 mL

251. The physician orders 50 mg of a drug for an infant. The drug on hand reads 250 mg/mL. How much drug would you administer to the infant?
    A. 0.02 mL
    B. 0.20 mL
    C. 1.20 mL
    D. 2.50 mL
    E. 5.0 mL

252. A bronchodilatory used in the treatment of bronchospasm is
    A. Feldene
    B. Timoptic
    C. Lopressor
    D. Seldane
    E. Proventil

253. The physician orders 0.1 mg. The drug on hand is 0.4 mg/mL. How much drug would you administer?
    A. 0.04 mL
    B. 0.10 mL
    C. 0.25 mL
    D. 0.40 mL
    E. 4.0 mL

254. A patient is to take 1 gram of a medication daily. The tablet strength is 250 mg. How many tablets should the patient take each day?
    A. 1/4
    B. 1.2
    C. 2
    D. 4
    E. 8

255. Which of the following injections will require the largest needle lumen?
    A. allergy testing
    B. allergy desensitization serum 1:10,000
    C. tetanus toxoid
    D. tetanus immune globulin
    E. cyanocobalamin (B_{12})

256. The recommended needle size for an intradermal injection is
    A. 25-gauge, 1/2 inch
    B. 25-gauge, 5/8 inch
    C. 26-gauge, 3/8 inch
    D. 26-gauge, 1/2 inch
    E. 27 gauge, 1/2 inch

257. How much of 90% stock isopropyl alcohol would you need to prepare 1 liter of 70% isopropyl alcohol?
    A. 223 mL
    B. 300 mL
    C. 700 mL
    D. 777 mL
    E. 937 mL

258. Massage after an injection is primarily to
    A. stop bleeding
    B. decrease pain
    C. refer pain to a wider area
    D. decrease the escape of medication
    E. protect the site from contamination

259. In treating infant diarrhea or severe vomiting, one of the minerals replaced by the use of formula Pedialyte is
    A. copper
    B. iodine
    C. phosphorus
    D. potassium
    E. iron

260. Pernicious anemia may be treated with injections of vitamin
    A. A
    B. B_1
    C. B_{12}
    D. D
    E. K

261. The patient should be isolated at home for each of the following conditions EXCEPT
    A. impetigo
    B. german measles
    C. chickenpox
    D. mononucleosis
    E. salmonellosis

262. When one is handling a blood specimen, each of the following is correct EXCEPT
    A. labeling the specimen with a biohazard label
    B. cleaning visible container contamination with household bleach
    C. wearing gloves
    D. placing the specimen in a sturdy container with a secure lid
    E. shipping the specimen in a collection tube inside a single shipping container

263. For which of the following routine situations should the medical assistant wear gloves?
    A. x-ray procedures
    B. electrocardiography procedures
    C. obtaining vital signs
    D. obtaining a throat culture
    E. assisting a patient after an examination of the upper respiratory tract

264. Gloves must be worn for each of the following EXCEPT
    A. rinsing instruments after use
    B. wrapping instruments for the autoclave
    C. immersing instruments in disinfectant solutions
    D. removing instruments from the autoclave
    E. removing instruments from the ultrasonic cleaner

265. Gloves must be worn for touching or handling each of the following EXCEPT
    A. mucous membranes
    B. cytology smears
    C. dressings
    D. blood tubes
    E. thermometers following oral temperatures

266. Monilia (Candida) is more likely to occur
    A. when patients take antibiotics
    B. during pregnancy
    C. in diabetics
    D. when patients take hormones
    E. after douching with OTC drugs

267. For which of the following procedures should a medical assistant have ready, on the sterile field, material for suturing an incision?
  A. needle biopsy
  B. incision and drainage
  C. cervical biopsy
  D. cyst removal
  E. wart removal

268. A 6-year-old patient comes into the office for a physical examination. Which of the following recordings indicates that illness may be present?
  A. T 101°F (38.3°C)
  B. BP 90/60
  C. P 110
  D. R 20
  E. Wt 45 pounds

269. The physician orders 600 mg of aspirin; the bottle is labeled: Aspirin tablets, 5 grains. How many grains is equal to 600 mg?
  A. 2.5 grains
  B. 5 grains
  C. 6 grains
  D. 10 grains
  E. 20 grains

270. The risk of drug toxicity is especially high
  A. during infancy
  B. during illness
  C. both A and B
  D. in the elderly
  E. both A and D

271. The ECG recording lead I measures the electrical activity angles of the
  A. right arm to left arm
  B. midpoint of left leg to left arm
  C. left arm to left leg
  D. right arm to left leg
  E. midpoint right arm to left leg

272. Symptoms that may indicate severe head injury include
  A. projectile vomiting
  B. increase in pulse rate
  C. absent pulse pressure
  D. decrease in blood pressure
  E. bleeding into the skin (hematoma)

273. The recurrent turn is preferred when bandaging the
  A. finger
  B. elbow
  C. ankle
  D. wrist
  E. chest

274. Emergency treatments for a child that has ingested 10 antihistamines include
  A. gastric lavage
  B. ipecac
  C. both A and B
  D. large amounts of orange or lemon juice
  E. both A and D

275. Each of the following is an instance when a peripheral blood specimen may be used for testing EXCEPT
  A. infectious mononucleosis test-slide method
  B. blood culture
  C. complete blood count
  D. hematocrit
  E. blood glucose

276. Each of the following procedures requires the patient to be in a state of fasting EXCEPT
  A. barium enema
  B. barium swallow
  C. upper GI series
  D. gallbladder series
  E. intravenous pyelography

277. Slide tests that are interpreted as positive in the presence of agglutination include
  A. infectious mononucleosis test
  B. rheumatoid arthritis test
  C. both A and B
  D. pregnancy test
  E. both A and D

278. Which of the following medications is contraindicated with milk?
  A. Motrin
  B. prednisone
  C. Macrodantin
  D. tetracycline
  E. Feldene

279. Unless otherwise directed, each of the following injections should be massaged EXCEPT
    A. penicillin G with procaine
    B. iron preparations
    C. tetanus toxoid
    D. insulin
    E. human immune serum globulin

280. Of the following, which is a nonnarcotic, anti-inflammatory, analgesic, antipyretic drug?
    A. Ecotrin
    B. Motrin
    C. Advil
    D. Demerol
    E. Tylenol

281. Infiltration anesthetics with epinephrine
    A. are contraindicated in patients with heart block
    B. increase systemic absorption of the anesthetic
    C. both A and B
    D. should be stored separately from plain infiltration anesthetics
    E. both A and D

282. Antimicrobial medications are appropriate for each of the following EXCEPT
    A. flu
    B. septicemia
    C. wound healing
    D. postoperatively
    E. endocarditis

283. A subcutaneous injection may be the preferred route if the drug is
    A. to be deposited in the muscle
    B. potent enough in small quantities
    C. a large amount
    D. a long-acting insoluble substance
    E. to be absorbed rapidly

284. Of the "rights" governing the administration of medications, the "right time" includes checking whether or not a medication is
    A. administered during a specific body cycle
    B. one of a series of administrations
    C. both A and B
    D. oral or parenteral
    E. both A and D

285. True statements concerning the administration of epinephrine (Adrenalin) include which?
    A. The subcutaneous route is preferred.
    B. The intramuscular route is preferred.
    C. Usually, a single dose is ordered.
    D. Do not massage after injection.
    E. The buttocks is preferred.

286. When one is preparing a medication to be given by injection, which of the following parts can never be touched?
    A. plunger
    B. needle cap opening
    C. both A and B
    D. barrel
    E. both A and D

287. A drug that neutralizes the hydrochloric acid in the stomach and acts as a laxative is
    A. Tums
    B. Rolaids
    C. Riopan
    D. milk of magnesia
    E. Mylanta

288. Asking a patient for specific allergies is important when administering
    A. tetanus antitoxins
    B. tetanus immune globulin
    C. both A and B
    D. live virus vaccines
    E. both A and D

289. Patients for whom influenza vaccines are recommended include
    A. the elderly
    B. children
    C. both A and B
    D. the chronically ill
    E. both A and D

290. Low dosages of salicylates are being given prophylactically in
    A. patients who have suffered heart attacks
    B. patients with Vitamin K deficiency
    C. both A and B
    D. post-operative patients at increased risk for thrombophlebitis
    E. both A and D

291. The B₃ vitamin, nicotinic acid, is now being used in patient treatment because it
     A. releases histamine and is a vasodilator
     B. may reduce asthmalike episodes
     C. decreases gastric acidity
     D. relieves skin rashes and pruritis
     E. helps maintain resistance to infections

292. Products that must be considered sterile include
     A. eyedrops
     B. ear wicks
     C. both A and B
     D. vaginal suppositories
     E. both A and D

293. Ingestion of large doses of vitamins is known to cause
     A. nutritional dependency
     B. mental retardation
     C. decrease in bone formation
     D. toxicity
     E. loss of appetite

294. During treatment of a patient for migraine headaches, concurrent use of tyramine-rich food substances is avoided. Foods containing tyramine-rich substances include
     A. aged cheeses
     B. coffee
     C. raw fruits
     D. liver
     E. leafy green vegetables

On the way home from work, a medical assistant stops to assist at the scene of an accident (Fig. 4–2). The patient appears to have a back injury and is bleeding from the head and a wound on her left leg.

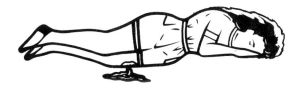

Figure 4–2. First-aid situation, accident victim.

Using this situation, answer the next five questions.

295. What is the first action the medical assistant should take?
     A. Open the airway.
     B. Search for additional wounds.
     C. Call for help.
     D. Assess the situation.
     E. Determine the victim's level of consciousness.

296. Because of the head injury, it is extremely important to observe the victim's
     A. pupils
     B. pulse
     C. respiration
     D. skin temperature
     E. coloring

297. The patient is bleeding profusely from an avulsed wound on her left leg above the ankle. On which artery should the medical assistant apply pressure?
     A. external iliac
     B. femoral
     C. greater saphenous
     D. popliteal
     E. posterior tibial

298. The victim's pulse rate is fast and scarcely perceptible. This pulse is called
     A. anacrotic
     B. dicrotic
     C. entopic
     D. jerky
     E. thready

299. For treatment of this patient for shock, the best position would be
     A. Trendelenburg position
     B. back-lying position
     C. side-lying position
     D. semisitting position
     E. face-down position

300. The instrument pictured in Figure 4–3 is used to test for
     A. Ménière's disease
     B. perception of sound
     C. both A and B
     D. mastoiditis
     E. both A and D

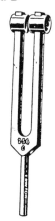

Figure 4–3. Tuning fork.

ANSWER KEY FOR SIMULATION TEST 4

1. **C.** Freely movable joints are diarthrotic; joints with limited motion, amphiarthrotic; and joints that are immovable, synarthrotic. ***Gylys & Wedding, p. 210.***

2. **B.** Blood serum from persons or animals whose bodies have built up antibodies is called antiserum or immune serum. ***Lane, Medications, p. 237.***

3. **C.** The nasopharynx is generally regarded as the back portion of the nasal cavity, where it meets the throat at the back of the oropharynx. ***Gylys & Wedding, p. 122.***

4. **A.** In hyperventilation, the patient breathes faster owing to anxiety. Hyperventilation results in hyperoxygenation of the blood with an accompanying depletion of carbon dioxide. Because carbon dioxide itself is the most important respiratory stimulant, immediate treatment is to have the patient breath into a paper bag to replace the "blown-off" carbon dioxide. Once the carbon dioxide is replaced, respirations will automatically become slower and more shallow. Left unattended, the patient's respiratory functions may become depressed with an accompanying alkalosis, a fall in blood pressure, vasoconstriction, and sometimes syncope. ***Tamparo & Lewis, p. 192.***

5. **A.** Mucous membranes line the body cavities that open to the outside of the body. ***Sheldon, pp. 111–112.***

6. **D.** Adipose tissue is a connective tissue that has the ability to store fat. ***Sheldon, p. 5.***

7. **B.** *Pneumocystis carinii* is a protozoan present in most normal individuals but causing a severe opportunistic pneumonia in AIDS patients. ***Sheldon, p. 147.***

8. **D.** Vitamin K is essential for the normal biosynthesis of prothrombin and coagulation factors VII, IX, and X. ***Sheldon, p. 508.***

9. **A.** Fingernails are formed from epithelial tissue in the outer part of the epidermis. ***Gylys & Wedding, p. 66.***

10. **C.** The intact skin is one of the body's most important barriers to infectious disease. ***Sheldon, p. 111.***

11. **A.** The cell is the basic structural unit of the human body. ***Sheldon, p. 5.***

12. **E.** The place where impulses cross between two nerves is called a synapse. ***Gylys & Wedding, p. 322.***

13. **C.** Platelets are small, colorless bodies that tend to agglutinate in shed blood; therefore, they play an important roll in clotting by releasing thrombokinase, which in the presence of calcium reacts with prothrombin to form thrombin. ***Sheldon, pp. 504; 505–506.***

14. **B.** The term for the adjustment of the lens for near and far vision is accommodation. ***Gylys & Wedding, p. 345.***

15. **E.** The sclera is the outer coating; the choroid, the middle; and the retina, the innermost coating of the eyeball. ***Gylys & Wedding, p. 344.***

16. **C.** The vagus is the longest nerve in the body and supplies sensations, movement, and secretions of the thoracic and abdominal viscera. ***Taber's, p. 2107.***

17. **B.** The healthy, normal tympanic membrane is pale gray and reflects a shiny cone of light when examined with the otoscope. ***Lane, Keenon, Coleman (eds.), p. 330.***

18. **D.** Equilibrium is maintained by the vestibular apparatus. The cochlear apparatus is concerned with hearing. The malleus, incus, and stapes are located in the middle ear and are concerned with the transmission of sound vibrations, although their functioning is not completely understood. ***Taber's, p. 597.***

19. **A.** Subacute bacterial endocarditis is an inflammation caused by the *Streptococcus viridans* group and usually involves the heart valves and the endocardium (the membrane lining the heart). ***Tamparo & Lewis, p. 208.***

20. C. The average, healthy man has 4.5 to 6 million red blood cells per cubic millimeter of blood. *Frew, Lane, Frew, p. 808.*

21. C. Vital functions of the body are controlled in the medulla oblongata. *Gylys & Wedding, p. 324.*

22. D. Vegetarian diets, without animal proteins, cannot supply all the necessary amino acids. Vegetables, fruits, and legumes each do not contain all amino acids. A vegetarian diet should include soybean, the one vegetable that does include all nine essential amino acids, and be carefully planned to include the full range of essential amino acids through a proper mix of nonanimal foods. *Frew, Lane, Frew, p. 513.*

23. C. Melanin is responsible for skin color, tanning, and freckles. *Taber's, p. 1186.*

24. B. The skull rests on the first cervical vertebra, the atlas. The second cervical vertebra is termed the axis, because it forms a pivot around which the atlas turns and carries the skull. The vertebra prominens is the 7th cervical vertebra. *Gylys & Wedding, p. 206.*

25. D. The sacrum is comprised of five fused vertebrae, located immediately below the lumbar spine. *Gylys & Wedding, p. 206.*

26. B. Cardiac muscle is composed of cross-striated fibers. Their activity is regulated by the autonomic nervous system. *Sheldon, p. 3.*

27. E. The anterior fontanel is composed of a fibrous membrane in which ossification is incomplete at birth. The larger of the fontanels, it usually fills in and closes between the eighth and fifteenth months of life. The posterior fontanel usually closes by the third or fourth month of life. *Taber's, p. 747.*

28. D. Most of the daily requirements for water are satisfied by ingested foods (vegetables and fruits are 80% water; meat, 40%–60%). Although no requirement for humans is set, 2 liters (about 8 glasses) is recommended. *Frew, Lane, Frew, p. 516(t).*

29. C. Ovulation is generally considered to occur 12 to 14 days before the next menstrual period. *Gylys & Wedding, pp. 266–267.*

30. A. A posterior convex curvature (primary curvature) is called kyphosis or hunchback, whereas a posterior concave curvature (secondary curvature) is termed lordosis or swayback. *Gylys & Wedding, p. 219.*

31. C. The organisms commonly responsible for causing subacute bacterial endocarditis (rheumatic fever) are *Staphylococcus aureus* and *Streptococcus viridans*. *Sheldon, p. 160(t).*

32. C. The distal portion of the sternum is termed the xiphoid process. *Taber's, p. 2171.*

33. A. Heartbeat originates in the sinoatrial node, which is located at the junction of the superior vena cava and the right atrium. *Gylys & Wedding, pp. 149–150.*

34. C. A temperature that is elevated at certain times within a 24-hour period but falls to normal within that time is called intermittent. *Frew, Lane, Frew, p. 347(t).*

35. C. The aqueous humor fills the anterior and posterior chambers of the eye. Its composition is protein-free plasma and normally creates an introocular pressure of 8–21 mm Hg. *Gylys & Wedding, p. 344(f).*

36. E. The deltoid is the triangular muscle that abducts the upper arm. It is often the site of injections. *Lane, Medications, pp. 202, 203(f).*

37. C. The fascia forms fibrous membranes that separate muscles from one another and invests them. Its functions include providing origins and insertions for muscles. *Scanlon, p. 132.*

38. D. A brief contraction is a twitch; a prolonged contraction is called tetany; a contraction that increases with warm-up is called treppe; and muscle tone is the constant, partially contracted state of muscles. *Taber's, p. 2059.*

39. D. During inhalation, the diaphragm contracts and moves downward, enlarging the thorax vertically. *Gylys & Wedding, pp. 122–123, 122(f).*

40. **C.** A subpoena is a legal order (writ) to appear at a given time and place to present evidence or to submit records, correspondence, and documents to the court as evidence. *Frew, Lane, Frew, p. 31.*

41. **B.** An informed consent implies an understanding of what is to be done, why it should be done, the risks involved, and alternative treatments, including the failure to treat and the attendant risks of alternative treatment(s). *Lewis & Tamparo, p. 98.*

42. **D.** The standard of conduct in determining a person's liability is the conduct of a reasonable person of ordinary prudence under the same or similar circumstances. Even if a patient's action was contributory, the patient can still recover damages if the medical assistant's negligence cannot be disproved. *Lewis & Tamparo, p. 59.*

43. **E.** Although the patient has a right to all the selections, a living will is designed to allow a person to make specific decisions concerning terminal care and death. *Lewis & Tamparo, pp. 197–198.*

44. **C.** A cancellation fee may be ethically assessed, if it is office policy and patients are informed of the policy. No account may be ethically turned over to a collection agency without the doctor's review. Use of office samples without the doctor's knowledge is unethical. Even innocuous-sounding statements about treatment promises or past treatments are not only unethical, but may have serious medicolegal repercussions. *Frew, Lane, Frew, p. 43.*

45. **C.** There are state statutes of limitations for the collection of an unpaid balance on a promissory note. Although there may be limitations on check cashing, these limitations are not by state laws. There are no time limitations on the usual real estate deed or power of attorney statement. *Frew, Lane, Frew, p. 258.*

46. **E.** Patients who state they wish they were dead should always be considered potentially depressed and a potential suicide. *Taber's, p. 1905.*

47. **B.** The first personality crisis, sometimes called the First Stage of Man, is trust versus mistrust. It occurs during the first year of life. It is especially during this time that infants need to be comforted with positive touch and sounds. *Davis, p. 19.*

48. **C.** A hypochondriac is a person affected by abnormal concern about one's health. *Taber's, p. 945.*

49. **E.** The communication of words is the patient's medical record; the other communications are nonverbal. *Lewis & Tamparo, p. 108.*

50. **A.** When there is a false personal belief based on an incorrect inference about external reality, this is a delusion. If the patient entered the bathroom and saw spiders, this would be a visual hallucination. If the patient saw specimen containers in the bathroom and thought the containers were spiders, this would be an illusion. *Taber's, p. 510.*

51. **E.** The medical assistant must be careful not to talk about the patient's problems, as it could make the patient more anxious and afraid. Laughing at a person's fears destroys trust in those who are there to help. The best way to communicate with mentally ill patients is to be on their own level of functioning and not to reveal annoyance, anger, or amusement through verbal or nonverbal reactions. *Davis, pp. 145–146.*

52. **A.** The primary reason women fear mastectomy is the loss of feeling feminine and attractive as a sex partner. *Taber's, p. 1170.*

53. **A.** The worried and afraid patient needs to be able to express those concerns. Ask the patient to talk about it, then be a good listener. *Davis, pp. 173–174.*

54. **E.** The medical assistant must report the patient's feelings to the physician, so it is important to gently let the patient know what you are going to do, why, and that it will be all right. *Davis, p. 174.*

55. **A.** Contusion. *Gylys & Wedding, p. 72.*

56. **E.** The food exchange list is a model originally developed for diabetics, and it is now widely used for personal diet menu planning. Foods are grouped with other foods that have similar calories and carbohydrate weight, so that individual food "exchanges" may be made without changing the goals of the diet. *Frew, Lane, Frew, pp. 536, 537–538(t).*

57. **E.** Asymptomatic. *Gylys & Wedding, p. 272.*

58. **A.** An invasive procedure is an intentional surgical entry into the human tissues, during which bleeding occurs or the potential for bleeding exists. *Frew, Lane, Frew, p. 417.*

59. **D.** The term for a fungal condition of the foot is tinea pedis. Both pediculosis and phthiriasis are terms for infestation with lice; pityriasis is a group of skin diseases with fine, branny patches, one of which is a condition termed tinea versicolor. *Tamparo & Lewis, p. 320.*

60. **B.** Mucus is the noun; mucous, the adjective. *Gylys & Wedding, p. 130.*

61. **E.** "Oligo" is the combining form from Latin meaning scanty, little; "meno" (from Gr.) is the word element for menstruation; and "rrhea" is a suffix meaning flow. *Gylys & Wedding, pp. 15, 244.*

62. **D.** Parathyroid. *Gylys & Wedding, pp. 297–298.*

63. **A.** Vascular hemophilia is also known as von Willebrand's disease. The patient's bleeding time is increased. Many times the cause is unknown. *Sheldon, p. 508.*

64. **A.** Bulimia is an eating disorder characterized by binge eating followed by purging. *Gylys & Wedding, p. 101.*

65. **A.** Petechia; pl. petechiae; pinpoint, non-raised, round, purplish red spot caused by intradermal or submucous hemorrhage. *Gylys & Wedding, p. 76.*

66. **B.** A cerebral vascular accident is a disorder of the blood vessels serving the cerebrum, resulting from an impaired blood supply to the brain; also called a stroke. *Tamparo & Lewis, pp. 255–260.*

67. **E.** Arrhythmia. *Taber's, p. 149.*

68. **A.** Aerobic is the adjectival form of aerobe, and means a microorganism that lives in the presence of free oxygen. *Taber's, p. 48.*

69. **B.** Desquamation means the shedding of epithelial cells. *Taber's, p. 528.*

70. **B.** Diabetes mellitus. *Taber's, p. 532.*

71. **D.** An avulsion is tissue separated from the body in a jagged or mutilated form, sometimes amputation. *Taber's, p. 185.*

72. **A.** Serum albumin in the urine is one type of increased urine protein. *Gylys & Wedding, pp. 244–245.*

73. **B.** Mydratics dilate the pupil; myopics constrict the pupil. *Gylys & Wedding, p. 356.*

74. **D.** Nuclear isotope. *Taber's, pp. 1029, 1324.*

75. **C.** Most lay persons use the term heart attack to mean a myocardial infarction. *Frew, Lane, Frew, p. 471.*

76. **C.** Decubitus ulcer. *Taber's, p. 503.*

77. **A.** Optician. *Taber's, p. 1365.*

78. **E.** White blood cells have the power to ingest bacteria and other small particles; they are important in both defensive and reparative functions of the body; and they form, with dead bacteria, suppurative material called pus. White blood cells do not function in regulating body metabolism. *Sheldon, pp. 113–114.*

79. **D.** A glioma is a malignant neoplasm of the glial tissue, the supporting tissue of the brain and spinal cord. *Taber's, p. 806.*

80. **A.** In an emergency situation, any implied agreement lasts only as long as the emergency. *Lewis & Tamparo, p. 97.*

81. **B.** The basis of the patient-physician relationship is usually an implied agreement that the physician will offer services; and in consideration, the patient will pay for those services. This implied contract must include capacity on the parts of both parties and legality of the agreed services. There is no written contract signed to begin the patient-physician relationship. The relationship usually begins when the patient first sees the physician. *Lewis & Tamparo, p. 63.*

82. **E.** Drainage of the paranasal sinuses may be through either ciliary action or by suction set up during blowing of the nose. *Tamparo & Lewis, p. 174.*

83. **C.** The sinuses referred to as the paranasal sinuses are: frontal, ethmoid, sphenoid, and maxillary. The mastoid sinuses are very small cavities within the mastoid process of the temporal bone and communicate with the middle ear. *Taber's, p. 1802.*

84. **D.** Cerumen, ear wax, is a mixture of the secretions of sebaceous and ceruminous glands. Auricular glands are the external otic lymph nodes and apocrine glands are mammary glands and sweat glands. *Gylys & Wedding, p. 347.*

85. **C.** A reflex that protects the body from injury is termed nociceptive. Sneezing, coughing, and gagging are reflexes to foreign bodies in the nose or throat. Winking is a reflex that protects the eye. *Taber's, p. 1313.*

86. **D.** On normal examination, cerebrospinal fluid contains 15–45 mg/100 mL of protein, small amounts of glucose, and approximately 120 mEq/L of chloride but no blood cells or bacteria. *Sheldon, p. 547.*

87. **B.** The gluteous maximus is important in the action of running, climbing, and rising from a sitting position. It is relaxed when the body is standing upright, and it has little function in ordinary walking. *Taber's, 2234.*

88. **E.** The skin holds the body together, protects the internal structures from harm, and regulates body temperature and waste elimination through perspiration. *Gylys & Wedding, p. 64.*

89. **D.** The spinal cord and nerve roots are contained in the dorsal cavity. *Gylys & Wedding, p. 48(t).*

90. **C.** The nasal cavity can be examined either through a nostril (anterior rhinoscopy) or through the nasopharynx (posterior rhinoscopy). *Gylys & Wedding, p. 122.*

91. **B.** The sternoclavicular joint is formed by the medial end of the clavicle, the sternum, and the first costal cartilage. It is a double gliding joint. *Taber's, p. 2237.*

92. **C.** The brain and spinal cord make up the central nervous system. *Gylys & Wedding, p. 318.*

93. **A.** Phosphorus and calcium are essential for bone growth and development. *Frew, Lane, Frew, p. 515(t).*

94. **C.** The implied contract between a patient and the physician does not include the patient giving notice to change physicians or a blanket release of information to third parties. A release of information must be obtained each time records are released. *Frew, Lane, Frew, pp. 34, 39.*

95. **A.** Only the physician can order prescription medications. *Lane, Medications, p. 37.*

96. **C.** The principal defenses to liability include the proving that a patient willingly assumed the risks of the known or foreseeable dangers (informed consent) or that the patient did not exercise a reasonable degree of caution and was the proximate cause of the injury (contributory negligence). Res ipsa loquitur is not a defense, but a shifting of the burden of proof from the plaintiff to the defendant. *Lewis & Tamparo, p. 61.*

97. **C.** A tort is a wrong committed by one person to another person or property of another person, with or without force, either by omission or wrongful act (negligence). An act for which the wrongdoer is subject to punishment by the state and is condemned by law is called a crime. *Lewis & Tamparo, pp. 64–65.*

98. **A.** Fibrinogen and prothrombin are synthesized by the liver cells. *Sheldon, p. 507.*

99. **D.** Diabetes mellitus is treated, in part, by restricting those calories that arise from carbohydrates, because it is an inherited disorder of carbohydrate metabolism. Anorexia nervosa, obesity, and bulimia, on the other hand, are behavioral disorders of weight control and eating habits, usually caused by emotional conflicts or psychotic states, rather than physical disease. ***Tamparo & Lewis, p. 281.***

100. **C.** "Cephalo" means brain; both "dynia" and "algia" are suffixes for pain. ***Gylys & Wedding, pp. 12, 213.***

101. **C.** It is generally recommended that women not douche for at least 1 to 2 days prior to examination, as the douching tends to wash away vaginal secretions that are required for specimen collection. ***Lane, Keenon, Coleman (eds.), p. 442.***

102. **E.** A complete physical examination on a new patient with a cardiovascular condition should be blocked for 1.5 hours, in order to accomplish the additional tests and procedures that will be required for this patient, such as pulmonary function studies, ECG, blood and urine testing, and chest radiography. ***Lane, Keenon, Coleman (eds.), p. 4.***

103. **A.** A database file is one specific form in the database collection; a document file is a word processing file; a field is a single information blank on a data file form; and working copy is the name given to a yet unnamed word processing document. ***Gylys, pp. 13, 43, 373.***

104. **C.** File name extensions are used to classify the kind of word processing documents stored, such as .DOC or .LET or .MEM. ***Gylys, p. 373; Frew, Lane, Frew, p. 221.***

105. **E.** The disk letter and colon locate the disk; a backslash is used to separate each directory, subdirectory, and file path name. ***Gylys, p. 18; Frew, Lane, Frew, p. 221.***

106. **C.** Exit the work, which will remove it from RAM; then pull it up again and start over. Do not rekey; the work is still saved on disk. Renaming the document will take up disk room storing an unusable file. Saving the current work will permanently alter the stored version with the deleted material. Deleting the current file will also delete the stored version because both are under the same name. ***Gylys, p. 7.***

107. **E.** A modem is necessary only to transmit information on-line, using telephone lines. ***Gylys, p. 374.***

108. **B.** "Stet" is used to reverse a proofreader mark and to alert the editor to let the material stand as originally typed. ***Fordney and Diehl, p. 361.***

109. **C.** The "#" mark tells the typesetter to insert a space. ***Fordney and Diehl, p. 361.***

110. **D.** The monthly Index Medicus and the annual Cumulated Index Medicus are published by the National Library of Medicine. ***Frew, Lane, Frew, p. 220.***

111. **B.** The computer equivalent to the Index Medicus is MEDLINE. MEDLINE/Health File is the equivalent to Hospital Index; EMBASE, Excerpta Medica; and EMPIRES, the GTE/AMA database. ***Frew, Lane, Frew, p. 220.***

112. **A.** If the CE key is depressed before striking the arithmetic function key, it will clear a number key that is entered in error, such as when you depress the wrong number. After pressing the CE key, you may reenter the correct number and continue with the calculation. ***Haverty & Rhodes, p. 272.***

113. **D.** Electronic fund transfer is a method of the bank internally debiting and crediting your account by computer without checks or deposit slips. It is available to any business account. ***Frew, Lane, Frew, p. 255.***

114. **D.** The original price ($20.00) − discount (0.05) = $1.00 off per item for buying in quantity, or a new price of $19.00 each × 6 = $114.00. ***No reference needed.***

115. **B.** Charges are posted from the daily log to the general ledger, which is the basic reference for the double-entry bookkeeping system. The daily log, or journal, is the book of original entry. A chart of accounts is a list of codes and descriptions that is used to categorize sources of income and expenses. *Frew, Lane, Frew, p. 268.*

116. **A.** Current assets are those resources that will be turned into cash or used in the operation of the practice within one business (operating) cycle or a 12-month period, whichever is longer. *Frew, Lane, Frew, p. 269.*

117. **B.** Whether or not the patient requests one, a receipt should be written for every cash payment. The completion of cash receipts assures the physician that cash is accounted for and also acts as protection for the medical assistant and the patient. *Frew, Lane, Frew, p. 261.*

118. **B.** A truth-in-lending statement must be completed with the patient when four or more payments are involved, whether or not there is an interest charge. *Frew, Lane, Frew, p. 259.*

119. **D.** $.03 \times 40.00 = 1.20$; $40.00 - 1.20 = 38.80$; or another way: $40.00 \times .97 = 38.80$. *No reference needed.*

120. **B.** Using the ordinary method for computing time, calculate Principal ($500) × Rate (12%) × Time (0.5 − one-half year) = $30.00. *Frew, Lane, Frew, p. 234.*

121. **B.** The physician may decide to reduce a fee for a patient who cannot afford the usual cost of care. The full fee should first be charged, then reduced to the agreed-on amount, and a written agreement should be drawn up limiting the time within which the account must be paid and with the term "without prejudice." A fee should not be reduced for a patient who has died, patients who are dissatisfied with care or the physician's charges, or to avoid sending a bill to collections. *Lane, Keenon, Coleman (eds.), p. 90.*

122. **C.** A service charge is a fee charged by a bank for services rendered. *Lane, Keenon, Coleman (eds.), pp. 106–107.*

123. **A.** A medical plan that provides both basic medical insurance and catastrophic coverage for costs of illness and injury beyond those covered in the basic medical portion is a major medical plan. *Frew, Lane, Frew, p. 300.*

124. **E.** CHAMPUS is always considered the secondary carrier, unless the patient has Medicaid and CHAMPUS-supplement type, in which case you would bill CHAMPUS first. *Gylys, p. 199.*

125. **E.** A copayment is a contribution the patient must make to cover some portion of each insurance claim. *Gylys, p. 186.*

126. **A.** Workers' compensation payments are made directly from the insurance carrier to the physician. The physician must accept the payment as payment in full and there are no deductible or copayment patient obligations. *Gylys, p. 104.*

127. **B.** CHAMPUS dependents are issued ID cards at age 10. *Lane, Keenon, Coleman (eds.), p. 166.*

128. **D.** Whenever a patient is referred to another physician or to a facility for special services for laboratory or x-ray workups, state it. This will establish a continuity of claims processing. *Lane, Keenon, Coleman (eds.), p. 177.*

129. **C.** A deductible must be met for each person. *Frew, Lane, Frew, p. 286.*

130. **E.** Nonduplication of benefits is the coordination of benefits between two separate insurance companies. *Frew, Lane, Frew, p. 290.*

131. **A.** The correct transcription of suture size is 4–0. Use only the number, hyphen, and the zero when the number is larger than three. *Forney and Diehl, p. 305.*

132. **D.** Some ICD-9 codes require three digits; however, others require four or five digits for proper coding. *Lane, Keenon, Coleman (eds.), pp. 189, 195.*

133. **E.** If the postoperative diagnosis differs from the preoperative diagnosis, the postoperative diagnosis is selected for coding. The first sequence of codes is the diagnosis, followed by descriptors of coexisting conditions. Previous conditions that are known no longer to exist are not coded. *Lane, Keenon, Coleman (eds.), p. 196.*

134. **E.** Because the diagnosis has not been confirmed, the correct code would be the condition, signs, symptoms, or abnormal test results, to the highest degree of certainty. There are no codes for "rule out" or "ruled out." If the term "rule out" is used in the diagnosis, code the case with codes that describe the condition to the highest degree of specificity, including whether or not it is suspected or confirmed. Only in the hospital setting may a suspected condition be coded as if it were present. *Lane, Keenon, Coleman (eds.), pp. 194, 196.*

135. **D.** For certain tax advantages, capital equipment is depreciated over 5 or 10 years, depending on its classification. *Lane, Keenon, Coleman (eds.), p. 56.*

136. **B.** Because the filing process is really a five-step process of records review and sorting, a certain time each day should be set aside for returning files to storage. This time should be used for quiet and concentration to avoid omission of notes or misfiles. Filling after each patient would increase the chances of filing errors during a busy, hectic day. *Frew, Lane, Frew, p. 110.*

137. **B.** The numeric system has no personal reference or relationship to the subject of the medical record. All other systems refer to some manner of patient classification. Because of this, a cross-reference system is needed to identify a patient name with the correct medical record number. *Frew, Lane, Frew, pp. 105–108.*

138. **A.** One should avoid confusing questions such as "Why are you here?" ("That's what I came to find out.") or "What brings you here?" ("My daughter's car.") When collecting data, ask the patient a direct question; for example, "For what reason have you come to see the doctor?" When you have completed the history, give the patient an opportunity to say anything still concerning him or her. *Frew, Lane, Frew, pp. 331–332.*

139. **E.** Permission to release records must be signed by the patient for each individual request. *Frew, Lane, Frew, p. 39.*

140. **A.** A medical history, as it is related by the patient, is subjective. It should be noted, however, that a medical history in the form of a report from another physician would be an example of objective information. *Frew, Lane, Frew, p. 323.*

141. **D.** The seriousness of a situation determines whether or not an appointment should be made immediately. A reciprocal understanding exists among physicians to accept referred patients outside of the regular scheduling. To ensure this patient fits into the system quickly, the medical assistant or the physician should make the appointment for him before he leaves the office. *Lane, Keenon, Coleman (eds.), p. 13.*

142. **D.** Patient allergies should be labeled clearly on every page of the medical record. The other methods are not safe, because the record may be separated from the folder-cover or the front page turned back and not reviewed. *Frew, Lane, Frew, p. 329.*

143. **B.** The Problem-Oriented Medical Record is the system of medical record-keeping that is based on the patient's health problems. The other selections are abbreviations used in banking and medical insurance. *Frew, Lane, Frew, p. 84.*

144. **A.** Inspecting the file for the necessary release marks that indicate that the document is cleared for filing is the same for all filing systems. The other four selections are performed differently, depending on the type of filing system used. *Frew, Lane, Frew, p. 105.*

145. **A.** The trend is to allow patients access to their medical records. Federally operated health agencies now make records available by federal law, and certain states have laws making it permissible for patients to see their records in private health facilities. *Frew, Lane, Frew, p. 92.*

146. **C.** The preferred filing systems for medical and scientific reports is either by subject or topic. *Frew, Lane, Frew, pp. 106–107.*

147. **B.** Hyphenated names are considered one unit. The name of a married woman is indexed by her legal name; that is, her husband's surname, her given name, and her middle name or maiden surname. *Frew, Lane, Frew, p. 108.*

148. **D.** The numbers are filed in groups from right to left, instead of from left to right. *Lane, Keenon, Coleman (eds.), p. 21.*

149. **D.** The abbreviations are used to describe the quadrants of the abdomen: right upper quadrant, left upper quadrant, right lower quadrant, left lower quadrant. *Lane, Keenon, Coleman (eds.), pp. 697–698.*

150. **B.** When a referring physician calls to refer a patient, the call is immediately put through to the physician. *Frew, Lane, Frew, p. 166.*

151. **A.** All files are first grouped together by the last two digits, then they are grouped by their middle digits, and then finally they are arranged by the first two digits, so that 88 34 23 precedes 89 34 23. *Lane, Keenon, Coleman (eds.), p. 21.*

152. **B.** Information that is gathered for the purpose of estimating how long a particular piece of equipment will be used should be gathered and saved under a file titled "Master List." "Purchases" usually refers to records of equipment already purchased. After purchase, maintenance agreements and invoice may be filed under "Receipts," "Maintenance and Repairs," and "Inventory." *Frew, Lane, Frew, p. 100.*

153. **C.** A recall system and tickler file is used to confirm or set regular appointments with patients. *Frew, Lane, Frew, pp. 198, 200.*

154. **D.** Bulk ordering materials, when there is the possibility that the equipment will be no longer used, is the cost effective concern here. If there is a chance that the physician will discontinue using the product before the existing supply has been consumed, it is impractical and costly to order a large quantity until a final decision is made. *Lane, Keenon, Coleman (eds.), p. 61.*

155. **A.** "Mister" is abbreviated "Mr." *Fordney & Diehl, p. 7.*

156. **D.** "As ever," "Best wishes," and "Kindest regards" are examples of first-name basis, informal complimentary closes. *Fordney and Diehl, p. 189.*

157. **B.** "Achilles" needs a capital letter. *Fordney and Diehl, pp. 43, 122.*

158. **E.** "Grade" is not capitalized; "four" is recorded as a capitalized Roman numeral. *Fordney and Diehl, p. 300.*

159. **E.** When both the post office box and the street address are given, use only the post office box. *Fordney and Diehl, p. 20.*

160. **D.** In mixed punctuation, a colon is used after the salutation. *Fordney and Diehl, p. 22.*

161. **B.** Blind carbon copies are no longer recommended. If the writer still insists, type "bcc:" and the names of the people who will receive the copies on the copies only, either in the same position as a regular "cc:" notation, or in the upper left-hand corner of the copies. *Lane, Keenon, Coleman (eds.), p. 39.*

162. **D.** The primary recipient should be noted first in the address, and the courtesy titles should be parallel (i.e., Dr. and Mr.). *Fordney and Diehl, p. 22.*

163. **B.** The employee does not receive a copy. *Frew, Lane, Frew, p. 297.*

164. **A.** For Medicaid, up to two diagnoses will be allowed. Past conditions are not coded if they have no impact on the current condition. For inpatient care, the principal diagnosis submitted by the physician and the hospital must be the same. Do not automatically send reports with claim forms unless they are specifically requested. *Lane, Keenon, Coleman (eds.), p. 177.*

165. **B.** It is necessary to keep receipts for business equipment only until the item is fully depreciated. Income tax returns, canceled checks, and liability insurance policies are kept in a fireproof file for three years, then stored in dead storage indefinitely. Patient records are kept permanently, or at least as long as the doctor is in practice. *Lane, Keenon, Coleman (eds.), p. 56.*

166. **B.** Patient records are admissible in a court of law. *Lewis & Tamparo, p. 111.*

167. **E.** The system requires more training, but once the system is mastered, fewer errors occur then in alphabetic filing and physical control over the system is easier. The other four selections are correct statements concerning numeric filing. *Frew, Lane, Frew, p. 106.*

168. **B.** Roll microfilm is not ideal for records that need frequent updating. *Lane, Keenon, Coleman (eds.), p. 23.*

169. **D.** The position of the patient during the examination is not relevant for the record. *Frew, Lane, Frew, pp. 87–88.*

170. **A.** The financial records are kept separate. All other patient contacts related to medical care, office visits, telephone conversations, and correspondence should be noted in the medical record. *Frew, Lane, Frew, pp. 86–88.*

171. **D.** You need to reinsert your DOS diskette to do the following external commands: format, diskcopy, compare disks, and select. *Gylys, p. 373.*

172. **C.** The patient's authorization to release records should be a permanent record. *Frew, Lane, Frew, p. 87.*

173. **E.** A return receipt provides the sender a record of delivery. Certified and registered mail prove an item was mailed and a record is kept at the post office. A certificate of mailing gives proof of mailing but does not give proof of receipt. Special delivery assures delivery the same day that the item is received at the post office, but no proof of receipt is provided the sender. *Frew, Lane, Frew, p. 137.*

174. **C.** Assets, liabilities, and owner's equity are the three major headings of a balance sheet. The income and expenses are listed on the profit and loss statement. *Lane, Keenon, Coleman (eds.), p. 79.*

175. **D.** Medicare part B does not cover routine physical examinations and tests, eye examinations and hearing examinations for the sole purpose of fitting for eyeglasses and hearing aids, immunizations for travel, or cosmetic surgery that is not to correct accidental injury. *Frew, Lane, Frew, p. 288.*

176. **D.** When the physician agrees to participate, the medical assistant must write off the difference between what was billed and what is *allowed*. The payment will be 80% of the allowable. The patient is always responsible for any copayment and the deductible amount due under the program. The patient completes the top half of Form 500 or 501. The bottom half is completed and submitted by the medical assistant if the physician agrees to participate. *Gylys, pp. 197–200.*

177. **B.** As mandated by the US Congress, Medicare covers *at any age* renal dialysis, kidney transplant donor expenses, blind persons, and the permanently disabled (if disabled for 2 years or longer). Medicare limits the coverge of heart bypass surgery. *Gylys, p. 185.*

178. **E.** The ICD-9 coding system is used to provide an accurate diagnosis for each item or service provided by a physician. *Lane, Keenon, Coleman (eds.), p. 187.*

179. **B.** Patients who have nonparticipating physicians must pay their charges, then apply for direct Medicare reimbursement. These patients do not have a waiting period before eligibility nor are they reimbursed at different rates. Medical assistants must be prepared to process all Medicare claims and assist the patients with filing their forms. Medicare may limit charges even on the nonparticipating physician. *Frew, Lane, Frew, p. 290.*

180. **E.** If there is a confirmed diagnosis, code the case with each specific. If the condition is both acute and chronic, code both with the acute sequenced first. *Lane, Keenon, Coleman (eds.), p. 196.*

181. **E.** When billing workers' compensation cases, x-ray charges must be supplemented with interpretations. *Gylys, p. 204.*

182. **C.** Workers who are not eligible for social security because they have not worked enough quarters to qualify for benefits may enroll by paying for both part A and part B. *Frew, Lane, Frew, p. 288.*

183. **C.** Every receipt of supplies should be checked against the original order to make sure the order is correct, and it should be inventoried with details of receipt date, amount received, unit cost, and total cost. *Lane, Keenon, Coleman (eds.), p. 63.*

184. **D.** Letters marked "personal" or "confidential" should not be opened by the assistant unless there is specific authority to do so. *Frew, Lane, Frew, p. 156.*

185. **D.** The U.S. Post Office offers a priority mail service in a "flat rate envelope" for $2.90. *Frew, Lane, Frew, p. 137.*

186. **B.** Record the cancellation by writing "cancelled" above the patient's name and whether or not a new appointment is scheduled. Record the cancellation in the patient's record. *Frew, Lane, Frew, p. 204.*

187. **B.** Physicians routinely send records with a referred patient; otherwise, a request for medical information must always be accompanied by a valid release-of-information document. The exceptions to this are workers' compensation cases, Social Security Administration examinations and reports, government entities, Medicare and Medicaid, and information about the commission of a crime to police departments. *Lane, Keenon, Coleman (eds.), pp. 30–33.*

188. **E.** A referral letter should contain the condition and findings for which the patient is being referred, and a description of any treatments that have been given so far for that condition. *Lane, Keenon, Coleman (eds.), p. 41.*

189. **E.** The patient owns her medical information; the physician owns the physical record. Omissions are as important in litigation as what is included in a medical record. Procedures that are omitted from the record are considered not performed by the courts. A signed release is not necessary when reporting communicable diseases required by law or for subpoenaed records. *Frew, Lane, Frew, pp. 88–89.*

190. **D.** Color-coding can decrease (not eliminate) the time required for indexing and make misfiles easier to locate. The color-coding of files does not constitute a filing system. The numeric system provides unlimited expansion without shifting of folders and confidentiality of records. Color-coded files are not necessarily numeric files. *Frew, Lane, Frew, p. 103.*

191. **A.** The abbreviation "Esq." is used after the surnames of professional persons, such as attorneys, architects, and consuls. The plural of "Esq." is "Esqs." and it is used with the surnames of multiple addressees. If a courtesy title such as "Ms., Miss, Mrs., Mr., Dr., Hon.," or "Rev." is used, "Esq." is omitted. *Fordney and Diehl, pp. 7, 15.*

192. **A.** A period is needed to punctuate the end of the line: "enc." A capital letter is needed to begin the line. *Fordney and Diehl, p. 194.*

193. **E.** In transcription, the medical assistant's duties include checking for errors in sentence structure, punctuation, and spelling, and then checking the work twice before presenting it for signature: once for typewriting accuracy and once to make sure that it makes grammatical sense, which includes flow of thought, correct sequencing of dates, and correct names. It is the physician's responsibility to ensure that the medical information makes sense. *Frew, Lane, Frew, p. 148.*

194. **C.** Drug trade names and the genus of microorganisms are capitalized. *Fordney and Diehl, pp. 43, 44.*

195. **D.** The modified semi-block style features a date line, complimentary close, and signature block either slightly to the right of dead center or flush right and paragraph indentations of five to ten spaces. *Frew, Lane, Frew, p. 125.*

196. **D.** The postscript is indented five to ten spaces to agree with the message paragraphing. Special mailing notations, on-arrival notations, and carbon copy notations are always flush left. Although it is often centered when using the Modified Semi-Block style, an attention line may be positioned flush left in any style. *Fordney and Diehl, p. 201.*

197. **C.** In a modified semi-block letter, the attention line is flush left two lines below the inside address. *Fordney and Diehl, p. 188.*

198. **E.** The second line of the signature block is reserved for the writer's professional position and/or department title. Professional rating abbreviations should only be included as initials on the first line, after the writer's name. If the courtesy title "Dr." is not used in the address, the academic or medical degree abbreviation follows the surname. The professional position and/or department title is never abbreviated. The title "Doctor" may be typed out in full or abbreviated in the salutation and in the body of the letter. *Fordney and Diehl, pp. 206–207.*

199. **D.** The reference line may be positioned one line above salutation and blocked with the date. A reference should not be positioned flush left when using the modified semi-block style. *Fordney and Diehl, p. 203.*

200. **B.** The Centers for Disease Control of the U.S. Public Health Service are the best source for information on the control of infection. *Lane, Keenon, Coleman (eds.), pp. 301–303, 352–353, 768–790.*

201. **B.** Steam and water may damage sharp edges; therefore, sharp cutting instruments should be autoclaved using the dry oven method. *Frew, Lane, Frew, pp. 599, 603–604.*

202. **B.** Disposable syringes and needles must be placed in puncture-resistant containers located as close as is practical to the area in which they were used. Disposable needles should not be recapped, purposefully bent or broken, removed from syringes, or otherwise manipulated by hand after use. For situations in which the needle must be preserved, intact, the use of one hand and a countertop is considered a safe technique that is not likely to increase the risk of needlestick injury from a laboratory specimen. *Frew, Lane, Frew, p. 649.*

203. **E.** Hold the lid of the container above and to the side of the Bard-Parker tray, with the inside of the lid downward, as you transfer sterile dressings to the field with your major hand and transfer forceps. *Lane, Keenon, Coleman (eds.), pp. 378–379; Frew, Lane, Frew, p. 620.*

204. **C.** $F - 32 \times 5/9 = C$; $103.8 - 32 \times 5/9 = 39.88$ which when rounded to the visible scale = 39.9. *Lane, Keenon, Coleman (eds.), p. 314; Frew, Lane, Frew, p. 350.*

205. **C.** Tilting the affected eye downward prevents the solution from flowing into the unaffected eye, therefore reducing the chances of cross-contamination. The downward gaze helps to protect the cornea as the assistant directs the flow from the inner contour of the eye. *Lane, Medications, pp. 196–97.*

206. **D.** Clamp the suture needle within the upper one third of the curve. Clamping midpoint will distort the curvature; too low may damage the point or not give the physician enough room to pass the needle through the skin; and too high may damage the thread connection or leave the physician with too little control of the suture. *Frew, Lane, Frew, p. 639.*

207. **E.** Radiographically, the compact substance is seen peripherally as a homogenous band of lime density. The spongy bone is seen particularly toward the ends of the shaft as a network of lime density. The bone marrow and periosteum present a soft-tissue density. Muscle is not visible in the ordinary radiogram. *Frew, Lane, Frew, p. 855.*

208. **E.** The instruments needed for an ear lavage are an otoscope, Reiner ear syringe, and a basin. *Lane, Keenon, Coleman (eds.), pp. 329–330; Frew, Lane, Frew, p. 449.*

209. **B.** The sense of touch to determine the size of a part or the presence of abnormal growth is called palpation. *Frew, Lane, Frew, p. 401.*

210. **D.** In ophthalmoscopy, or fundoscopy, the physician uses an ophthalmoscope to examine the retina. *Lane, Keenon, Coleman (eds.), p. 327.*

211. **C.** Some physicians call the change at phase IV the "fading sound" and want the point of change recorded between the systolic and diastolic recordings. It should be noted, however, that opinions vary and some physicians consider the "fading sound" the true diastolic reading, especially for children. *Lane, Keenon, Coleman (eds.), pp. 317–318; Frew, Lane, Frew, p. 359.*

212. **E.** Carotid stenosis is the result of a narrowing of the carotid arteries in the neck and head. *Frew, Lane, Frew, p. 473.*

213. **B.** A pulse pressure is the difference between the systolic and diastolic pressures. *Frew, Lane, Frew, p. 357.*

214. **B.** During phase II, the blood pressure sounds may disappear completely for as much as 30 mm, before the beginning of phase III. *Lane, Keenon, Coleman (eds.), pp. 317–318; Frew, Lane, Frew, p. 359.*

215. **D.** A systolic change greater than 10 mm Hg from the lying to the standing position should be reported immediately. *Frew, Lane, Frew, p. 381.*

216. **A.** An oral thermometer does not have a safety bulb and could, therefore, injure the rectal mucosa. All thermometers register the same, regardless of the site used. *Frew, Lane, Frew, p. 347.*

217. **C.** Rectal examination most often detects prostatic cancer or benign prostatic hypertrophy at the early stages. It is recommended annually for men over age 45. *Frew, Lane, Frew, p. 484.*

218. **A.** The frontal and paranasal sinuses are first examined by palpation above and below the eyes. *Frew, Lane, Frew, p. 405.*

219. **D.** Fibrocystic disease appears to predispose a patient to breast cancer, as well as hereditary factors. Childbearing, breast-feeding, and milk abscesses do not appear to predispose a patient to breast cancer. *Lane, Keenon, Coleman (eds.), p. 452.*

220. **C.** First palpate the radial artery and inflate until pulse disappears. Mentally add 30 mm to the measurement at disappearance. Deflate and wait 1 minute. Then palpate the brachial artery and place the disc of the stethoscope over the artery. *Lane, Keenon, Coleman (eds.), p. 318; Frew, Lane, Frew, pp. 378–379.*

221. **D.** One minute is the recommended time for counting the irregular pulse rate. *Frew, Lane, Frew, p. 375.*

222. **B.** With the decrease in hormone production the reproductive organs atrophy, secretion production decreases, the vagina shortens, and examination may be painful, requiring the use of additional lubricating substances. *Frew, Lane, Frew, pp. 485–486.*

223. **E.** A rash, fever, and chills are the most common reactions, although any of the other selections may result from penicillin allergy. *Lane, Medications, pp. 102–104; 275–276.*

224. **A.** Sensor-produced artifacts are distinguished by a wandering or drifting baseline. *Frew, Lane, Frew, pp. 843–844.*

225. **C.** A negative deflection of the R wave indicates that you have connected a lead wire to an incorrect sensor. *Lane, Keenon, Coleman (eds.), p. 501.*

226. **B.** The common electrode on both leads I and III is the patient's left arm. The most likely source of interference will be the left arm. *Frew, Lane, Frew, p. 844.*

227. **E.** Unlike standard leads, chest lead placement must be at precise points in order to record accurate pictures of the heart. *Lane, Keenon, Coleman (eds.), p. 500; Frew, Lane, Frew, p. 843.*

228. **A.** The first waveform to appear is the P wave and represents the impulse that causes the atria to contract. In medical terminology, the P wave, therefore, represents atrial depolarization. *Frew, Lane, Frew, p. 840; Lane, Keenon, Coleman (eds.), p. 501.*

229. **A.** Leads I, II, and III are the standard or bipolar limb leads. *Frew, Lane, Frew, p. 842.*

230. **E.** When there is one rescuer, two rescue breaths should be given after every fifteen compressions. *Frew, Lane, Frew, p. 700; Lane, Keenon, Coleman (eds.), p. 666.*

231. **C.** The carotid artery is the most accessible and easily palpated because it is so large. The femoral artery is large but not easily accessible. *Frew, Lane, Frew, p. 699; Lane, Keenon, Coleman (eds.), p. 666.*

232. **E.** The preferred position is the patient standing and allowed to fall over the arms of the rescuer. The maneuver may also be performed with the patient recumbent. *Frew, Lane, Frew, p. 680; Lane, Keenon, Coleman (eds.), p. 668.*

233. **A.** Confirmatory tests for albuminuria include the sulfosalicylic acid test, the acetic acid test, and microscopic examination. *Frew, Lane, Frew, p. 762.*

234. **B.** Eosin-methylene blue (EMB) agar and MacConkey are two examples of selective media for urine culturing. Although blood agar is also used for urine culturing, it is a nonselective media. *Frew, Lane, Frew, p. 778.*

235. **D.** *Neisseria gonorrhoeae* is a gram-negative bacterium. *Wedding and Toenjes, p. 384.*

236. **C.** A patient is to limit fat intake 12 hours prior to a cholecystogram. *Frew, Lane, Frew, p. 857.*

237. **E.** Ketones evaporate at room temperature, and they should be tested immediately. *Lane, Keenon, Coleman (eds.), p. 555.*

238. **C.** The refractometer measures the density of a liquid by the refraction of light. This density is the same as specific gravity. *Wedding and Toenjes, p. 84.*

239. **B.** Acetest tablets may be used to test for ketones (acetones). *Wedding and Toenjes, p. 103.*

240. **D.** The individual color of urine varies with the concentration of urine. *Wedding and Toenjes, p. 80.*

241. **E.** A green urine usually indicates a *Pseudomonas* infection. *Frew, Lane, Frew, p. 756.*

242. **C.** Protective eyewear or face shields should be worn during procedures that are likely to generate droplets of blood or other body fluids, to prevent exposure to the mucous membranes of the mouth, nose, and eyes. Procedures that have a high potential for creating aerosols or infectious droplets include centrifuging, blending, sonication, and vigorous mixing of human tissues. *Frew, Lane, Frew, pp. 737–738; 750; Lane, Keenon, Coleman (eds.), pp. 773–774.*

243. **E.** PKU screening is required by law in most states in the United States and in all provinces of Canada for all babies. It is performed with a wet diaper or collected urine and a Phenistix at birth and then a second time a few weeks later, during a well-baby checkup. Simple screening must be followed by more extensive laboratory testing for all positive cases. *Frew, Lane, Frew, p. 763.*

244. **D.** A test meal is ordered in preparation for a glucose tolerance test. *Lane, Keenon, Coleman (eds.), pp. 605–606; Frew, Lane, Frew, p. 816.*

245. **B.** Reagent-strip testing is specific for glucose. Clinitest tablets detect other sugars as well as glucose. *Wedding and Toenjes, p. 103.*

246. **A.** Food inhibits the absorption of penicillin. The other drugs are irritating to the stomach and should be taken with milk or meals. *Lane, Medications, p. 191.*

247. **A.** When an original label becomes separated from its container, the medical assistant would discard the medication. It is never safe to assume that a detached label belongs to a certain bottle. *Lane, Medications, p. 101.*

248. **B.** A 1:750 solution is the same as a 0.13%. Using 128 ounces (1 gallon), add one ounce of Zephiran 17% concentrate, then add 127 ounces distilled water q.s. to equal 128 ounces. *Lane, Medications, pp. 169–171.*

249. **E.** Because the vastus lateralis is the first muscle developed by the infant, it is considered the correct site for all infant intramuscular injections. *Lane, Medications, p. 202.*

250. **B.** The dose on hand is 1 g (1000 mg)/mL. Because 500 mg is one-half the drug strength on hand, you would give half of the available amount, or 0.5 mL. *Lane, Medications, p. 158.*

251. **B.** 50 mg is 1/5 of 250; therefore, administer 0.20 mL of medication. *Lane, Medications, p. 154.*

252. **E.** Proventil is classified as a bronchodilator for bronchospasm associated with reversible obstructive airway disease. *Lane, Medications, p. 289.*

253. **C.** 0.25 mL. *Lane, Medications, p. 154.*

254. **D.** There are 1000 mg in a gram; 250 mg goes into 1000 mg four times. *Lane, Medications, p. 155.*

255. **D.** Tetanus immune globulin would require the largest needle because it is a thick substance and is given intramuscularly. *Lane, Medications, p. 133.*

256. **C.** The recommended needle size for an intradermal injection is 26- or 27-gauge, 3/8 inch. *Lane, Medications, p. 133.*

257. **D.** 70% / 90% = x / 1000 mL; x = 777 mL. To make a 70% solution of isopropyl alcohol from a 90% isopropyl stock solution, you would add 777 mL of alcohol and 223 mL of diluent. *Lane, Medications, p. 171.*

258. **B.** Gentle pressure following an injection reduces pain and increases absorption of the medication. *Lane, Medications, p. 209.*

259. **D.** In the treatment of infant dehydration, therapy may include the replacement of depleted electrolytes, such as potassium, sodium, calcium, magnesium, chloride, and bicarbonate. *Lane, Keenon, Coleman (eds.), p. 599.*

260. **C.** Vitamine B_{12} is needed for the manufacture of red blood cells. If persons cannot properly absorb vitamin B_{12} from the digestive tract, it must be supplemented by injection. *Lane, Medications, p. 253.*

261. **D.** A patient with mononucleosis need not be isolated from others. Intimate exposure is needed to transfer the disease. *Lane, Keenon, Coleman (eds.), pp. 429–434.*

262. **E.** Treat all specimens as potentially infectious. All blood specimens in a collection tube are first placed in a sturdy container, then placed in a second container, such as an impervious bag, for transport. All containers should be checked for leaks. *Frew, Lane, Frew, p. 718.*

263. **D.** New CDC Universal Blood and Body-Fluid precautions recommend wearing gloves in any situation in which the medical assistant may come into contact with the patient's blood or body fluids. *Lane, Keenon, Coleman (eds.), pp. 532, 787–788; Frew, Lane, Frew, pp. 717, 900.*

264. **D.** Standard sterilization and high-level disinfection procedures are adequate to sterilize or disinfect instruments or other items contaminated with blood or other body fluids from persons infected with blood-borne pathogens. Until all items have undergone high-level disinfection or sterilization, existing recommendations are to consider all equipment "worst-case"; consequently, appropriate barrier conditions include wearing gloves. *Frew, Lane, Frew, p. 597.*

265. **E.** Gloves should be worn in any situation where there may be contact with a patient's blood or other body fluid. Saliva is not considered a category I body fluid, except in dentistry where saliva is considered mixed with blood. *Frew, Lane, Frew, pp. 716–717.*

266. **A.** Monilia is more common when antibiotics disturb the normal flora of the vagina and cause new infections called "superinfections." *Lane, Medications, p. 245.*

267. **D.** To perform a cyst removal, a small incision is made. Suturing is used to close the incision. *Lane, Keenon, Coleman (eds.), p. 385.*

268. **A.** P, R, BP, and weight are normal for a patient this age. The temperature does indicate that there is infection occurring somewhere in the body. *Lane, Keenon, Coleman (eds.), pp. 421, 427–428.*

269. **D.** 60 mg = 1 grain; 600 mg = 10 grains. *Lane, Medications, p. 12.*

270. **E.** Increased body metabolism during infancy and decreased metabolism in the elderly put both age groups at higher risk for drug toxicity than any other age group. *Lane, Medications, pp. 106–109.*

271. **A.** The "picture" given from lead I is right arm to left arm. *Frew, Lane, Frew, p. 843.*

272. **A.** Symptoms of severe head injury include projectile vomiting, unequal pupil size, a decrease in the pulse rate, and an increase in blood pressure and pulse pressure. *Frew, Lane, Frew, p. 676.*

273. **A.** A recurrent bandage is most useful when bandaging a finger. *Lane, Keenon, Coleman (eds.), p. 396.*

274. **C.** Appropriate first aid for the ingestion of 10 antihistamines could include induced vomiting or gastric lavage. *Frew, Lane, Frew, p. 683.*

275. **B.** The peripheral blood specimen can be used for complete blood counts, hematocrits, and slide tests, to name a few. Venipuncture is necessary when collecting blood that must be sterile or in a large volume for testing. *Wedding and Toenjes, p. 332.*

276. **A.** A patient may have a clear liquid breakfast the day of a barium enema. For each of the other tests listed, a patient is to have nothing by mouth after midnight the day of the test. *Frew, Lane, Frew, pp. 857–858.*

277. **C.** Mononc[sic]uleosis and rheumatoid arthritis slide tests are rapid slide tests using an agglutination reaction. If there is agglutination, the test result is positive. The rapid slide test for pregnancy is an agglutination inhibition test: agglutination only appears if the result is negative. *Wedding and Toenjes, pp. 318, 333, 345.*

278. **D.** Medications that are irritating to the digestive tract should be taken with food or milk. Tetracycline is one medication that must not be taken with dairy products (substances high in calcium). *Lane, Medications, p. 191.*

279. **B.** The injection site should not be massaged after Z-tract injections of irritating medications. *Lane, Medications, pp. 204, 209.*

280. **A.** Motrin and Advil are anti-inflammatory and analgesic but not antipyretic. Demerol is a narcotic analgesic. Tylenol is an analgesic and antipyretic but has no significant anti-inflammatory effects. *Lane, Medications, p. 244.*

281. **E.** The use of epinephrine keeps anesthesia locally longer. Epinephrine can cause severe hypotension or hypertension and cardiac arrhythmias, and therefore, should be stored away from plain anesthetics. *Lane, Medications, p. 244.*

282. **A.** Antimicrobials are used to treat infections caused by bacteria, some of the rickettsial organisms, and a few viruses. Antimicrobials are not effective against most viruses, especially those that cause the common cold, influenza, hepatitis, and AIDS. In addition to their curative effects, antimicrobials may be given prophylactically following injury or surgery. *Lane, Medications, p. 245.*

283. **B.** Subcutaneous injections must be soluble drugs less than 2.0 mL. Therefore, subcutaneous drugs must be quickly absorbable and potent enough in small quantities to be effective. *Lane, Medications, pp. 200, 201–202.*

284. C. The "right time" includes the correct time in a series of medication administration, the correct time in a body cycle, and the correct time within a 24-hour period. The method of administration must be decided under the rule "Is this the right route?" *Lane, Medications, p. 99.*

285. A. Epinephrine is a vasopressor that increases blood pressure and increases heart rate and cardiac output. It is used for cardiac emergencies, usually in repeated doses of 0.2 to 0.5 mg sc. The buttocks should be avoided. Massage after injection counteracts vasoconstriction. *Lane, Medications, pp. 256–257.*

286. B. The plunger, barrel, and outside of the needle cap are the only parts that may be touched. The needle cap opening and the needle are sterile. *Lane, Medications, pp. 131, 208.*

287. D. Milk of magnesia acts as an antacid and as a laxative. *Lane, Medications, p. 43, 83.*

288. E. Virus vaccines and certain antitoxins and immune sera (antisera) grown in animals cannot be washed free of the foreign protein of the living animals in which they were grown; thus, patients known to be sensitive to eggs or horsehair, or who have had previous exposures to horse serum, should be closely questioned and evaluated. *Lane, Medications, pp. 237, 239.*

289. E. Influenza vaccines have frequently proven useful in short-term prophylaxis for the elderly and people of all ages with conditions that might make them more likely to suffer from influenza complications. *Lane, Medications, p. 259.*

290. D. Salicylates are frequently used prophylactically for reduction of myocardial infarction risk after previous heart attack and post-operatively or in post-partum patients at increased risk for thrombophlebitis or to prevent blood platelet aggregation. *Lane, Medications, p. 242.*

291. A. Niacin, in the form of nicotinic acid, is used clinically as a vasodilator because it releases histamine, causing a flushing of the skin, and sometimes a fall in blood pressure. Side effects of niacin include GI disturbances, skin rashes, pruritis, and asthma-like episodes. *Frew, Lane, Frew, p. 521.*

292. A. The eyes are treated with sterile solutions or sterile ointments. *Lane, Medications, p. 196.*

293. D. Documented side effects of vitamin overdose include toxicity. In addition, women who have taken high doses of Vitamin C during pregnancy have given birth to babies with a dependency on high doses and who develop scurvy when deprived of those high doses. *Lane, Medications, p. 43.*

294. A. Foods rich in tyramine include aged cheeses, red wine, beer, cream, chocolate, and yeast. *Frew, Lane, Frew, p. 534.*

295. D. The rescuer must first keep herself from harm. The first action is to assess the area for live wires, fire, or any other danger to either the patient or the rescuers, then call for help. Next, determine the consciousness of the patient, then clear the airway and begin CPR, if necessary. After it is determined that the patient is breathing, search for additional wounds and care for bleeding. *Lane, Keenon, Coleman (eds.), p. 664.*

296. A. In a case of head injury, it is important to check the pupils: how they react to light and the evenness of reaction. The patient would be in a life-threatening situation if the pupils remained dilated or were unequal in size. *Frew, Lane, Frew, p. 676.*

297. B. To control bleeding of the lower leg, pressure should be placed on the femoral artery. *Frew, Lane, Frew, p. 675.*

298. E. A thready pulse is very fine and scarcely perceptible. A jerky pulse is one in which the vessel suddenly becomes distended. *Frew, Lane, Frew, p. 352.*

299. C. The Trendelenburg position should never be used in cases of head injury; and because there is a suspected back injury, the patient should not be moved. *Frew, Lane, Frew, p. 672.*

300. C. The tuning fork is used to test the perception of hearing (by tapping the instrument and moving it around the patient's ear) and for differentiating deafness owing to sound conduction or damage to the acoustic nerve (by striking the instrument and holding it against the patient's mastoid bone). *Frew, Lane, Frew, p. 403.*

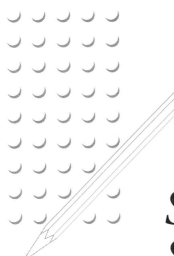

Sample Examination Simulation 5

- The following pages contain 300 test items.

- The examination is divided into:
    Part 1 - General Medical Knowledge
    Part 2 - Administrative Procedures
    Part 3 - Clinical Procedures.

- Answer sheets are provided for your use.

- The answer key immediately follows the test items and includes references with page numbers.

- References and suggested readings are at the end of the book.

Last   First   Middle

Directions for Marking Answers

- Use a black lead pencil (No. 2 or softer). Do NOT use pen or a pencil with hard lead.
- Make each mark heavy and black enough to completely obliterate the letter within the circle. Marks should fill the circles.
- Erase clearly any answer you wish to change.
- Make no stray marks on this answer sheet.
- Mark one and only one answer for each question. Multiple answers will be counted as wrong.

Example

WRONG   Ⓐ Ⓑ̷ Ⓒ Ⓓ Ⓔ

WRONG   Ⓐ Ⓑ̶ Ⓒ Ⓓ Ⓔ

WRONG   Ⓐ Ⓑ Ⓒ Ⓓ Ⓔ

RIGHT   Ⓐ Ⓑ Ⓒ ● Ⓔ

1 Ⓐ Ⓑ Ⓒ Ⓓ Ⓔ	26 Ⓐ Ⓑ Ⓒ Ⓓ Ⓔ	51 Ⓐ Ⓑ Ⓒ Ⓓ Ⓔ	76 Ⓐ Ⓑ Ⓒ Ⓓ Ⓔ
2 Ⓐ Ⓑ Ⓒ Ⓓ Ⓔ	27 Ⓐ Ⓑ Ⓒ Ⓓ Ⓔ	52 Ⓐ Ⓑ Ⓒ Ⓓ Ⓔ	77 Ⓐ Ⓑ Ⓒ Ⓓ Ⓔ
3 Ⓐ Ⓑ Ⓒ Ⓓ Ⓔ	28 Ⓐ Ⓑ Ⓒ Ⓓ Ⓔ	53 Ⓐ Ⓑ Ⓒ Ⓓ Ⓔ	78 Ⓐ Ⓑ Ⓒ Ⓓ Ⓔ
4 Ⓐ Ⓑ Ⓒ Ⓓ Ⓔ	29 Ⓐ Ⓑ Ⓒ Ⓓ Ⓔ	54 Ⓐ Ⓑ Ⓒ Ⓓ Ⓔ	79 Ⓐ Ⓑ Ⓒ Ⓓ Ⓔ
5 Ⓐ Ⓑ Ⓒ Ⓓ Ⓔ	30 Ⓐ Ⓑ Ⓒ Ⓓ Ⓔ	55 Ⓐ Ⓑ Ⓒ Ⓓ Ⓔ	80 Ⓐ Ⓑ Ⓒ Ⓓ Ⓔ
6 Ⓐ Ⓑ Ⓒ Ⓓ Ⓔ	31 Ⓐ Ⓑ Ⓒ Ⓓ Ⓔ	56 Ⓐ Ⓑ Ⓒ Ⓓ Ⓔ	81 Ⓐ Ⓑ Ⓒ Ⓓ Ⓔ
7 Ⓐ Ⓑ Ⓒ Ⓓ Ⓔ	32 Ⓐ Ⓑ Ⓒ Ⓓ Ⓔ	57 Ⓐ Ⓑ Ⓒ Ⓓ Ⓔ	82 Ⓐ Ⓑ Ⓒ Ⓓ Ⓔ
8 Ⓐ Ⓑ Ⓒ Ⓓ Ⓔ	33 Ⓐ Ⓑ Ⓒ Ⓓ Ⓔ	58 Ⓐ Ⓑ Ⓒ Ⓓ Ⓔ	83 Ⓐ Ⓑ Ⓒ Ⓓ Ⓔ
9 Ⓐ Ⓑ Ⓒ Ⓓ Ⓔ	34 Ⓐ Ⓑ Ⓒ Ⓓ Ⓔ	59 Ⓐ Ⓑ Ⓒ Ⓓ Ⓔ	84 Ⓐ Ⓑ Ⓒ Ⓓ Ⓔ
10 Ⓐ Ⓑ Ⓒ Ⓓ Ⓔ	35 Ⓐ Ⓑ Ⓒ Ⓓ Ⓔ	60 Ⓐ Ⓑ Ⓒ Ⓓ Ⓔ	85 Ⓐ Ⓑ Ⓒ Ⓓ Ⓔ
11 Ⓐ Ⓑ Ⓒ Ⓓ Ⓔ	36 Ⓐ Ⓑ Ⓒ Ⓓ Ⓔ	61 Ⓐ Ⓑ Ⓒ Ⓓ Ⓔ	86 Ⓐ Ⓑ Ⓒ Ⓓ Ⓔ
12 Ⓐ Ⓑ Ⓒ Ⓓ Ⓔ	37 Ⓐ Ⓑ Ⓒ Ⓓ Ⓔ	62 Ⓐ Ⓑ Ⓒ Ⓓ Ⓔ	87 Ⓐ Ⓑ Ⓒ Ⓓ Ⓔ
13 Ⓐ Ⓑ Ⓒ Ⓓ Ⓔ	38 Ⓐ Ⓑ Ⓒ Ⓓ Ⓔ	63 Ⓐ Ⓑ Ⓒ Ⓓ Ⓔ	88 Ⓐ Ⓑ Ⓒ Ⓓ Ⓔ
14 Ⓐ Ⓑ Ⓒ Ⓓ Ⓔ	39 Ⓐ Ⓑ Ⓒ Ⓓ Ⓔ	64 Ⓐ Ⓑ Ⓒ Ⓓ Ⓔ	89 Ⓐ Ⓑ Ⓒ Ⓓ Ⓔ
15 Ⓐ Ⓑ Ⓒ Ⓓ Ⓔ	40 Ⓐ Ⓑ Ⓒ Ⓓ Ⓔ	65 Ⓐ Ⓑ Ⓒ Ⓓ Ⓔ	90 Ⓐ Ⓑ Ⓒ Ⓓ Ⓔ
16 Ⓐ Ⓑ Ⓒ Ⓓ Ⓔ	41 Ⓐ Ⓑ Ⓒ Ⓓ Ⓔ	66 Ⓐ Ⓑ Ⓒ Ⓓ Ⓔ	91 Ⓐ Ⓑ Ⓒ Ⓓ Ⓔ
17 Ⓐ Ⓑ Ⓒ Ⓓ Ⓔ	42 Ⓐ Ⓑ Ⓒ Ⓓ Ⓔ	67 Ⓐ Ⓑ Ⓒ Ⓓ Ⓔ	92 Ⓐ Ⓑ Ⓒ Ⓓ Ⓔ
18 Ⓐ Ⓑ Ⓒ Ⓓ Ⓔ	43 Ⓐ Ⓑ Ⓒ Ⓓ Ⓔ	68 Ⓐ Ⓑ Ⓒ Ⓓ Ⓔ	93 Ⓐ Ⓑ Ⓒ Ⓓ Ⓔ
19 Ⓐ Ⓑ Ⓒ Ⓓ Ⓔ	44 Ⓐ Ⓑ Ⓒ Ⓓ Ⓔ	69 Ⓐ Ⓑ Ⓒ Ⓓ Ⓔ	94 Ⓐ Ⓑ Ⓒ Ⓓ Ⓔ
20 Ⓐ Ⓑ Ⓒ Ⓓ Ⓔ	45 Ⓐ Ⓑ Ⓒ Ⓓ Ⓔ	70 Ⓐ Ⓑ Ⓒ Ⓓ Ⓔ	95 Ⓐ Ⓑ Ⓒ Ⓓ Ⓔ
21 Ⓐ Ⓑ Ⓒ Ⓓ Ⓔ	46 Ⓐ Ⓑ Ⓒ Ⓓ Ⓔ	71 Ⓐ Ⓑ Ⓒ Ⓓ Ⓔ	96 Ⓐ Ⓑ Ⓒ Ⓓ Ⓔ
22 Ⓐ Ⓑ Ⓒ Ⓓ Ⓔ	47 Ⓐ Ⓑ Ⓒ Ⓓ Ⓔ	72 Ⓐ Ⓑ Ⓒ Ⓓ Ⓔ	97 Ⓐ Ⓑ Ⓒ Ⓓ Ⓔ
23 Ⓐ Ⓑ Ⓒ Ⓓ Ⓔ	48 Ⓐ Ⓑ Ⓒ Ⓓ Ⓔ	73 Ⓐ Ⓑ Ⓒ Ⓓ Ⓔ	98 Ⓐ Ⓑ Ⓒ Ⓓ Ⓔ
24 Ⓐ Ⓑ Ⓒ Ⓓ Ⓔ	49 Ⓐ Ⓑ Ⓒ Ⓓ Ⓔ	74 Ⓐ Ⓑ Ⓒ Ⓓ Ⓔ	99 Ⓐ Ⓑ Ⓒ Ⓓ Ⓔ
25 Ⓐ Ⓑ Ⓒ Ⓓ Ⓔ	50 Ⓐ Ⓑ Ⓒ Ⓓ Ⓔ	75 Ⓐ Ⓑ Ⓒ Ⓓ Ⓔ	100 Ⓐ Ⓑ Ⓒ Ⓓ Ⓔ

Name _____ Date _____

Last   First   Middle

Directions for Marking Answers

101 Ⓐ Ⓑ Ⓒ Ⓓ Ⓔ
102 Ⓐ Ⓑ Ⓒ Ⓓ Ⓔ
103 Ⓐ Ⓑ Ⓒ Ⓓ Ⓔ
104 Ⓐ Ⓑ Ⓒ Ⓓ Ⓔ
105 Ⓐ Ⓑ Ⓒ Ⓓ Ⓔ
106 Ⓐ Ⓑ Ⓒ Ⓓ Ⓔ
107 Ⓐ Ⓑ Ⓒ Ⓓ Ⓔ
108 Ⓐ Ⓑ Ⓒ Ⓓ Ⓔ
109 Ⓐ Ⓑ Ⓒ Ⓓ Ⓔ
110 Ⓐ Ⓑ Ⓒ Ⓓ Ⓔ
111 Ⓐ Ⓑ Ⓒ Ⓓ Ⓔ
112 Ⓐ Ⓑ Ⓒ Ⓓ Ⓔ
113 Ⓐ Ⓑ Ⓒ Ⓓ Ⓔ
114 Ⓐ Ⓑ Ⓒ Ⓓ Ⓔ
115 Ⓐ Ⓑ Ⓒ Ⓓ Ⓔ
116 Ⓐ Ⓑ Ⓒ Ⓓ Ⓔ
117 Ⓐ Ⓑ Ⓒ Ⓓ Ⓔ
118 Ⓐ Ⓑ Ⓒ Ⓓ Ⓔ
119 Ⓐ Ⓑ Ⓒ Ⓓ Ⓔ
120 Ⓐ Ⓑ Ⓒ Ⓓ Ⓔ
121 Ⓐ Ⓑ Ⓒ Ⓓ Ⓔ
122 Ⓐ Ⓑ Ⓒ Ⓓ Ⓔ
123 Ⓐ Ⓑ Ⓒ Ⓓ Ⓔ
124 Ⓐ Ⓑ Ⓒ Ⓓ Ⓔ
125 Ⓐ Ⓑ Ⓒ Ⓓ Ⓔ

126 Ⓐ Ⓑ Ⓒ Ⓓ Ⓔ
127 Ⓐ Ⓑ Ⓒ Ⓓ Ⓔ
128 Ⓐ Ⓑ Ⓒ Ⓓ Ⓔ
129 Ⓐ Ⓑ Ⓒ Ⓓ Ⓔ
130 Ⓐ Ⓑ Ⓒ Ⓓ Ⓔ
131 Ⓐ Ⓑ Ⓒ Ⓓ Ⓔ
132 Ⓐ Ⓑ Ⓒ Ⓓ Ⓔ
133 Ⓐ Ⓑ Ⓒ Ⓓ Ⓔ
134 Ⓐ Ⓑ Ⓒ Ⓓ Ⓔ
135 Ⓐ Ⓑ Ⓒ Ⓓ Ⓔ
136 Ⓐ Ⓑ Ⓒ Ⓓ Ⓔ
137 Ⓐ Ⓑ Ⓒ Ⓓ Ⓔ
138 Ⓐ Ⓑ Ⓒ Ⓓ Ⓔ
139 Ⓐ Ⓑ Ⓒ Ⓓ Ⓔ
140 Ⓐ Ⓑ Ⓒ Ⓓ Ⓔ
141 Ⓐ Ⓑ Ⓒ Ⓓ Ⓔ
142 Ⓐ Ⓑ Ⓒ Ⓓ Ⓔ
143 Ⓐ Ⓑ Ⓒ Ⓓ Ⓔ
144 Ⓐ Ⓑ Ⓒ Ⓓ Ⓔ
145 Ⓐ Ⓑ Ⓒ Ⓓ Ⓔ
146 Ⓐ Ⓑ Ⓒ Ⓓ Ⓔ
147 Ⓐ Ⓑ Ⓒ Ⓓ Ⓔ
148 Ⓐ Ⓑ Ⓒ Ⓓ Ⓔ
149 Ⓐ Ⓑ Ⓒ Ⓓ Ⓔ
150 Ⓐ Ⓑ Ⓒ Ⓓ Ⓔ

151 Ⓐ Ⓑ Ⓒ Ⓓ Ⓔ
152 Ⓐ Ⓑ Ⓒ Ⓓ Ⓔ
153 Ⓐ Ⓑ Ⓒ Ⓓ Ⓔ
154 Ⓐ Ⓑ Ⓒ Ⓓ Ⓔ
155 Ⓐ Ⓑ Ⓒ Ⓓ Ⓔ
156 Ⓐ Ⓑ Ⓒ Ⓓ Ⓔ
157 Ⓐ Ⓑ Ⓒ Ⓓ Ⓔ
158 Ⓐ Ⓑ Ⓒ Ⓓ Ⓔ
159 Ⓐ Ⓑ Ⓒ Ⓓ Ⓔ
160 Ⓐ Ⓑ Ⓒ Ⓓ Ⓔ
161 Ⓐ Ⓑ Ⓒ Ⓓ Ⓔ
162 Ⓐ Ⓑ Ⓒ Ⓓ Ⓔ
163 Ⓐ Ⓑ Ⓒ Ⓓ Ⓔ
164 Ⓐ Ⓑ Ⓒ Ⓓ Ⓔ
165 Ⓐ Ⓑ Ⓒ Ⓓ Ⓔ
166 Ⓐ Ⓑ Ⓒ Ⓓ Ⓔ
167 Ⓐ Ⓑ Ⓒ Ⓓ Ⓔ
168 Ⓐ Ⓑ Ⓒ Ⓓ Ⓔ
169 Ⓐ Ⓑ Ⓒ Ⓓ Ⓔ
170 Ⓐ Ⓑ Ⓒ Ⓓ Ⓔ
171 Ⓐ Ⓑ Ⓒ Ⓓ Ⓔ
172 Ⓐ Ⓑ Ⓒ Ⓓ Ⓔ
173 Ⓐ Ⓑ Ⓒ Ⓓ Ⓔ
174 Ⓐ Ⓑ Ⓒ Ⓓ Ⓔ
175 Ⓐ Ⓑ Ⓒ Ⓓ Ⓔ

176 Ⓐ Ⓑ Ⓒ Ⓓ Ⓔ
177 Ⓐ Ⓑ Ⓒ Ⓓ Ⓔ
178 Ⓐ Ⓑ Ⓒ Ⓓ Ⓔ
179 Ⓐ Ⓑ Ⓒ Ⓓ Ⓔ
180 Ⓐ Ⓑ Ⓒ Ⓓ Ⓔ
181 Ⓐ Ⓑ Ⓒ Ⓓ Ⓔ
182 Ⓐ Ⓑ Ⓒ Ⓓ Ⓔ
183 Ⓐ Ⓑ Ⓒ Ⓓ Ⓔ
184 Ⓐ Ⓑ Ⓒ Ⓓ Ⓔ
185 Ⓐ Ⓑ Ⓒ Ⓓ Ⓔ
186 Ⓐ Ⓑ Ⓒ Ⓓ Ⓔ
187 Ⓐ Ⓑ Ⓒ Ⓓ Ⓔ
188 Ⓐ Ⓑ Ⓒ Ⓓ Ⓔ
189 Ⓐ Ⓑ Ⓒ Ⓓ Ⓔ
190 Ⓐ Ⓑ Ⓒ Ⓓ Ⓔ
191 Ⓐ Ⓑ Ⓒ Ⓓ Ⓔ
192 Ⓐ Ⓑ Ⓒ Ⓓ Ⓔ
193 Ⓐ Ⓑ Ⓒ Ⓓ Ⓔ
194 Ⓐ Ⓑ Ⓒ Ⓓ Ⓔ
195 Ⓐ Ⓑ Ⓒ Ⓓ Ⓔ
196 Ⓐ Ⓑ Ⓒ Ⓓ Ⓔ
197 Ⓐ Ⓑ Ⓒ Ⓓ Ⓔ
198 Ⓐ Ⓑ Ⓒ Ⓓ Ⓔ
199 Ⓐ Ⓑ Ⓒ Ⓓ Ⓔ
200 Ⓐ Ⓑ Ⓒ Ⓓ Ⓔ

Directions for Marking Answers

- Use a black lead pencil (No. 2 or softer). Do NOT use pen or a pencil with hard lead.
- Make each mark heavy and black enough to completely obliterate the letter within the circle. Marks should fill the circles.
- Erase clearly any answer you wish to change.
- Make no stray marks on this answer sheet.
- Mark one and only one answer for each question. Multiple answers will be counted as wrong.

Example

WRONG Ⓐ Ⓑ Ⓒ Ⓓ Ⓔ
WRONG Ⓐ Ⓑ Ⓒ Ⓓ Ⓔ
WRONG Ⓐ Ⓑ Ⓒ Ⓓ Ⓔ
RIGHT Ⓐ Ⓑ Ⓒ ● Ⓔ

201 Ⓐ Ⓑ Ⓒ Ⓓ Ⓔ   226 Ⓐ Ⓑ Ⓒ Ⓓ Ⓔ   251 Ⓐ Ⓑ Ⓒ Ⓓ Ⓔ   276 Ⓐ Ⓑ Ⓒ Ⓓ Ⓔ
202 Ⓐ Ⓑ Ⓒ Ⓓ Ⓔ   227 Ⓐ Ⓑ Ⓒ Ⓓ Ⓔ   252 Ⓐ Ⓑ Ⓒ Ⓓ Ⓔ   277 Ⓐ Ⓑ Ⓒ Ⓓ Ⓔ
203 Ⓐ Ⓑ Ⓒ Ⓓ Ⓔ   228 Ⓐ Ⓑ Ⓒ Ⓓ Ⓔ   253 Ⓐ Ⓑ Ⓒ Ⓓ Ⓔ   278 Ⓐ Ⓑ Ⓒ Ⓓ Ⓔ
204 Ⓐ Ⓑ Ⓒ Ⓓ Ⓔ   229 Ⓐ Ⓑ Ⓒ Ⓓ Ⓔ   254 Ⓐ Ⓑ Ⓒ Ⓓ Ⓔ   279 Ⓐ Ⓑ Ⓒ Ⓓ Ⓔ
205 Ⓐ Ⓑ Ⓒ Ⓓ Ⓔ   230 Ⓐ Ⓑ Ⓒ Ⓓ Ⓔ   255 Ⓐ Ⓑ Ⓒ Ⓓ Ⓔ   280 Ⓐ Ⓑ Ⓒ Ⓓ Ⓔ
206 Ⓐ Ⓑ Ⓒ Ⓓ Ⓔ   231 Ⓐ Ⓑ Ⓒ Ⓓ Ⓔ   256 Ⓐ Ⓑ Ⓒ Ⓓ Ⓔ   281 Ⓐ Ⓑ Ⓒ Ⓓ Ⓔ
207 Ⓐ Ⓑ Ⓒ Ⓓ Ⓔ   232 Ⓐ Ⓑ Ⓒ Ⓓ Ⓔ   257 Ⓐ Ⓑ Ⓒ Ⓓ Ⓔ   282 Ⓐ Ⓑ Ⓒ Ⓓ Ⓔ
208 Ⓐ Ⓑ Ⓒ Ⓓ Ⓔ   233 Ⓐ Ⓑ Ⓒ Ⓓ Ⓔ   258 Ⓐ Ⓑ Ⓒ Ⓓ Ⓔ   283 Ⓐ Ⓑ Ⓒ Ⓓ Ⓔ
209 Ⓐ Ⓑ Ⓒ Ⓓ Ⓔ   234 Ⓐ Ⓑ Ⓒ Ⓓ Ⓔ   259 Ⓐ Ⓑ Ⓒ Ⓓ Ⓔ   284 Ⓐ Ⓑ Ⓒ Ⓓ Ⓔ
210 Ⓐ Ⓑ Ⓒ Ⓓ Ⓔ   235 Ⓐ Ⓑ Ⓒ Ⓓ Ⓔ   260 Ⓐ Ⓑ Ⓒ Ⓓ Ⓔ   285 Ⓐ Ⓑ Ⓒ Ⓓ Ⓔ
211 Ⓐ Ⓑ Ⓒ Ⓓ Ⓔ   236 Ⓐ Ⓑ Ⓒ Ⓓ Ⓔ   261 Ⓐ Ⓑ Ⓒ Ⓓ Ⓔ   286 Ⓐ Ⓑ Ⓒ Ⓓ Ⓔ
212 Ⓐ Ⓑ Ⓒ Ⓓ Ⓔ   237 Ⓐ Ⓑ Ⓒ Ⓓ Ⓔ   262 Ⓐ Ⓑ Ⓒ Ⓓ Ⓔ   287 Ⓐ Ⓑ Ⓒ Ⓓ Ⓔ
213 Ⓐ Ⓑ Ⓒ Ⓓ Ⓔ   238 Ⓐ Ⓑ Ⓒ Ⓓ Ⓔ   263 Ⓐ Ⓑ Ⓒ Ⓓ Ⓔ   288 Ⓐ Ⓑ Ⓒ Ⓓ Ⓔ
214 Ⓐ Ⓑ Ⓒ Ⓓ Ⓔ   239 Ⓐ Ⓑ Ⓒ Ⓓ Ⓔ   264 Ⓐ Ⓑ Ⓒ Ⓓ Ⓔ   289 Ⓐ Ⓑ Ⓒ Ⓓ Ⓔ
215 Ⓐ Ⓑ Ⓒ Ⓓ Ⓔ   240 Ⓐ Ⓑ Ⓒ Ⓓ Ⓔ   265 Ⓐ Ⓑ Ⓒ Ⓓ Ⓔ   290 Ⓐ Ⓑ Ⓒ Ⓓ Ⓔ
216 Ⓐ Ⓑ Ⓒ Ⓓ Ⓔ   241 Ⓐ Ⓑ Ⓒ Ⓓ Ⓔ   266 Ⓐ Ⓑ Ⓒ Ⓓ Ⓔ   291 Ⓐ Ⓑ Ⓒ Ⓓ Ⓔ
217 Ⓐ Ⓑ Ⓒ Ⓓ Ⓔ   242 Ⓐ Ⓑ Ⓒ Ⓓ Ⓔ   267 Ⓐ Ⓑ Ⓒ Ⓓ Ⓔ   292 Ⓐ Ⓑ Ⓒ Ⓓ Ⓔ
218 Ⓐ Ⓑ Ⓒ Ⓓ Ⓔ   243 Ⓐ Ⓑ Ⓒ Ⓓ Ⓔ   268 Ⓐ Ⓑ Ⓒ Ⓓ Ⓔ   293 Ⓐ Ⓑ Ⓒ Ⓓ Ⓔ
219 Ⓐ Ⓑ Ⓒ Ⓓ Ⓔ   244 Ⓐ Ⓑ Ⓒ Ⓓ Ⓔ   269 Ⓐ Ⓑ Ⓒ Ⓓ Ⓔ   294 Ⓐ Ⓑ Ⓒ Ⓓ Ⓔ
220 Ⓐ Ⓑ Ⓒ Ⓓ Ⓔ   245 Ⓐ Ⓑ Ⓒ Ⓓ Ⓔ   270 Ⓐ Ⓑ Ⓒ Ⓓ Ⓔ   295 Ⓐ Ⓑ Ⓒ Ⓓ Ⓔ
221 Ⓐ Ⓑ Ⓒ Ⓓ Ⓔ   246 Ⓐ Ⓑ Ⓒ Ⓓ Ⓔ   271 Ⓐ Ⓑ Ⓒ Ⓓ Ⓔ   296 Ⓐ Ⓑ Ⓒ Ⓓ Ⓔ
222 Ⓐ Ⓑ Ⓒ Ⓓ Ⓔ   247 Ⓐ Ⓑ Ⓒ Ⓓ Ⓔ   272 Ⓐ Ⓑ Ⓒ Ⓓ Ⓔ   297 Ⓐ Ⓑ Ⓒ Ⓓ Ⓔ
223 Ⓐ Ⓑ Ⓒ Ⓓ Ⓔ   248 Ⓐ Ⓑ Ⓒ Ⓓ Ⓔ   273 Ⓐ Ⓑ Ⓒ Ⓓ Ⓔ   298 Ⓐ Ⓑ Ⓒ Ⓓ Ⓔ
224 Ⓐ Ⓑ Ⓒ Ⓓ Ⓔ   249 Ⓐ Ⓑ Ⓒ Ⓓ Ⓔ   274 Ⓐ Ⓑ Ⓒ Ⓓ Ⓔ   299 Ⓐ Ⓑ Ⓒ Ⓓ Ⓔ
225 Ⓐ Ⓑ Ⓒ Ⓓ Ⓔ   250 Ⓐ Ⓑ Ⓒ Ⓓ Ⓔ   275 Ⓐ Ⓑ Ⓒ Ⓓ Ⓔ   300 Ⓐ Ⓑ Ⓒ Ⓓ Ⓔ

Directions for Marking Answers

- Use a black lead pencil (No. 2 or softer). Do NOT use pen or a pencil with hard lead.
- Make each mark heavy and black enough to completely obliterate the letter within the circle. Marks should fill the circles.
- Erase clearly any answer you wish to change.
- Make no stray marks on this answer sheet.
- Mark one and only one answer for each question. Multiple answers will be counted as wrong.

Example

WRONG   Ⓐ Ⓑ̸ Ⓒ Ⓓ Ⓔ

WRONG   Ⓐ ⊠ Ⓒ Ⓓ Ⓔ

WRONG   Ⓐ Ⓑ Ⓒ Ⓓ Ⓔ

RIGHT   Ⓐ Ⓑ Ⓒ ● Ⓔ

1 Ⓐ Ⓑ Ⓒ Ⓓ Ⓔ	26 Ⓐ Ⓑ Ⓒ Ⓓ Ⓔ	51 Ⓐ Ⓑ Ⓒ Ⓓ Ⓔ	76 Ⓐ Ⓑ Ⓒ Ⓓ Ⓔ
2 Ⓐ Ⓑ Ⓒ Ⓓ Ⓔ	27 Ⓐ Ⓑ Ⓒ Ⓓ Ⓔ	52 Ⓐ Ⓑ Ⓒ Ⓓ Ⓔ	77 Ⓐ Ⓑ Ⓒ Ⓓ Ⓔ
3 Ⓐ Ⓑ Ⓒ Ⓓ Ⓔ	28 Ⓐ Ⓑ Ⓒ Ⓓ Ⓔ	53 Ⓐ Ⓑ Ⓒ Ⓓ Ⓔ	78 Ⓐ Ⓑ Ⓒ Ⓓ Ⓔ
4 Ⓐ Ⓑ Ⓒ Ⓓ Ⓔ	29 Ⓐ Ⓑ Ⓒ Ⓓ Ⓔ	54 Ⓐ Ⓑ Ⓒ Ⓓ Ⓔ	79 Ⓐ Ⓑ Ⓒ Ⓓ Ⓔ
5 Ⓐ Ⓑ Ⓒ Ⓓ Ⓔ	30 Ⓐ Ⓑ Ⓒ Ⓓ Ⓔ	55 Ⓐ Ⓑ Ⓒ Ⓓ Ⓔ	80 Ⓐ Ⓑ Ⓒ Ⓓ Ⓔ
6 Ⓐ Ⓑ Ⓒ Ⓓ Ⓔ	31 Ⓐ Ⓑ Ⓒ Ⓓ Ⓔ	56 Ⓐ Ⓑ Ⓒ Ⓓ Ⓔ	81 Ⓐ Ⓑ Ⓒ Ⓓ Ⓔ
7 Ⓐ Ⓑ Ⓒ Ⓓ Ⓔ	32 Ⓐ Ⓑ Ⓒ Ⓓ Ⓔ	57 Ⓐ Ⓑ Ⓒ Ⓓ Ⓔ	82 Ⓐ Ⓑ Ⓒ Ⓓ Ⓔ
8 Ⓐ Ⓑ Ⓒ Ⓓ Ⓔ	33 Ⓐ Ⓑ Ⓒ Ⓓ Ⓔ	58 Ⓐ Ⓑ Ⓒ Ⓓ Ⓔ	83 Ⓐ Ⓑ Ⓒ Ⓓ Ⓔ
9 Ⓐ Ⓑ Ⓒ Ⓓ Ⓔ	34 Ⓐ Ⓑ Ⓒ Ⓓ Ⓔ	59 Ⓐ Ⓑ Ⓒ Ⓓ Ⓔ	84 Ⓐ Ⓑ Ⓒ Ⓓ Ⓔ
10 Ⓐ Ⓑ Ⓒ Ⓓ Ⓔ	35 Ⓐ Ⓑ Ⓒ Ⓓ Ⓔ	60 Ⓐ Ⓑ Ⓒ Ⓓ Ⓔ	85 Ⓐ Ⓑ Ⓒ Ⓓ Ⓔ
11 Ⓐ Ⓑ Ⓒ Ⓓ Ⓔ	36 Ⓐ Ⓑ Ⓒ Ⓓ Ⓔ	61 Ⓐ Ⓑ Ⓒ Ⓓ Ⓔ	86 Ⓐ Ⓑ Ⓒ Ⓓ Ⓔ
12 Ⓐ Ⓑ Ⓒ Ⓓ Ⓔ	37 Ⓐ Ⓑ Ⓒ Ⓓ Ⓔ	62 Ⓐ Ⓑ Ⓒ Ⓓ Ⓔ	87 Ⓐ Ⓑ Ⓒ Ⓓ Ⓔ
13 Ⓐ Ⓑ Ⓒ Ⓓ Ⓔ	38 Ⓐ Ⓑ Ⓒ Ⓓ Ⓔ	63 Ⓐ Ⓑ Ⓒ Ⓓ Ⓔ	88 Ⓐ Ⓑ Ⓒ Ⓓ Ⓔ
14 Ⓐ Ⓑ Ⓒ Ⓓ Ⓔ	39 Ⓐ Ⓑ Ⓒ Ⓓ Ⓔ	64 Ⓐ Ⓑ Ⓒ Ⓓ Ⓔ	89 Ⓐ Ⓑ Ⓒ Ⓓ Ⓔ
15 Ⓐ Ⓑ Ⓒ Ⓓ Ⓔ	40 Ⓐ Ⓑ Ⓒ Ⓓ Ⓔ	65 Ⓐ Ⓑ Ⓒ Ⓓ Ⓔ	90 Ⓐ Ⓑ Ⓒ Ⓓ Ⓔ
16 Ⓐ Ⓑ Ⓒ Ⓓ Ⓔ	41 Ⓐ Ⓑ Ⓒ Ⓓ Ⓔ	66 Ⓐ Ⓑ Ⓒ Ⓓ Ⓔ	91 Ⓐ Ⓑ Ⓒ Ⓓ Ⓔ
17 Ⓐ Ⓑ Ⓒ Ⓓ Ⓔ	42 Ⓐ Ⓑ Ⓒ Ⓓ Ⓔ	67 Ⓐ Ⓑ Ⓒ Ⓓ Ⓔ	92 Ⓐ Ⓑ Ⓒ Ⓓ Ⓔ
18 Ⓐ Ⓑ Ⓒ Ⓓ Ⓔ	43 Ⓐ Ⓑ Ⓒ Ⓓ Ⓔ	68 Ⓐ Ⓑ Ⓒ Ⓓ Ⓔ	93 Ⓐ Ⓑ Ⓒ Ⓓ Ⓔ
19 Ⓐ Ⓑ Ⓒ Ⓓ Ⓔ	44 Ⓐ Ⓑ Ⓒ Ⓓ Ⓔ	69 Ⓐ Ⓑ Ⓒ Ⓓ Ⓔ	94 Ⓐ Ⓑ Ⓒ Ⓓ Ⓔ
20 Ⓐ Ⓑ Ⓒ Ⓓ Ⓔ	45 Ⓐ Ⓑ Ⓒ Ⓓ Ⓔ	70 Ⓐ Ⓑ Ⓒ Ⓓ Ⓔ	95 Ⓐ Ⓑ Ⓒ Ⓓ Ⓔ
21 Ⓐ Ⓑ Ⓒ Ⓓ Ⓔ	46 Ⓐ Ⓑ Ⓒ Ⓓ Ⓔ	71 Ⓐ Ⓑ Ⓒ Ⓓ Ⓔ	96 Ⓐ Ⓑ Ⓒ Ⓓ Ⓔ
22 Ⓐ Ⓑ Ⓒ Ⓓ Ⓔ	47 Ⓐ Ⓑ Ⓒ Ⓓ Ⓔ	72 Ⓐ Ⓑ Ⓒ Ⓓ Ⓔ	97 Ⓐ Ⓑ Ⓒ Ⓓ Ⓔ
23 Ⓐ Ⓑ Ⓒ Ⓓ Ⓔ	48 Ⓐ Ⓑ Ⓒ Ⓓ Ⓔ	73 Ⓐ Ⓑ Ⓒ Ⓓ Ⓔ	98 Ⓐ Ⓑ Ⓒ Ⓓ Ⓔ
24 Ⓐ Ⓑ Ⓒ Ⓓ Ⓔ	49 Ⓐ Ⓑ Ⓒ Ⓓ Ⓔ	74 Ⓐ Ⓑ Ⓒ Ⓓ Ⓔ	99 Ⓐ Ⓑ Ⓒ Ⓓ Ⓔ
25 Ⓐ Ⓑ Ⓒ Ⓓ Ⓔ	50 Ⓐ Ⓑ Ⓒ Ⓓ Ⓔ	75 Ⓐ Ⓑ Ⓒ Ⓓ Ⓔ	100 Ⓐ Ⓑ Ⓒ Ⓓ Ⓔ

Name _____ **Date** _____
         Last   First   Middle

Directions for Marking Answers

- Use a black lead pencil (No. 2 or softer). Do NOT use pen or a pencil with hard lead.
- Make each mark heavy and black enough to completely obliterate the letter within the circle. Marks should fill the circles.
- Erase clearly any answer you wish to change.
- Make no stray marks on this answer sheet.
- Mark one and only one answer for each question. Multiple answers will be counted as wrong.

Example

WRONG   Ⓐ Ⓑ Ⓒ Ⓓ Ⓔ
WRONG   Ⓐ Ⓑ Ⓒ Ⓓ Ⓔ
WRONG   Ⓐ Ⓑ Ⓒ Ⓓ Ⓔ
RIGHT   Ⓐ Ⓑ Ⓒ ● Ⓔ

101 Ⓐ Ⓑ Ⓒ Ⓓ Ⓔ	126 Ⓐ Ⓑ Ⓒ Ⓓ Ⓔ	151 Ⓐ Ⓑ Ⓒ Ⓓ Ⓔ	176 Ⓐ Ⓑ Ⓒ Ⓓ Ⓔ
102 Ⓐ Ⓑ Ⓒ Ⓓ Ⓔ	127 Ⓐ Ⓑ Ⓒ Ⓓ Ⓔ	152 Ⓐ Ⓑ Ⓒ Ⓓ Ⓔ	177 Ⓐ Ⓑ Ⓒ Ⓓ Ⓔ
103 Ⓐ Ⓑ Ⓒ Ⓓ Ⓔ	128 Ⓐ Ⓑ Ⓒ Ⓓ Ⓔ	153 Ⓐ Ⓑ Ⓒ Ⓓ Ⓔ	178 Ⓐ Ⓑ Ⓒ Ⓓ Ⓔ
104 Ⓐ Ⓑ Ⓒ Ⓓ Ⓔ	129 Ⓐ Ⓑ Ⓒ Ⓓ Ⓔ	154 Ⓐ Ⓑ Ⓒ Ⓓ Ⓔ	179 Ⓐ Ⓑ Ⓒ Ⓓ Ⓔ
105 Ⓐ Ⓑ Ⓒ Ⓓ Ⓔ	130 Ⓐ Ⓑ Ⓒ Ⓓ Ⓔ	155 Ⓐ Ⓑ Ⓒ Ⓓ Ⓔ	180 Ⓐ Ⓑ Ⓒ Ⓓ Ⓔ
106 Ⓐ Ⓑ Ⓒ Ⓓ Ⓔ	131 Ⓐ Ⓑ Ⓒ Ⓓ Ⓔ	156 Ⓐ Ⓑ Ⓒ Ⓓ Ⓔ	181 Ⓐ Ⓑ Ⓒ Ⓓ Ⓔ
107 Ⓐ Ⓑ Ⓒ Ⓓ Ⓔ	132 Ⓐ Ⓑ Ⓒ Ⓓ Ⓔ	157 Ⓐ Ⓑ Ⓒ Ⓓ Ⓔ	182 Ⓐ Ⓑ Ⓒ Ⓓ Ⓔ
108 Ⓐ Ⓑ Ⓒ Ⓓ Ⓔ	133 Ⓐ Ⓑ Ⓒ Ⓓ Ⓔ	158 Ⓐ Ⓑ Ⓒ Ⓓ Ⓔ	183 Ⓐ Ⓑ Ⓒ Ⓓ Ⓔ
109 Ⓐ Ⓑ Ⓒ Ⓓ Ⓔ	134 Ⓐ Ⓑ Ⓒ Ⓓ Ⓔ	159 Ⓐ Ⓑ Ⓒ Ⓓ Ⓔ	184 Ⓐ Ⓑ Ⓒ Ⓓ Ⓔ
110 Ⓐ Ⓑ Ⓒ Ⓓ Ⓔ	135 Ⓐ Ⓑ Ⓒ Ⓓ Ⓔ	160 Ⓐ Ⓑ Ⓒ Ⓓ Ⓔ	185 Ⓐ Ⓑ Ⓒ Ⓓ Ⓔ
111 Ⓐ Ⓑ Ⓒ Ⓓ Ⓔ	136 Ⓐ Ⓑ Ⓒ Ⓓ Ⓔ	161 Ⓐ Ⓑ Ⓒ Ⓓ Ⓔ	186 Ⓐ Ⓑ Ⓒ Ⓓ Ⓔ
112 Ⓐ Ⓑ Ⓒ Ⓓ Ⓔ	137 Ⓐ Ⓑ Ⓒ Ⓓ Ⓔ	162 Ⓐ Ⓑ Ⓒ Ⓓ Ⓔ	187 Ⓐ Ⓑ Ⓒ Ⓓ Ⓔ
113 Ⓐ Ⓑ Ⓒ Ⓓ Ⓔ	138 Ⓐ Ⓑ Ⓒ Ⓓ Ⓔ	163 Ⓐ Ⓑ Ⓒ Ⓓ Ⓔ	188 Ⓐ Ⓑ Ⓒ Ⓓ Ⓔ
114 Ⓐ Ⓑ Ⓒ Ⓓ Ⓔ	139 Ⓐ Ⓑ Ⓒ Ⓓ Ⓔ	164 Ⓐ Ⓑ Ⓒ Ⓓ Ⓔ	189 Ⓐ Ⓑ Ⓒ Ⓓ Ⓔ
115 Ⓐ Ⓑ Ⓒ Ⓓ Ⓔ	140 Ⓐ Ⓑ Ⓒ Ⓓ Ⓔ	165 Ⓐ Ⓑ Ⓒ Ⓓ Ⓔ	190 Ⓐ Ⓑ Ⓒ Ⓓ Ⓔ
116 Ⓐ Ⓑ Ⓒ Ⓓ Ⓔ	141 Ⓐ Ⓑ Ⓒ Ⓓ Ⓔ	166 Ⓐ Ⓑ Ⓒ Ⓓ Ⓔ	191 Ⓐ Ⓑ Ⓒ Ⓓ Ⓔ
117 Ⓐ Ⓑ Ⓒ Ⓓ Ⓔ	142 Ⓐ Ⓑ Ⓒ Ⓓ Ⓔ	167 Ⓐ Ⓑ Ⓒ Ⓓ Ⓔ	192 Ⓐ Ⓑ Ⓒ Ⓓ Ⓔ
118 Ⓐ Ⓑ Ⓒ Ⓓ Ⓔ	143 Ⓐ Ⓑ Ⓒ Ⓓ Ⓔ	168 Ⓐ Ⓑ Ⓒ Ⓓ Ⓔ	193 Ⓐ Ⓑ Ⓒ Ⓓ Ⓔ
119 Ⓐ Ⓑ Ⓒ Ⓓ Ⓔ	144 Ⓐ Ⓑ Ⓒ Ⓓ Ⓔ	169 Ⓐ Ⓑ Ⓒ Ⓓ Ⓔ	194 Ⓐ Ⓑ Ⓒ Ⓓ Ⓔ
120 Ⓐ Ⓑ Ⓒ Ⓓ Ⓔ	145 Ⓐ Ⓑ Ⓒ Ⓓ Ⓔ	170 Ⓐ Ⓑ Ⓒ Ⓓ Ⓔ	195 Ⓐ Ⓑ Ⓒ Ⓓ Ⓔ
121 Ⓐ Ⓑ Ⓒ Ⓓ Ⓔ	146 Ⓐ Ⓑ Ⓒ Ⓓ Ⓔ	171 Ⓐ Ⓑ Ⓒ Ⓓ Ⓔ	196 Ⓐ Ⓑ Ⓒ Ⓓ Ⓔ
122 Ⓐ Ⓑ Ⓒ Ⓓ Ⓔ	147 Ⓐ Ⓑ Ⓒ Ⓓ Ⓔ	172 Ⓐ Ⓑ Ⓒ Ⓓ Ⓔ	197 Ⓐ Ⓑ Ⓒ Ⓓ Ⓔ
123 Ⓐ Ⓑ Ⓒ Ⓓ Ⓔ	148 Ⓐ Ⓑ Ⓒ Ⓓ Ⓔ	173 Ⓐ Ⓑ Ⓒ Ⓓ Ⓔ	198 Ⓐ Ⓑ Ⓒ Ⓓ Ⓔ
124 Ⓐ Ⓑ Ⓒ Ⓓ Ⓔ	149 Ⓐ Ⓑ Ⓒ Ⓓ Ⓔ	174 Ⓐ Ⓑ Ⓒ Ⓓ Ⓔ	199 Ⓐ Ⓑ Ⓒ Ⓓ Ⓔ
125 Ⓐ Ⓑ Ⓒ Ⓓ Ⓔ	150 Ⓐ Ⓑ Ⓒ Ⓓ Ⓔ	175 Ⓐ Ⓑ Ⓒ Ⓓ Ⓔ	200 Ⓐ Ⓑ Ⓒ Ⓓ Ⓔ

Last   First   Middle

Directions for Marking Answers

- Use a black lead pencil (No. 2 or softer). Do NOT use pen or a pencil with hard lead.
- Make each mark heavy and black enough to completely obliterate the letter within the circle. Marks should fill the circles.
- Erase clearly any answer you wish to change.
- Make no stray marks on this answer sheet.
- Mark one and only one answer for each question. Multiple answers will be counted as wrong.

Example

WRONG   Ⓐ Ⓑ Ⓒ Ⓓ Ⓔ

WRONG   Ⓐ Ⓑ Ⓒ Ⓓ Ⓔ

WRONG   Ⓐ Ⓑ Ⓒ Ⓓ Ⓔ

RIGHT   Ⓐ Ⓑ Ⓒ ● Ⓔ

201 Ⓐ Ⓑ Ⓒ Ⓓ Ⓔ	226 Ⓐ Ⓑ Ⓒ Ⓓ Ⓔ	251 Ⓐ Ⓑ Ⓒ Ⓓ Ⓔ	276 Ⓐ Ⓑ Ⓒ Ⓓ Ⓔ
202 Ⓐ Ⓑ Ⓒ Ⓓ Ⓔ	227 Ⓐ Ⓑ Ⓒ Ⓓ Ⓔ	252 Ⓐ Ⓑ Ⓒ Ⓓ Ⓔ	277 Ⓐ Ⓑ Ⓒ Ⓓ Ⓔ
203 Ⓐ Ⓑ Ⓒ Ⓓ Ⓔ	228 Ⓐ Ⓑ Ⓒ Ⓓ Ⓔ	253 Ⓐ Ⓑ Ⓒ Ⓓ Ⓔ	278 Ⓐ Ⓑ Ⓒ Ⓓ Ⓔ
204 Ⓐ Ⓑ Ⓒ Ⓓ Ⓔ	229 Ⓐ Ⓑ Ⓒ Ⓓ Ⓔ	254 Ⓐ Ⓑ Ⓒ Ⓓ Ⓔ	279 Ⓐ Ⓑ Ⓒ Ⓓ Ⓔ
205 Ⓐ Ⓑ Ⓒ Ⓓ Ⓔ	230 Ⓐ Ⓑ Ⓒ Ⓓ Ⓔ	255 Ⓐ Ⓑ Ⓒ Ⓓ Ⓔ	280 Ⓐ Ⓑ Ⓒ Ⓓ Ⓔ
206 Ⓐ Ⓑ Ⓒ Ⓓ Ⓔ	231 Ⓐ Ⓑ Ⓒ Ⓓ Ⓔ	256 Ⓐ Ⓑ Ⓒ Ⓓ Ⓔ	281 Ⓐ Ⓑ Ⓒ Ⓓ Ⓔ
207 Ⓐ Ⓑ Ⓒ Ⓓ Ⓔ	232 Ⓐ Ⓑ Ⓒ Ⓓ Ⓔ	257 Ⓐ Ⓑ Ⓒ Ⓓ Ⓔ	282 Ⓐ Ⓑ Ⓒ Ⓓ Ⓔ
208 Ⓐ Ⓑ Ⓒ Ⓓ Ⓔ	233 Ⓐ Ⓑ Ⓒ Ⓓ Ⓔ	258 Ⓐ Ⓑ Ⓒ Ⓓ Ⓔ	283 Ⓐ Ⓑ Ⓒ Ⓓ Ⓔ
209 Ⓐ Ⓑ Ⓒ Ⓓ Ⓔ	234 Ⓐ Ⓑ Ⓒ Ⓓ Ⓔ	259 Ⓐ Ⓑ Ⓒ Ⓓ Ⓔ	284 Ⓐ Ⓑ Ⓒ Ⓓ Ⓔ
210 Ⓐ Ⓑ Ⓒ Ⓓ Ⓔ	235 Ⓐ Ⓑ Ⓒ Ⓓ Ⓔ	260 Ⓐ Ⓑ Ⓒ Ⓓ Ⓔ	285 Ⓐ Ⓑ Ⓒ Ⓓ Ⓔ
211 Ⓐ Ⓑ Ⓒ Ⓓ Ⓔ	236 Ⓐ Ⓑ Ⓒ Ⓓ Ⓔ	261 Ⓐ Ⓑ Ⓒ Ⓓ Ⓔ	286 Ⓐ Ⓑ Ⓒ Ⓓ Ⓔ
212 Ⓐ Ⓑ Ⓒ Ⓓ Ⓔ	237 Ⓐ Ⓑ Ⓒ Ⓓ Ⓔ	262 Ⓐ Ⓑ Ⓒ Ⓓ Ⓔ	287 Ⓐ Ⓑ Ⓒ Ⓓ Ⓔ
213 Ⓐ Ⓑ Ⓒ Ⓓ Ⓔ	238 Ⓐ Ⓑ Ⓒ Ⓓ Ⓔ	263 Ⓐ Ⓑ Ⓒ Ⓓ Ⓔ	288 Ⓐ Ⓑ Ⓒ Ⓓ Ⓔ
214 Ⓐ Ⓑ Ⓒ Ⓓ Ⓔ	239 Ⓐ Ⓑ Ⓒ Ⓓ Ⓔ	264 Ⓐ Ⓑ Ⓒ Ⓓ Ⓔ	289 Ⓐ Ⓑ Ⓒ Ⓓ Ⓔ
215 Ⓐ Ⓑ Ⓒ Ⓓ Ⓔ	240 Ⓐ Ⓑ Ⓒ Ⓓ Ⓔ	265 Ⓐ Ⓑ Ⓒ Ⓓ Ⓔ	290 Ⓐ Ⓑ Ⓒ Ⓓ Ⓔ
216 Ⓐ Ⓑ Ⓒ Ⓓ Ⓔ	241 Ⓐ Ⓑ Ⓒ Ⓓ Ⓔ	266 Ⓐ Ⓑ Ⓒ Ⓓ Ⓔ	291 Ⓐ Ⓑ Ⓒ Ⓓ Ⓔ
217 Ⓐ Ⓑ Ⓒ Ⓓ Ⓔ	242 Ⓐ Ⓑ Ⓒ Ⓓ Ⓔ	267 Ⓐ Ⓑ Ⓒ Ⓓ Ⓔ	292 Ⓐ Ⓑ Ⓒ Ⓓ Ⓔ
218 Ⓐ Ⓑ Ⓒ Ⓓ Ⓔ	243 Ⓐ Ⓑ Ⓒ Ⓓ Ⓔ	268 Ⓐ Ⓑ Ⓒ Ⓓ Ⓔ	293 Ⓐ Ⓑ Ⓒ Ⓓ Ⓔ
219 Ⓐ Ⓑ Ⓒ Ⓓ Ⓔ	244 Ⓐ Ⓑ Ⓒ Ⓓ Ⓔ	269 Ⓐ Ⓑ Ⓒ Ⓓ Ⓔ	294 Ⓐ Ⓑ Ⓒ Ⓓ Ⓔ
220 Ⓐ Ⓑ Ⓒ Ⓓ Ⓔ	245 Ⓐ Ⓑ Ⓒ Ⓓ Ⓔ	270 Ⓐ Ⓑ Ⓒ Ⓓ Ⓔ	295 Ⓐ Ⓑ Ⓒ Ⓓ Ⓔ
221 Ⓐ Ⓑ Ⓒ Ⓓ Ⓔ	246 Ⓐ Ⓑ Ⓒ Ⓓ Ⓔ	271 Ⓐ Ⓑ Ⓒ Ⓓ Ⓔ	296 Ⓐ Ⓑ Ⓒ Ⓓ Ⓔ
222 Ⓐ Ⓑ Ⓒ Ⓓ Ⓔ	247 Ⓐ Ⓑ Ⓒ Ⓓ Ⓔ	272 Ⓐ Ⓑ Ⓒ Ⓓ Ⓔ	297 Ⓐ Ⓑ Ⓒ Ⓓ Ⓔ
223 Ⓐ Ⓑ Ⓒ Ⓓ Ⓔ	248 Ⓐ Ⓑ Ⓒ Ⓓ Ⓔ	273 Ⓐ Ⓑ Ⓒ Ⓓ Ⓔ	298 Ⓐ Ⓑ Ⓒ Ⓓ Ⓔ
224 Ⓐ Ⓑ Ⓒ Ⓓ Ⓔ	249 Ⓐ Ⓑ Ⓒ Ⓓ Ⓔ	274 Ⓐ Ⓑ Ⓒ Ⓓ Ⓔ	299 Ⓐ Ⓑ Ⓒ Ⓓ Ⓔ
225 Ⓐ Ⓑ Ⓒ Ⓓ Ⓔ	250 Ⓐ Ⓑ Ⓒ Ⓓ Ⓔ	275 Ⓐ Ⓑ Ⓒ Ⓓ Ⓔ	300 Ⓐ Ⓑ Ⓒ Ⓓ Ⓔ

Last   First   Middle

Directions for Marking Answers

- Use a black lead pencil (No. 2 or softer). Do NOT use pen or a pencil with hard lead.
- Make each mark heavy and black enough to completely obliterate the letter within the circle. Marks should fill the circles.
- Erase clearly any answer you wish to change.
- Make no stray marks on this answer sheet.
- Mark one and only one answer for each question. Multiple answers will be counted as wrong.

Example

WRONG   Ⓐ Ⓑ̸ Ⓒ Ⓓ Ⓔ

WRONG   Ⓐ Ⓧ Ⓒ Ⓓ Ⓔ

WRONG   Ⓐ Ⓑ ◎ Ⓓ Ⓔ

RIGHT   Ⓐ Ⓑ Ⓒ ● Ⓔ

1 Ⓐ Ⓑ Ⓒ Ⓓ Ⓔ	26 Ⓐ Ⓑ Ⓒ Ⓓ Ⓔ	51 Ⓐ Ⓑ Ⓒ Ⓓ Ⓔ	76 Ⓐ Ⓑ Ⓒ Ⓓ Ⓔ
2 Ⓐ Ⓑ Ⓒ Ⓓ Ⓔ	27 Ⓐ Ⓑ Ⓒ Ⓓ Ⓔ	52 Ⓐ Ⓑ Ⓒ Ⓓ Ⓔ	77 Ⓐ Ⓑ Ⓒ Ⓓ Ⓔ
3 Ⓐ Ⓑ Ⓒ Ⓓ Ⓔ	28 Ⓐ Ⓑ Ⓒ Ⓓ Ⓔ	53 Ⓐ Ⓑ Ⓒ Ⓓ Ⓔ	78 Ⓐ Ⓑ Ⓒ Ⓓ Ⓔ
4 Ⓐ Ⓑ Ⓒ Ⓓ Ⓔ	29 Ⓐ Ⓑ Ⓒ Ⓓ Ⓔ	54 Ⓐ Ⓑ Ⓒ Ⓓ Ⓔ	79 Ⓐ Ⓑ Ⓒ Ⓓ Ⓔ
5 Ⓐ Ⓑ Ⓒ Ⓓ Ⓔ	30 Ⓐ Ⓑ Ⓒ Ⓓ Ⓔ	55 Ⓐ Ⓑ Ⓒ Ⓓ Ⓔ	80 Ⓐ Ⓑ Ⓒ Ⓓ Ⓔ
6 Ⓐ Ⓑ Ⓒ Ⓓ Ⓔ	31 Ⓐ Ⓑ Ⓒ Ⓓ Ⓔ	56 Ⓐ Ⓑ Ⓒ Ⓓ Ⓔ	81 Ⓐ Ⓑ Ⓒ Ⓓ Ⓔ
7 Ⓐ Ⓑ Ⓒ Ⓓ Ⓔ	32 Ⓐ Ⓑ Ⓒ Ⓓ Ⓔ	57 Ⓐ Ⓑ Ⓒ Ⓓ Ⓔ	82 Ⓐ Ⓑ Ⓒ Ⓓ Ⓔ
8 Ⓐ Ⓑ Ⓒ Ⓓ Ⓔ	33 Ⓐ Ⓑ Ⓒ Ⓓ Ⓔ	58 Ⓐ Ⓑ Ⓒ Ⓓ Ⓔ	83 Ⓐ Ⓑ Ⓒ Ⓓ Ⓔ
9 Ⓐ Ⓑ Ⓒ Ⓓ Ⓔ	34 Ⓐ Ⓑ Ⓒ Ⓓ Ⓔ	59 Ⓐ Ⓑ Ⓒ Ⓓ Ⓔ	84 Ⓐ Ⓑ Ⓒ Ⓓ Ⓔ
10 Ⓐ Ⓑ Ⓒ Ⓓ Ⓔ	35 Ⓐ Ⓑ Ⓒ Ⓓ Ⓔ	60 Ⓐ Ⓑ Ⓒ Ⓓ Ⓔ	85 Ⓐ Ⓑ Ⓒ Ⓓ Ⓔ
11 Ⓐ Ⓑ Ⓒ Ⓓ Ⓔ	36 Ⓐ Ⓑ Ⓒ Ⓓ Ⓔ	61 Ⓐ Ⓑ Ⓒ Ⓓ Ⓔ	86 Ⓐ Ⓑ Ⓒ Ⓓ Ⓔ
12 Ⓐ Ⓑ Ⓒ Ⓓ Ⓔ	37 Ⓐ Ⓑ Ⓒ Ⓓ Ⓔ	62 Ⓐ Ⓑ Ⓒ Ⓓ Ⓔ	87 Ⓐ Ⓑ Ⓒ Ⓓ Ⓔ
13 Ⓐ Ⓑ Ⓒ Ⓓ Ⓔ	38 Ⓐ Ⓑ Ⓒ Ⓓ Ⓔ	63 Ⓐ Ⓑ Ⓒ Ⓓ Ⓔ	88 Ⓐ Ⓑ Ⓒ Ⓓ Ⓔ
14 Ⓐ Ⓑ Ⓒ Ⓓ Ⓔ	39 Ⓐ Ⓑ Ⓒ Ⓓ Ⓔ	64 Ⓐ Ⓑ Ⓒ Ⓓ Ⓔ	89 Ⓐ Ⓑ Ⓒ Ⓓ Ⓔ
15 Ⓐ Ⓑ Ⓒ Ⓓ Ⓔ	40 Ⓐ Ⓑ Ⓒ Ⓓ Ⓔ	65 Ⓐ Ⓑ Ⓒ Ⓓ Ⓔ	90 Ⓐ Ⓑ Ⓒ Ⓓ Ⓔ
16 Ⓐ Ⓑ Ⓒ Ⓓ Ⓔ	41 Ⓐ Ⓑ Ⓒ Ⓓ Ⓔ	66 Ⓐ Ⓑ Ⓒ Ⓓ Ⓔ	91 Ⓐ Ⓑ Ⓒ Ⓓ Ⓔ
17 Ⓐ Ⓑ Ⓒ Ⓓ Ⓔ	42 Ⓐ Ⓑ Ⓒ Ⓓ Ⓔ	67 Ⓐ Ⓑ Ⓒ Ⓓ Ⓔ	92 Ⓐ Ⓑ Ⓒ Ⓓ Ⓔ
18 Ⓐ Ⓑ Ⓒ Ⓓ Ⓔ	43 Ⓐ Ⓑ Ⓒ Ⓓ Ⓔ	68 Ⓐ Ⓑ Ⓒ Ⓓ Ⓔ	93 Ⓐ Ⓑ Ⓒ Ⓓ Ⓔ
19 Ⓐ Ⓑ Ⓒ Ⓓ Ⓔ	44 Ⓐ Ⓑ Ⓒ Ⓓ Ⓔ	69 Ⓐ Ⓑ Ⓒ Ⓓ Ⓔ	94 Ⓐ Ⓑ Ⓒ Ⓓ Ⓔ
20 Ⓐ Ⓑ Ⓒ Ⓓ Ⓔ	45 Ⓐ Ⓑ Ⓒ Ⓓ Ⓔ	70 Ⓐ Ⓑ Ⓒ Ⓓ Ⓔ	95 Ⓐ Ⓑ Ⓒ Ⓓ Ⓔ
21 Ⓐ Ⓑ Ⓒ Ⓓ Ⓔ	46 Ⓐ Ⓑ Ⓒ Ⓓ Ⓔ	71 Ⓐ Ⓑ Ⓒ Ⓓ Ⓔ	96 Ⓐ Ⓑ Ⓒ Ⓓ Ⓔ
22 Ⓐ Ⓑ Ⓒ Ⓓ Ⓔ	47 Ⓐ Ⓑ Ⓒ Ⓓ Ⓔ	72 Ⓐ Ⓑ Ⓒ Ⓓ Ⓔ	97 Ⓐ Ⓑ Ⓒ Ⓓ Ⓔ
23 Ⓐ Ⓑ Ⓒ Ⓓ Ⓔ	48 Ⓐ Ⓑ Ⓒ Ⓓ Ⓔ	73 Ⓐ Ⓑ Ⓒ Ⓓ Ⓔ	98 Ⓐ Ⓑ Ⓒ Ⓓ Ⓔ
24 Ⓐ Ⓑ Ⓒ Ⓓ Ⓔ	49 Ⓐ Ⓑ Ⓒ Ⓓ Ⓔ	74 Ⓐ Ⓑ Ⓒ Ⓓ Ⓔ	99 Ⓐ Ⓑ Ⓒ Ⓓ Ⓔ
25 Ⓐ Ⓑ Ⓒ Ⓓ Ⓔ	50 Ⓐ Ⓑ Ⓒ Ⓓ Ⓔ	75 Ⓐ Ⓑ Ⓒ Ⓓ Ⓔ	100 Ⓐ Ⓑ Ⓒ Ⓓ Ⓔ

Name _____ **Date** _____

Last   First   Middle

Directions for Marking Answers

- Use a black lead pencil (No. 2 or softer). Do NOT use pen or a pencil with hard lead.
- Make each mark heavy and black enough to completely obliterate the letter within the circle. Marks should fill the circles.
- Erase clearly any answer you wish to change.
- Make no stray marks on this answer sheet.
- Mark one and only one answer for each question. Multiple answers will be counted as wrong.

Example

WRONG   (A) (B̸) (C) (D) (E)
WRONG   (A) (X̶) (C) (D) (E)
WRONG   (A) (B) (Ⓒ) (D) (E)
RIGHT   (A) (B) (C) (●) (E)

101 Ⓐ Ⓑ Ⓒ Ⓓ Ⓔ	126 Ⓐ Ⓑ Ⓒ Ⓓ Ⓔ	151 Ⓐ Ⓑ Ⓒ Ⓓ Ⓔ	176 Ⓐ Ⓑ Ⓒ Ⓓ Ⓔ
102 Ⓐ Ⓑ Ⓒ Ⓓ Ⓔ	127 Ⓐ Ⓑ Ⓒ Ⓓ Ⓔ	152 Ⓐ Ⓑ Ⓒ Ⓓ Ⓔ	177 Ⓐ Ⓑ Ⓒ Ⓓ Ⓔ
103 Ⓐ Ⓑ Ⓒ Ⓓ Ⓔ	128 Ⓐ Ⓑ Ⓒ Ⓓ Ⓔ	153 Ⓐ Ⓑ Ⓒ Ⓓ Ⓔ	178 Ⓐ Ⓑ Ⓒ Ⓓ Ⓔ
104 Ⓐ Ⓑ Ⓒ Ⓓ Ⓔ	129 Ⓐ Ⓑ Ⓒ Ⓓ Ⓔ	154 Ⓐ Ⓑ Ⓒ Ⓓ Ⓔ	179 Ⓐ Ⓑ Ⓒ Ⓓ Ⓔ
105 Ⓐ Ⓑ Ⓒ Ⓓ Ⓔ	130 Ⓐ Ⓑ Ⓒ Ⓓ Ⓔ	155 Ⓐ Ⓑ Ⓒ Ⓓ Ⓔ	180 Ⓐ Ⓑ Ⓒ Ⓓ Ⓔ
106 Ⓐ Ⓑ Ⓒ Ⓓ Ⓔ	131 Ⓐ Ⓑ Ⓒ Ⓓ Ⓔ	156 Ⓐ Ⓑ Ⓒ Ⓓ Ⓔ	181 Ⓐ Ⓑ Ⓒ Ⓓ Ⓔ
107 Ⓐ Ⓑ Ⓒ Ⓓ Ⓔ	132 Ⓐ Ⓑ Ⓒ Ⓓ Ⓔ	157 Ⓐ Ⓑ Ⓒ Ⓓ Ⓔ	182 Ⓐ Ⓑ Ⓒ Ⓓ Ⓔ
108 Ⓐ Ⓑ Ⓒ Ⓓ Ⓔ	133 Ⓐ Ⓑ Ⓒ Ⓓ Ⓔ	158 Ⓐ Ⓑ Ⓒ Ⓓ Ⓔ	183 Ⓐ Ⓑ Ⓒ Ⓓ Ⓔ
109 Ⓐ Ⓑ Ⓒ Ⓓ Ⓔ	134 Ⓐ Ⓑ Ⓒ Ⓓ Ⓔ	159 Ⓐ Ⓑ Ⓒ Ⓓ Ⓔ	184 Ⓐ Ⓑ Ⓒ Ⓓ Ⓔ
110 Ⓐ Ⓑ Ⓒ Ⓓ Ⓔ	135 Ⓐ Ⓑ Ⓒ Ⓓ Ⓔ	160 Ⓐ Ⓑ Ⓒ Ⓓ Ⓔ	185 Ⓐ Ⓑ Ⓒ Ⓓ Ⓔ
111 Ⓐ Ⓑ Ⓒ Ⓓ Ⓔ	136 Ⓐ Ⓑ Ⓒ Ⓓ Ⓔ	161 Ⓐ Ⓑ Ⓒ Ⓓ Ⓔ	186 Ⓐ Ⓑ Ⓒ Ⓓ Ⓔ
112 Ⓐ Ⓑ Ⓒ Ⓓ Ⓔ	137 Ⓐ Ⓑ Ⓒ Ⓓ Ⓔ	162 Ⓐ Ⓑ Ⓒ Ⓓ Ⓔ	187 Ⓐ Ⓑ Ⓒ Ⓓ Ⓔ
113 Ⓐ Ⓑ Ⓒ Ⓓ Ⓔ	138 Ⓐ Ⓑ Ⓒ Ⓓ Ⓔ	163 Ⓐ Ⓑ Ⓒ Ⓓ Ⓔ	188 Ⓐ Ⓑ Ⓒ Ⓓ Ⓔ
114 Ⓐ Ⓑ Ⓒ Ⓓ Ⓔ	139 Ⓐ Ⓑ Ⓒ Ⓓ Ⓔ	164 Ⓐ Ⓑ Ⓒ Ⓓ Ⓔ	189 Ⓐ Ⓑ Ⓒ Ⓓ Ⓔ
115 Ⓐ Ⓑ Ⓒ Ⓓ Ⓔ	140 Ⓐ Ⓑ Ⓒ Ⓓ Ⓔ	165 Ⓐ Ⓑ Ⓒ Ⓓ Ⓔ	190 Ⓐ Ⓑ Ⓒ Ⓓ Ⓔ
116 Ⓐ Ⓑ Ⓒ Ⓓ Ⓔ	141 Ⓐ Ⓑ Ⓒ Ⓓ Ⓔ	166 Ⓐ Ⓑ Ⓒ Ⓓ Ⓔ	191 Ⓐ Ⓑ Ⓒ Ⓓ Ⓔ
117 Ⓐ Ⓑ Ⓒ Ⓓ Ⓔ	142 Ⓐ Ⓑ Ⓒ Ⓓ Ⓔ	167 Ⓐ Ⓑ Ⓒ Ⓓ Ⓔ	192 Ⓐ Ⓑ Ⓒ Ⓓ Ⓔ
118 Ⓐ Ⓑ Ⓒ Ⓓ Ⓔ	143 Ⓐ Ⓑ Ⓒ Ⓓ Ⓔ	168 Ⓐ Ⓑ Ⓒ Ⓓ Ⓔ	193 Ⓐ Ⓑ Ⓒ Ⓓ Ⓔ
119 Ⓐ Ⓑ Ⓒ Ⓓ Ⓔ	144 Ⓐ Ⓑ Ⓒ Ⓓ Ⓔ	169 Ⓐ Ⓑ Ⓒ Ⓓ Ⓔ	194 Ⓐ Ⓑ Ⓒ Ⓓ Ⓔ
120 Ⓐ Ⓑ Ⓒ Ⓓ Ⓔ	145 Ⓐ Ⓑ Ⓒ Ⓓ Ⓔ	170 Ⓐ Ⓑ Ⓒ Ⓓ Ⓔ	195 Ⓐ Ⓑ Ⓒ Ⓓ Ⓔ
121 Ⓐ Ⓑ Ⓒ Ⓓ Ⓔ	146 Ⓐ Ⓑ Ⓒ Ⓓ Ⓔ	171 Ⓐ Ⓑ Ⓒ Ⓓ Ⓔ	196 Ⓐ Ⓑ Ⓒ Ⓓ Ⓔ
122 Ⓐ Ⓑ Ⓒ Ⓓ Ⓔ	147 Ⓐ Ⓑ Ⓒ Ⓓ Ⓔ	172 Ⓐ Ⓑ Ⓒ Ⓓ Ⓔ	197 Ⓐ Ⓑ Ⓒ Ⓓ Ⓔ
123 Ⓐ Ⓑ Ⓒ Ⓓ Ⓔ	148 Ⓐ Ⓑ Ⓒ Ⓓ Ⓔ	173 Ⓐ Ⓑ Ⓒ Ⓓ Ⓔ	198 Ⓐ Ⓑ Ⓒ Ⓓ Ⓔ
124 Ⓐ Ⓑ Ⓒ Ⓓ Ⓔ	149 Ⓐ Ⓑ Ⓒ Ⓓ Ⓔ	174 Ⓐ Ⓑ Ⓒ Ⓓ Ⓔ	199 Ⓐ Ⓑ Ⓒ Ⓓ Ⓔ
125 Ⓐ Ⓑ Ⓒ Ⓓ Ⓔ	150 Ⓐ Ⓑ Ⓒ Ⓓ Ⓔ	175 Ⓐ Ⓑ Ⓒ Ⓓ Ⓔ	200 Ⓐ Ⓑ Ⓒ Ⓓ Ⓔ

Directions for Marking Answers

- Use a black lead pencil (No. 2 or softer). Do NOT use pen or a pencil with hard lead.
- Make each mark heavy and black enough to completely obliterate the letter within the circle. Marks should fill the circles.
- Erase clearly any answer you wish to change.
- Make no stray marks on this answer sheet.
- Mark one and only one answer for each question. Multiple answers will be counted as wrong.

Example

WRONG Ⓐ Ⓑ̷ Ⓒ Ⓓ Ⓔ
WRONG Ⓐ ⓧ Ⓒ Ⓓ Ⓔ
WRONG Ⓐ Ⓑ Ⓞ Ⓓ Ⓔ
RIGHT Ⓐ Ⓑ Ⓒ ● Ⓔ

201 Ⓐ Ⓑ Ⓒ Ⓓ Ⓔ
202 Ⓐ Ⓑ Ⓒ Ⓓ Ⓔ
203 Ⓐ Ⓑ Ⓒ Ⓓ Ⓔ
204 Ⓐ Ⓑ Ⓒ Ⓓ Ⓔ
205 Ⓐ Ⓑ Ⓒ Ⓓ Ⓔ
206 Ⓐ Ⓑ Ⓒ Ⓓ Ⓔ
207 Ⓐ Ⓑ Ⓒ Ⓓ Ⓔ
208 Ⓐ Ⓑ Ⓒ Ⓓ Ⓔ
209 Ⓐ Ⓑ Ⓒ Ⓓ Ⓔ
210 Ⓐ Ⓑ Ⓒ Ⓓ Ⓔ
211 Ⓐ Ⓑ Ⓒ Ⓓ Ⓔ
212 Ⓐ Ⓑ Ⓒ Ⓓ Ⓔ
213 Ⓐ Ⓑ Ⓒ Ⓓ Ⓔ
214 Ⓐ Ⓑ Ⓒ Ⓓ Ⓔ
215 Ⓐ Ⓑ Ⓒ Ⓓ Ⓔ
216 Ⓐ Ⓑ Ⓒ Ⓓ Ⓔ
217 Ⓐ Ⓑ Ⓒ Ⓓ Ⓔ
218 Ⓐ Ⓑ Ⓒ Ⓓ Ⓔ
219 Ⓐ Ⓑ Ⓒ Ⓓ Ⓔ
220 Ⓐ Ⓑ Ⓒ Ⓓ Ⓔ
221 Ⓐ Ⓑ Ⓒ Ⓓ Ⓔ
222 Ⓐ Ⓑ Ⓒ Ⓓ Ⓔ
223 Ⓐ Ⓑ Ⓒ Ⓓ Ⓔ
224 Ⓐ Ⓑ Ⓒ Ⓓ Ⓔ
225 Ⓐ Ⓑ Ⓒ Ⓓ Ⓔ

226 Ⓐ Ⓑ Ⓒ Ⓓ Ⓔ
227 Ⓐ Ⓑ Ⓒ Ⓓ Ⓔ
228 Ⓐ Ⓑ Ⓒ Ⓓ Ⓔ
229 Ⓐ Ⓑ Ⓒ Ⓓ Ⓔ
230 Ⓐ Ⓑ Ⓒ Ⓓ Ⓔ
231 Ⓐ Ⓑ Ⓒ Ⓓ Ⓔ
232 Ⓐ Ⓑ Ⓒ Ⓓ Ⓔ
233 Ⓐ Ⓑ Ⓒ Ⓓ Ⓔ
234 Ⓐ Ⓑ Ⓒ Ⓓ Ⓔ
235 Ⓐ Ⓑ Ⓒ Ⓓ Ⓔ
236 Ⓐ Ⓑ Ⓒ Ⓓ Ⓔ
237 Ⓐ Ⓑ Ⓒ Ⓓ Ⓔ
238 Ⓐ Ⓑ Ⓒ Ⓓ Ⓔ
239 Ⓐ Ⓑ Ⓒ Ⓓ Ⓔ
240 Ⓐ Ⓑ Ⓒ Ⓓ Ⓔ
241 Ⓐ Ⓑ Ⓒ Ⓓ Ⓔ
242 Ⓐ Ⓑ Ⓒ Ⓓ Ⓔ
243 Ⓐ Ⓑ Ⓒ Ⓓ Ⓔ
244 Ⓐ Ⓑ Ⓒ Ⓓ Ⓔ
245 Ⓐ Ⓑ Ⓒ Ⓓ Ⓔ
246 Ⓐ Ⓑ Ⓒ Ⓓ Ⓔ
247 Ⓐ Ⓑ Ⓒ Ⓓ Ⓔ
248 Ⓐ Ⓑ Ⓒ Ⓓ Ⓔ
249 Ⓐ Ⓑ Ⓒ Ⓓ Ⓔ
250 Ⓐ Ⓑ Ⓒ Ⓓ Ⓔ

251 Ⓐ Ⓑ Ⓒ Ⓓ Ⓔ
252 Ⓐ Ⓑ Ⓒ Ⓓ Ⓔ
253 Ⓐ Ⓑ Ⓒ Ⓓ Ⓔ
254 Ⓐ Ⓑ Ⓒ Ⓓ Ⓔ
255 Ⓐ Ⓑ Ⓒ Ⓓ Ⓔ
256 Ⓐ Ⓑ Ⓒ Ⓓ Ⓔ
257 Ⓐ Ⓑ Ⓒ Ⓓ Ⓔ
258 Ⓐ Ⓑ Ⓒ Ⓓ Ⓔ
259 Ⓐ Ⓑ Ⓒ Ⓓ Ⓔ
260 Ⓐ Ⓑ Ⓒ Ⓓ Ⓔ
261 Ⓐ Ⓑ Ⓒ Ⓓ Ⓔ
262 Ⓐ Ⓑ Ⓒ Ⓓ Ⓔ
263 Ⓐ Ⓑ Ⓒ Ⓓ Ⓔ
264 Ⓐ Ⓑ Ⓒ Ⓓ Ⓔ
265 Ⓐ Ⓑ Ⓒ Ⓓ Ⓔ
266 Ⓐ Ⓑ Ⓒ Ⓓ Ⓔ
267 Ⓐ Ⓑ Ⓒ Ⓓ Ⓔ
268 Ⓐ Ⓑ Ⓒ Ⓓ Ⓔ
269 Ⓐ Ⓑ Ⓒ Ⓓ Ⓔ
270 Ⓐ Ⓑ Ⓒ Ⓓ Ⓔ
271 Ⓐ Ⓑ Ⓒ Ⓓ Ⓔ
272 Ⓐ Ⓑ Ⓒ Ⓓ Ⓔ
273 Ⓐ Ⓑ Ⓒ Ⓓ Ⓔ
274 Ⓐ Ⓑ Ⓒ Ⓓ Ⓔ
275 Ⓐ Ⓑ Ⓒ Ⓓ Ⓔ

276 Ⓐ Ⓑ Ⓒ Ⓓ Ⓔ
277 Ⓐ Ⓑ Ⓒ Ⓓ Ⓔ
278 Ⓐ Ⓑ Ⓒ Ⓓ Ⓔ
279 Ⓐ Ⓑ Ⓒ Ⓓ Ⓔ
280 Ⓐ Ⓑ Ⓒ Ⓓ Ⓔ
281 Ⓐ Ⓑ Ⓒ Ⓓ Ⓔ
282 Ⓐ Ⓑ Ⓒ Ⓓ Ⓔ
283 Ⓐ Ⓑ Ⓒ Ⓓ Ⓔ
284 Ⓐ Ⓑ Ⓒ Ⓓ Ⓔ
285 Ⓐ Ⓑ Ⓒ Ⓓ Ⓔ
286 Ⓐ Ⓑ Ⓒ Ⓓ Ⓔ
287 Ⓐ Ⓑ Ⓒ Ⓓ Ⓔ
288 Ⓐ Ⓑ Ⓒ Ⓓ Ⓔ
289 Ⓐ Ⓑ Ⓒ Ⓓ Ⓔ
290 Ⓐ Ⓑ Ⓒ Ⓓ Ⓔ
291 Ⓐ Ⓑ Ⓒ Ⓓ Ⓔ
292 Ⓐ Ⓑ Ⓒ Ⓓ Ⓔ
293 Ⓐ Ⓑ Ⓒ Ⓓ Ⓔ
294 Ⓐ Ⓑ Ⓒ Ⓓ Ⓔ
295 Ⓐ Ⓑ Ⓒ Ⓓ Ⓔ
296 Ⓐ Ⓑ Ⓒ Ⓓ Ⓔ
297 Ⓐ Ⓑ Ⓒ Ⓓ Ⓔ
298 Ⓐ Ⓑ Ⓒ Ⓓ Ⓔ
299 Ⓐ Ⓑ Ⓒ Ⓓ Ⓔ
300 Ⓐ Ⓑ Ⓒ Ⓓ Ⓔ

SIMULATION TEST 5

Part 1—General Medical Knowledge

Directions: *Each of the following questions or incomplete statements precedes five suggested answers or completions. Select the ONE answer or completion that is BEST in each case and fill in the circle containing the corresponding letter on the answer sheet.*

1. An infection of the respiratory bronchioles, alveolar ducts, alveolar sacs, and alveoli is termed
   A. pleurisy
   B. pleural effusion
   C. chronic obstructive pulmonary disease
   D. chronic bronchitis
   E. pneumonia

2. Repair of a dislocation by manipulation is termed
   A. osteoplasty
   B. arthrodesis
   C. subluxation
   D. closed reduction
   E. open reduction

3. The family of a child with sickle-cell anemia wishes to take the child on a vacation. Which of the following vacation sites would NOT be suitable?
   A. the sea shore
   B. the Rocky Mountains
   C. theme parks
   D. a cruise on an ocean liner
   E. zoos

4. A pulmonary embolism would most likely be caused by a blood clot breaking away from the
   A. coronary artery
   B. aorta
   C. carotid artery
   D. pulmonary vein
   E. lower limb vein

5. In the urinary tract, a calculus is a
   A. stricture of the ureter
   B. stricture of the urethra
   C. twisting of the ureter upon itself
   D. stonelike formation
   E. tumor of the renal pelvis

6. A common injury in older people with osteoarthritis following a slight fall or stumble is a fracture of the
   A. olecranon process
   B. ilium
   C. ischium
   D. neck of the femur
   E. patella

7. The presence of air in the spaces of the membrane covering the lungs and the chest wall is called
   A. mediastinum
   B. pneumonia
   C. pneumothorax
   D. thoracentesis
   E. pleurisy

8. Vital capacity is the
   A. difference between quiet inspiration and quiet expiration
   B. maximum volume of air that can be inhaled after forcibly exhaling
   C. volume of air entering or leaving with each normal breath
   D. air volume remaining after as much air as possible has been expelled
   E. maximal air volume that can be forcibly expelled after a maximum inspiration

9. In the presence of a boil, severe pain in the external ear is due mainly to the fact that the skin of the external canal is so closely adherent to the
   A. parotid gland
   B. surfaces of the bone and cartilage
   C. tympanic membrane
   D. cochlea
   E. eustachian tube

10. Conditions associated with hyperthyroidism include:
    A. goiters
    B. exophthalmos
    C. goiters and exophthalmos
    D. myxedema
    E. goiters and myxedema

11. Mitral stenosis is an impeded blood flow from the
    A. right atrium to the right ventricle
    B. right ventricle to the pulmonary artery
    C. inferior vena cava into the right atrium
    D. left atrium to the left ventricle
    E. left ventricle to the aorta

12. The largest artery in the body is the
    A. carotid artery
    B. pulmonary artery
    C. aorta
    D. superior vena cava
    E. inferior vena cava

13. Cracking of joints, which may occur when the fingers are suddenly pulled, is generally due to
    A. a partial vacuum that is created in the joint cavity
    B. the grinding of the two articulated bone surfaces
    C. a sudden slipping of a tendon over a bony prominence
    D. a sudden slipping of a ligament over cartilage
    E. calcification of articular cartilage

14. Electromyography (EMG) is defined as
    A. an ultrasound test to visualize cardiac muscle
    B. a test to evaluate blood flow
    C. the recording of electrical currents emanating from the heart muscle
    D. the recording of the changes in the electrical potential of muscles
    E. x-ray examination of the muscles following an injection of radioactive materials

15. A pathologic or accentuated posterior, concave curvature of the spine, also known as "swayback," is referred to as
    A. kyphosis
    B. lordosis
    C. functional scoliosis
    D. structural scoliosis
    E. spondylolisthesis

16. A condition called torticollis (wryneck) usually is a result of an injury to which muscle?
    A. deltoid
    B. trapezius
    C. latissimus dorsi
    D. sternocleidomastoid
    E. pectoralis major

17. A protrusion of the stomach through the esophageal opening of the diaphragm is
    A. esophageal aneurism
    B. hiatal hernia
    C. umbilical hernia
    D. esophageal varices
    E. gastro-esophageal reflux disease

18. Body temperature and appetite are controlled by the
    A. hypothalamus
    B. medulla oblongata
    C. encephalon
    D. cerebrum
    E. cerebellum

19. A term that indicates an increase or worsening in a disease or any of its symptoms is
    A. exacerbation
    B. morbidity
    C. prodromal
    D. proliferation
    E. disseminated

20. Local anesthesia to a body part is caused by the interruption of the functioning of
    A. motor nerves
    B. sensory nerves
    C. cranial nerves
    D. efferent nerves
    E. the cerebral cortex

21. Supraspinatus ("painful arc") syndrome occurs during the midrange abduction of the
    A. wrist
    B. elbow
    C. shoulder
    D. knee
    E. hip

22. A patient with a heart murmur has experienced each of the following past conditions. Which condition is associated with structural changes of the valves of the heart?
    A. rheumatic fever
    B. German measles
    C. mononucleosis
    D. diphtheria
    E. pneumonia

23. The most distinguishing characteristic of a spore is that it
    A. grows in chains
    B. grows in clusters
    C. requires light to survive
    D. is destroyed by cold
    E. is difficult to destroy

24. A joint dysfunction marked by a clicking or grinding sensation in the joint, pain in or about the ears, and tiredness and soreness of the jaw muscles involves which of the following bones?
    A. maxilla
    B. mandible
    C. maxilla and mandible
    D. temporal bone
    E. mandible and temporal bone

25. The term proximal means
    A. toward the front
    B. toward the back
    C. nearest to the point of origin
    D. away from the point of origin
    E. nearest to the midline of a structure

26. A drug that is used to dilate the pupil and render it unable to accommodate for near and distant vision affects which part of the eye?
    A. ciliary muscles
    B. iris
    C. cornea
    D. retinal arteries
    E. optic nerve

27. The membrane lining a joint is called
    A. serous
    B. synovial
    C. fibrous
    D. cartilaginous
    E. fascia

28. The body area that is incised during a vaginal delivery is the
    A. periosteum
    B. peritoneum
    C. perineum
    D. periorchium
    E. perinephrium

29. Organisms that have either deoxyribonucleic acid (DNA) or ribonucleic acid (RNA) but never both are
    A. fungi
    B. bacteria
    C. rickettsiae
    D. viruses
    E. helminths

30. An abnormal, tubelike passage leading from an internal organ to the body surface is called a
    A. cleft
    B. cyst
    C. fissure
    D. fistula
    E. ulcer

31. The posterior portion of the hip is formed by the
    A. femur
    B. pubis
    C. ilium
    D. ischium
    E. coccyx

32. A stoma created in the small intestine and brought to the surface of the abdomen for the purpose of evacuating feces is termed
    A. colostomy
    B. ileostomy
    C. duodenojejunostomy
    D. coloproctostomy
    E. colosigmoidostomy

33. The genus of organisms responsible for Lyme disease is
    A. *Borrelia*
    B. *Yersinia*
    C. *Plasmodia*
    D. *Pediculus*
    E. *Rickettsia*

34. The portal vein functions to
    A. bring oxygenated blood to the liver cells
    B. bring blood rich in the products of digestion to the liver
    C. bring blood rich in oxygen and the products of digestion to the liver
    D. carry blood rich in nutrients from the liver to the inferior vena cava
    E. carry blood rich in oxygen from the liver to the inferior vena cava

35. Bones are connected to other bones by
    A. bursae
    B. synovium
    C. muscles
    D. tendons
    E. ligaments

36. Angina pectoris is
    A. caused by an increased myocardial oxygen demand
    B. caused by a reduced oxygen supply
    C. caused by either an increased myocardial oxygen demand or a reduced oxygen supply
    D. irreversible ischemia of the myocardium
    E. an irreversible ischemia of the myocardium caused by an increased oxygen supply

37. One cause of the inability of the body to concentrate bile, leading to fat intolerance, dyspepsia, and flatulence, is an impaction of a gallstone in the
    A. liver
    B. gallbladder
    C. cystic duct
    D. pancreatic duct
    E. duodenum

38. The crescent-shaped area of the nail is called the
    A. uvula
    B. root
    C. lamina dura
    D. lunula
    E. frenum

39. A medical assistant fails to turn on the answering machine with a message of what to do in an emergency. A patient cannot reach the physician and suffers permanent damage from a cast applied that day. Damages may be awarded under
    A. abandonment
    B. assault
    C. battery
    D. breach of contract
    E. trespass

40. Administrative laws that govern the medical assistant's right to practice originate in
    A. nurse practice acts
    B. state boards of nursing
    C. medical practice acts
    D. the United States Congress
    E. state legislatures

41. A patient wishes to discontinue a treatment prescribed by the physician, without the physician's consent. What procedure must the medical assistant follow?
    A. Refer the patient to another physician.
    B. Bill the patient immediately.
    C. Have the patient sign an appropriate release form.
    D. Ask the patient to discuss his decision with his family.
    E. Call the patient's family and inform them of his decision.

42. A state law that does not allow a health care provider to perform a specific task is an example of
    A. common law
    B. statutory law
    C. constitutional law
    D. administrative law
    E. a court ruling

43. Which of the following is applicable in any case of professional negligence wherein the medical assistant may be liable?
    A. doctrine of respondeat superior
    B. the law of agency
    C. contributory negligence
    D. strict liability
    E. personal liability

44. When a medical assistant fails to return a call to a patient or report the call to the physician to return, the medical assistant and the physician risk being legally accused of
    A. slander
    B. libel
    C. negligence
    D. battery
    E. assault

45. Which of the following vitamins is likely to turn the urine bright yellow?
    A. vitamin A
    B. vitamin B
    C. vitamin C
    D. vitamin D
    E. vitamin E

46. Of the following needs described by Maslow, which is the psychosocial need that must be met FIRST?
    A. love and emotional security
    B. self-esteem
    C. recognition
    D. achievement
    E. self-actualization

47. If a patient in the waiting room becomes unruly, the medical assistant should
    A. talk with the patient
    B. ask the physician to talk with the patient
    C. ignore the fact that the patient is upset
    D. remove the patient to a private room
    E. ask the patient to leave the office

48. Which of the following is the most helpful to a patient coming to terms with his own impending death?
    A. books and literature on death
    B. isolated contemplation
    C. listening to others who have personally experienced losing a loved one
    D. talking with others about feelings about death
    E. finding new interests to take his mind off the situation

49. According to Kubler-Ross, a patient who has been diagnosed with a terminal illness but is sure the test results are incorrect is most likely in which of the following stages?
    A. anger
    B. denial
    C. bargaining
    D. depression
    E. acceptance

50. The medical assistant is caring for a patient who is angry and arguing about the diagnosis. The medical assistant should
    A. agree with whatever the patient says
    B. calmly disagree with a point if the patient is wrong
    C. listen and allow the patient to vent feelings
    D. gain control of the situation by using a firm voice
    E. use more physical contact for communication

51. Daydreaming is an example of
    A. unrealistic self-concept
    B. fear of reality
    C. fantasy
    D. identification
    E. infantile behavior

52. When caring for terminal patients, the attitude that is most recommended for the medical assistant is
    A. sorrow
    B. sympathy
    C. empathy
    D. hopefulness
    E. cheerfulness

53. Which of the following statements concerning pain is always true?
    A. Pain is subjective.
    B. Pain occurs only after tissues have been permanently damaged.
    C. Pain is in direct proportion to the size of an area injured.
    D. Pain is in direct proportion to the weight and amount of body surface.
    E. Environmental and cultural factors have little influence on pain.

54. A middle-aged man with benign prostatic hypertrophy is to have a transurethral resection of the prostate. Where would this patient have a surgical incision?
    A. anterior to the anus
    B. on the anterior surface of the penis
    C. on the lower abdominal wall
    D. in the left or right groin area
    E. internally in the urinary tract

55. Suture repair of a torn or lacerated perineum is called
    A. episioplasty
    B. episiotomy
    C. perineoplasty
    D. perineorrhaphy
    E. perineotomy

56. Which of the following is spelled correctly?
    A. exopthalmas
    B. exopthalmos
    C. exophthalmas
    D. exophthalmis
    E. exophthalmos

57. The prescription order reads: Sig: ii qd. 1. h. h.s. Refil p.r.n. The medication is taken
    A. four times a day
    B. 1 hour after meals
    C. every hour
    D. at bedtime
    E. when needed

58. Which of the following is spelled correctly?
    A. ishcemia
    B. ishcimia
    C. ischemia
    D. ischemea
    E. ischimea

59. Which of the following is spelled correctly?
    A. phlebitis
    B. phlebites
    C. phlebetis
    D. phlebitas
    E. phlebitus

60. Which of the following is spelled correctly?
    A. bifourcate
    B. byfurcate
    C. bifurcate
    D. biforcate
    E. byfourcate

61. A noncancerous growth may also be called a
    A. malignancy
    B. benign neoplasm
    C. sarcoma
    D. carcinoma
    E. necrosis

62. The symbol used in clinical practice that means "moderate amount of reaction" is
    A. ++
    B. +++
    C. ++++
    D. ↑
    E. 2°

63. A patient whose condition is characterized by a decrease in the number of platelets in the circulating blood would have
    A. thrombocytopenia
    B. hemolytic anemia
    C. pernicious anemia
    D. hemophilia
    E. hemoglobinemia

64. An abnormal increase in the size of an organ is called
    A. atrophy
    B. dystrophy
    C. hypertrophy
    D. hypertropia
    E. hypotrophy

65. The word dorsal means
    A. near the brain
    B. back or behind
    C. toward the bottom
    D. divided in half
    E. divided top and bottom

66. Which of the following is spelled correctly?
    A. mycedema
    B. myxedema
    C. myxedemia
    D. mixedema
    E. mixedemia

67. Which of the following is spelled correctly?
    A. contrandication
    B. contraindicatian
    C. contraindication
    D. contradication
    E. contrindication

68. Which of the following is spelled correctly?
    A. goiter
    B. goitre
    C. goitar
    D. goitor
    E. goitur

69. Which of the following is spelled correctly?
    A. pharynx
    B. pharnix
    C. pharnyx
    D. pharinx
    E. pharyncs

70. Each of the following is a function of the autonomic nervous system EXCEPT:
    A. integrating behavioral mechanisms
    B. maintaining body temperature
    C. maintaining fluid balance
    D. maintaining the ionic composition of blood
    E. controlling activities associated with the special senses

71. When taking a patient history about pain, each of the following questions is an open-ended question EXCEPT:
    A. "When did the pain begin?"
    B. "What seems to bring on the pain?"
    C. "How long have you had the pain?"
    D. "Where is your pain most severe?"
    E. "Do you think you need treatment for your pain?"

72. Transillumination of the maxillary sinus is imaging using
    A. a contrast medium
    B. light
    C. ionizing radiation
    D. computers
    E. photosensitive film

73. The dermis is made up of
    A. muscle tissue
    B. epithelial tissue
    C. osseous tissue
    D. connective tissue
    E. nervous tissue

74. Normal flora in the digestive tract commonly cause infections in the
    A. respiratory tract
    B. circulatory system
    C. nervous system
    D. genitourinary system
    E. colon and rectum

75. The central nervous system activates
    A. skeletal muscle movement
    B. functions of learning and language
    C. both A and B
    D. stress reaction
    E. both A and D

76. Blistering of the nerve roots following inflammation of the nerve roots and the spinal ganglia results in
    A. herpes zoster
    B. herpes simplex-1
    C. both A and B
    D. herpes simplex-2
    E. both A and D

77. When patients travel out of the United States, diseases that are commonly spread by contaminated water include
    A. typhoid fever
    B. malaria
    C. both A and B
    D. amebic dysentery
    E. both A and D

78. Procedures for which the sternum is an anatomic landmark include:
    A. cardiopulmonary resuscitation
    B. electrocardiograms
    C. both A and B
    D. chest measurement
    E. both A and D

79. Medications that are smooth muscle relaxants affect the
    A. uterus
    B. skeletal muscle
    C. both A and B
    D. blood vessels
    E. both A and D

80. A discolored spot of skin that is neither elevated above nor depressed below the surrounding skin surface is called a
    A. bulla
    B. comedo
    C. macule
    D. papule
    E. wheal

81. Varices is a term related to
    A. hernias
    B. tumors
    C. severe constipation
    D. inhibition of peristalsis
    E. blood vessels

82. Which of the following statements about cerebrospinal fluid are true?
    A. It is a food source to brain tissues.
    B. It serves to carry away waste products from the brain.
    C. It equalizes fluid pressure around the brain.
    D. It minimizes damage from blows to the head and neck.
    E. It filters blood.

83. The most common type of kidney disease is
    A. glomerulonephritis
    B. pyelonephritis
    C. nephrotic syndrome
    D. uremia
    E. urinary tract infection

84. *Monilia* is normal flora of the
    A. vagina
    B. mouth
    C. both A and B
    D. urethra
    E. both A and D

85. The radiographic view from the left to right side is the
    A. PA
    B. AP
    C. lateral
    D. oblique
    E. coronal

86. Constriction of the pupil in reaction to light results from the contraction of the
    A. cornea
    B. iris
    C. lens
    D. aqueous humor
    E. vitreous humor

87. The functions of the liver include
    A. blood formation
    B. blood storage
    C. bile storage
    D. antibody formation
    E. glucose storage

88. During examination, the simple knee jerk is a
    A. contracture
    B. reflux
    C. reflex
    D. contraction
    E. nuchal rigidity

89. True statements concerning the peritoneum include:
    A. It tends to localize or wall off infections.
    B. In the female, it is a completely closed sac.
    C. both A and B
    D. Residual air enters it following the test for tubal patency.
    E. both A and D

90. Collateral circulation functions to
    A. control the conduction system of the heart
    B. allow individuals to survive myocardial infarctions
    C. both A and B
    D. decrease cardiac pain
    E. both A and D

91. Under the doctrine of informed consent, liability for negligence can occur if
    A. the doctor fails to discuss the procedure and how it is to be performed
    B. treatment exceeds the scope of the consent
    C. both A and B
    D. the patient is unhappy with the result
    E. both A and D

92. Benefits of corporate medical practice over noncorporate practice include
    A. an increased number of referrals
    B. a decrease in time required for being on call
    C. both A and B
    D. a decrease in personal liability
    E. both A and D

93. Without the physician's order, a medical assistant administers to a friend a controlled substance that results in the friend's injury. This incident represents
    A. liability for negligence on the part of the physician
    B. cause for revocation of the physician's license
    C. both A and B
    D. criminal liability on the part of the medical assistant
    E. both A and D

94. The Principles of Medical Ethics of the American Medical Association include
    A. using the talents of other health professionals when indicated
    B. volunteering services to the community
    C. both A and B
    D. accepting every patient who seeks his or her services
    E. both A and D

95. Specific elements of a doctor's liability in a tort include
    A. a duty owed to a patient
    B. compensation
    C. premeditation
    D. intention
    E. incorrect diagnosis

96. An autistic child is one who
    A. has language problems
    B. is frequently retarded
    C. both A and B
    D. is overly sensitive to stimulation to the sensory organs
    E. both A and D

97. Examples of nonverbal communications include
    A. working with papers while a patient is talking to you
    B. looking up or to the side during a conversation with a coworker
    C. both A and B
    D. writing directions for a patient to follow
    E. both A and D

98. Meanings for the symbol "++" include:
    A. positive
    B. excess
    C. plus
    D. acid reaction
    E. trace or notable reaction

99. In immunity, the body reacts to harmful pollens or drugs by producing
    A. agglutinogens
    B. antitoxins
    C. toxins
    D. antigens
    E. anticoagulants

100. A yeast infection may also be called
    A. candidiasis
    B. moniliasis
    C. both A and B
    D. trichomoniasis
    E. both A and D

SIMULATION TEST 5

Part 2—Administrative Procedures

Directions: *Each of the following questions or incomplete statements precedes five suggested answers or completions. Select the ONE best answer or completion in each case and fill in the circle containing the corresponding letter on the answer sheet.*

101. A patient calls at 8:00 AM and reports a fever that has lasted for more than 3 days. You have a full day booked, starting at 9:00 AM, and two small blocks left open for emergencies at 11:00 AM and 4:00 PM. When would you schedule this patient?
    A. before 9:00 AM
    B. 9:00 AM
    C. 11:00 AM
    D. 4:00 PM
    E. at the next regular opening

102. In word processing, the generic coding system used to represent all text characters and control codes that a computer is capable of generating is called
    A. ASCII
    B. DOS
    C. macros
    D. RAM
    E. ROM

103. While saving a revised document, your computer screen displayed the message "Disk is write-protected." You would
    A. contact the manufacturer for further copyright permission
    B. make a copy of the disk, then save on the second copy
    C. remove the tab from the upper right corner of your floppy disk
    D. format the disk before proceeding with the save command
    E. choose another unused disk

104. In computer terminology, "default" is
    A. a general error in processing
    B. an omission in a sequence of commands
    C. a basic setting the computer looks for or returns to automatically
    D. a file error message
    E. a password protection and access code

105. Date   Charge   Payment   Balance
    1/1/99 $345.00 $175.00 $170.00
    On 3/1/99, a payment of $178.00 is received from the insurance company. Make the next charge/payment entries for this insurance company payment.
    A. 3/1/99: 0.00 charge; 178.00 payment; <8.00> balance
    B. 3/1/99: 8.00 charge; 178.00 payment; 0 balance
    C. 3/1/99: <8.00> charge; 178.00 payment; 0 balance
    D. 3/1/99: <8.00> charge; 170.00 payment, 0 balance
    E. 1/1/99: 353.00 charge; 175 payment; 178.00 balance
    3/1/99: 0 charge; 178.00 payment; 0 balance

106. A new employee must complete which of the following federal income tax forms?
    A. W2
    B. W4
    C. 1099
    D. 940
    E. 941

107. What percentage is 12 of 96?
    A. 8%
    B. 0.125%
    C. 12%
    D. 12.5%
    E. 80%

108. Using the ordinary method of calculating interest, calculate the amount of interest on $5000.00 borrowed for 12 days at 13.5%.
    A. $2.25
    B. $22.50
    C. $81.00
    D. $225.00
    E. $675.00

109. When one is reconciling the bank account, outstanding checks are
    A. added to the previous balance
    B. added to the new bank balance
    C. deducted from the new bank balance
    D. added to the checkbook balance
    E. deducted from the checkbook balance

110. If the total income for 1 month is $17,420 and the total expenses for the same month are $15,910, the profit and loss statement would show a
    A. gross profit of $17,420
    B. gross profit of $1510
    C. net profit of $17,420
    D. net profit of $1510
    E. net loss of $15,910

111. The physician wishes to extend a 20% professional courtesy discount on a $25.00 patient charge. The ledger card has no adjustment column. Which of the following is the proper entry?
    A. $20.00 charge column
    B. $25.00 charge column; 5.00 payment column
    C. $25.00 charge column; <5.00> payment column
    D. $25.00 charge column; <5.00> (in the next charge row)
    E. $25.00 charge column; 5.00 (in the next charge row)

112. In addition to the judgment already owed in a small claims court, the plaintiff may recover
    A. the costs of filing the suit
    B. interest
    C. both A and B
    D. compensatory damages
    E. both A and D

113. To properly void a check, you would write "VOID" across the check and then
    A. cut off the signature area
    B. file the check with canceled checks
    C. return it to the bank
    D. destroy it after the bank statement arrives
    E. immediately shred and destroy the check

114. If the physician's fee is recorded as income at the time of the service, rather than at the time of payment, the accounting basis being used is
    A. cash
    B. accrual
    C. single-entry
    D. double-entry
    E. the pegboard accounting system

115. The statement for services rendered to a patient now deceased should be addressed to the
    A. deceased
    B. spouse or nearest relative
    C. estate of the deceased
    D. social security administration
    E. probate department of the Superior Court of your county or city

116. The judgment in a small claims court action may be appealed by
    A. the defendant
    B. the plaintiff
    C. legal aid attorneys
    D. a referee
    E. an arbitrator

117. Which of the following checking endorsements is "deposit only"?
    A. blank
    B. restrictive
    C. special
    D. qualified
    E. full

118. Checks that are returned, unpaid, from the bank are called
    A. canceled
    B. outstanding
    C. nonsufficient funds
    D. deposits-in-transit
    E. stop payments

119. Bankruptcy claims are handled by
    A. sending a final bill to the patient's attorney
    B. completing a special form and mailing it to a referee
    C. taking the patient to small claims court
    D. turning the account over to a collection agency
    E. turning the account over to the physician's attorney

120. Which of the following collection practices is ethical?
    A. misrepresenting why you are calling, in order to get the patient to come to the phone
    B. sending postcards saying "call me" with your first name signature
    C. calling the patient at his or her place of work
    D. calling before 8 AM
    E. calling after 8 PM

121. The special form that is completed after a worker who has been injured on the job is examined by the physician is
    A. attending physician's statement
    B. workers' compensation bill
    C. doctor's first report of occupational injury
    D. report back to work
    E. on-the-job injury report

122. A CHAMPUS-dependent child receives a $10 DPT immunization. The parent does not have a form DD1251. The family lives on base and has paid a deductible of $50. What will CHAMPUS most likely pay?
    A. 0
    B. 20% of the allowable
    C. 20% of the allowable, less $50
    D. 80% of the allowable
    E. 80% of the allowable, less $50

123. A patient is seeking medical care from his own attending physician for a work-related injury. Which of the following statements is true?
    A. Workers' compensation policy will not allow this.
    B. A separate chart must be established.
    C. A separate ledger card must be established.
    D. Both a separate chart and a separate ledger card must be established.
    E. Care is allowed if the physician includes prior medical information in reporting.

124. In the ICD-9-CM system,
    A. unlisted conditions may not be reported
    B. unlisted conditions should be matched as closely as possible to another code
    C. unlisted conditions have specific codes designated for reporting them
    D. listed conditions may not be altered
    E. listed conditions do not need descriptions

125. The portion of a service fee that the patient must pay is called
    A. copayment
    B. cost of coverage
    C. premium
    D. capitation rate
    E. coordination of benefits

126. The index that gives diagnoses in an alphabetical sequence, using standard nomenclature, and with appropriate code numbers following the descriptive terms is the
    A. Physicians' Current Procedural Terminology (CPT)
    B. Health Care Financing Administration Common Procedure Coding System
    C. International Classification of Disease, Volume 1
    D. International Classification of Disease, Volume 2
    E. International Classification of Disease, Volume 3

127. If a retired patient over age 65 has both private insurance and Medicare, the medical assistant should send the claim to
    A. Medicare
    B. the private insurance carrier
    C. both the private insurance carrier and Medicare
    D. the patient's previous employer
    E. the patient

128. Which of the following statements about workers' compensation is correct?
    A. It covers medical expenses for employees whose jobs are terminated.
    B. It covers medical expenses for nonoccupational injuries and illnesses.
    C. It covers medical expenses for occupational injuries.
    D. It pays a partial salary for nonoccupational injuries and illnesses.
    E. It pays a full salary for employees who are unable to work.

129. If the physician "accepts assignment" on Medicare claims, the physician will
    A. receive less than the 80% of the allowable charges from Medicare
    B. receive 100% of the charges from Medicare
    C. accept the Medicare payment as payment in full
    D. bill the patient for 20% of the allowable charges
    E. not be eligible to receive payment from a supplemental carrier

130. Which of the following is an insurance claim processing error?
    A. attaching operative reports to all claims for minor office surgery
    B. stating he physician's UCR fee on all claims
    C. listing all preoperative and postoperative care
    D. billing the insurance company an additional 20% to cover patient fees
    E. entering amounts that have been paid by the patient or another carrier

131. To be considered for payment, Medicare claims must be filed
    A. within 72 hours of the initial treatment
    B. at the time the patient is discharged
    C. within 90 days
    D. within 90 days after the year services were rendered
    E. by December 31st the year after the year services were rendered

132. An individual practice association contract with a group plan includes which of the following payment plans?
    A. a set amount per patient
    B. a set amount per month
    C. a small copayment for each visit
    D. payments based on a predetermined list of charges
    E. prepaid care

133. If a Medicaid patient is injured in an accident, assignment authorization is requested on Form
    A. XIX-TPD-1-76
    B. 500 or 501
    C. HCFA 1500
    D. HCFA 1490-SC
    E. 5021

134. The time limit on refiling a denied Medicare charge is
    A. 10 days
    B. 30 days
    C. 90 days
    D. 6 months
    E. 1 year

135. When obtaining consents for surgery, which of the following religious groups' beliefs will prevent patients from receiving whole blood plasma?
    A. Christian Scientists
    B. Seventh-Day Adventists
    C. Christian Scientists and Seventh-Day Adventists
    D. Jehovah's Witnesses
    E. Christian Scientists and Jehovah's Witnesses

136. Using slide presentations to medical students about medical cases is unethical if the discussion involves
    A. case studies
    B. treatments
    C. specific statistics
    D. names
    E. x-rays

137. A patient record abbreviation indicating a
    patient has had a "little" stroke lasting
    from a few minutes to almost 24 hours is
    A. CVA
    B. CVP
    C. TIA
    D. CSF
    E. MI

138. A medical record abbreviation indicating a
    condition in which the heart's pumping
    capability is impaired is
    A. CHF
    B. ASHD
    C. COPD
    D. CSF
    E. CVA

139. In the terminal-digit filing system, a folder
    is number 87 34 23. This number would be
    filed in
    A. section 23, guide 34, 87th in sequence
    B. section 87, guide 34, 23rd in sequence
    C. section 23, guide 87, 34th in sequence
    D. section 87, guide 23, 34th in sequence
    E. section 34, guide 23, 87th in sequence

140. A patient record entry noting the number
    of live births would begin
    A. LMP
    B. DOB
    C. PROM
    D. para
    E. gravida

141. Under which filing guide should new
    equipment brochures be filed?
    A. Administration-Contracts
    B. Administration-Budget
    C. Equipment-Inventory
    D. Equipment-Maintenance and Repairs
    E. Equipment-Purchases

142. In terminal-digit filing, which number
    would come after 87 34 23?
    A. 87 34 24
    B. 87 34 33
    C. 87 35 23
    D. 88 34 23
    E. 88 34 24

143. Which of the following is a medical record
    entry noting an objective symptom?
    A. headache
    B. stiff neck
    C. urinary frequency
    D. shuffling gait
    E. numbness in the right hand

144. The filing system that uses index dividers
    by month and day is called a(n)
    A. recall file
    B. reminder file
    C. follow-up file
    D. tickler file
    E. appointment file

145. A patient record abbreviation indicating
    the removal of foreign material from a
    traumatic or infected lesion is
    A. Bx
    B. D&C
    C. expl lap
    D. FB
    E. I&D

146. A file needs to be created for reports
    received from the Centers for Disease
    Control of the U.S. Department of Health
    and Human Services. The third indexing
    unit would be
    A. Human
    B. Department
    C. Health
    D. Services
    E. Government

147. Records may be released without patient
    signature
    A. after a patient has transferred care to a
       new physician
    B. after a patient has died
    C. to insurance companies
    D. if there is a blanket release signed and
       on file
    E. to a court of law

148. In addition to patient record entries,
    physicians who regularly engage in
    dispensing narcotic drugs are required to
    keep a record of
    A. dispensing
    B. inventory
    C. dispensing and inventory
    D. prescriptions written
    E. dispensing and prescriptions written

149. A laboratory calls with a urinalysis report. Which of the following indicates that the physician will call the patient with an abnormal report?
     A. RBC, 1–2 at high-power field
     B. WBC, 0–4 at high-power field
     C. casts, 0–1 hyaline
     D. mucous, few
     E. bacteria, moderate

150. A patient record abbreviation indicating a bladder infection is
     A. KUB
     B. UTI
     C. TUR
     D. UR
     E. URI

151. Telephone calls that require the immediate attention of the physician include:
     A. personal callers
     B. hospital staff nurses
     C. pharmacists
     D. laboratory technologists
     E. consulting physicians

152. Telephone calls that should be returned only by the physician include inquiries regarding
     A. normal test results
     B. abnormal test results
     C. both normal and abnormal test results
     D. medication refills
     E. abnormal test results and medication refills

153. A patient calls and tells the medical assistant she is worried about the cost of her illness. The medical assistant would
     A. have the physician return the patient's call
     B. review the patient's insurance policy with her
     C. tell the patient not to worry until she is well again
     D. refer the patient to social services
     E. refer the patient to her insurance carrier

154. While the physician is having office hours, the medical assistant is having difficulty interpreting a "garbled" piece of dictation. The medical assistant should FIRST
     A. transcribe the material based on a similar report
     B. omit the dictation, leaving it for the physician to interpret
     C. have another medical assistant interpret the dictation
     D. type the material as correctly as possible
     E. ask the physician to listen to the material

155. Which letter style is preferred for open punctuation letters?
     A. official
     B. modified semiblock
     C. semiblock
     D. modified block
     E. block

156. A subject line, if used, is
     A. typed two spaces above the salutation
     B. positioned flush right
     C. underscored with the first letter of each word capitalized
     D. typed in all capitals and underscored
     E. typed four lines below the date line and two lines above the inside address

157. Which of the following statements about microfilming is true?
     A. It reduces time searching for files.
     B. It reduces space required for storage.
     C. Its best benefits are its use with active records.
     D. It is less expensive than other forms of storage.
     E. It eliminates lost files or misfiles.

158. When a politely neutral (neither formal nor informal) tone is desired, which of the following is an acceptable complimentary close?
     A. Respectfully yours
     B. Very respectfully
     C. Fondly
     D. Sincerely yours
     E. Kindest regards

159. Before the medical assistant places an incoming caller on hold, each of the following steps should be completed EXCEPT:
    A. a greeting
    B. stating the office name
    C. stating the caller's name
    D. asking the reason for the call
    E. asking the caller for a return phone number

160. Each of the following statements about numeric filing is true EXCEPT
    A. Numeric filing allows unlimited expansion without folder shifting.
    B. Shelving or drawers are filled evenly.
    C. Filing activity is greatest at the end of the numeric series.
    D. The system is recommended for offices with greater than 15,000 files.
    E. Filing is direct and without reference.

161. Each of the following statements concerning the patient medical record is true EXCEPT
    A. They are used for research purposes.
    B. They are inadmissible in a court of law.
    C. They are used by review committees for evaluating the quality of care.
    D. They are used for exchanging information among medical assisting staff.
    E. They are used to teach medical and allied health students.

162. Each of the following is an essential element of the business letter EXCEPT:
    A. date line
    B. inside address
    C. salutation
    D. signature
    E. signature block

163. A 14-year-old patient, referred to the office by another physician, is to have medical photographs taken. To prevent possible patient claims of invasion of privacy, the medical assistant MUST obtain written permission.
    A. before the photographs are taken
    B. before the patient leaves the office
    C. after the photographs are processed and developed
    D. before the photographs are published
    E. after the photographs are published

164. In the previous question, the medical assistant must obtain written permission from the
    A. patient
    B. guardian
    C. patient and guardian
    D. referring physician
    E. guardian and referring physician

165. After adding a new document, computer storage options include output to a
    A. modem
    B. screen
    C. disk
    D. parallel printer
    E. serial printer

166. A macro is
    A. a circuit board
    B. a large file of 10 or more megabytes of storage
    C. a two-keystroke combination for executing commands
    D. a file located on the root directory
    E. a large directory that branches off the root directory

167. For retrieving computer information, "wildcard" commands include
    A. a:*.bat
    B. a:dir/p
    C. cd\win
    D. cd\root
    E. dir/p/w

168. You have just created a new document from one that is in storage. Which command keeps this new file separate from the original?
    A. "save" the document on the screen to a new directory
    B. "save" the document on the screen with a new extension.
    C. both A and B
    D. "copy" the document on the screen to another directory
    E. both A and D

169. The goal is to copy the file named "template.ltr" from C drive to A drive. The command is
    A. C:\>a:copy template.ltr
    B. C:\>copy template.ltr a:
    C. A:\>copy c:template.ltr
    D. A:\>copy c:template.ltr a:
    E. A:\>copy a:template.ltr c:

170. Passport applications may be obtained from
    A. embassies
    B. consulates
    C. travel agents
    D. libraries
    E. the Department of Transportation

171. The theft of controlled substances is reported to the
    A. local police department
    B. Drug Enforcement Agency
    C. both A and B
    D. Federal Bureau of Investigation
    E. both A and D

172. Which of the following is deposited quarterly?
    A. employee social security withheld
    B. federal income tax withheld
    C. employer contribution to social security
    D. federal unemployment tax
    E. all of the above

173. Credit adjustments on the patient ledger card are necessary for which of the following?
    A. correction of an undercharge for a service
    B. returned nonsufficient funds check
    C. both A and B
    D. refund
    E. both A and D

174. A pegboard system of record-keeping can be used to provide the patient
    A. a statement of account
    B. an itemization of charges
    C. both A and B
    D. a notation of the next appointment
    E. both A and D

175. In which of the following practices is the physician included on the staff payroll?
    A. closed-panel HMO
    B. IPA
    C. partnerships
    D. solo practice
    E. PPO

176. The preprinted banking "MICR" code number includes the
    A. check number
    B. checking account number
    C. both A and B
    D. check amount
    E. both A and D

177. A credit balance occurs in which of the following circumstances?
    A. a patient has paid in advance of a service
    B. a professional discount is offered to a patient
    C. both A and B
    D. an insurance company disallows a charge
    E. both A and D

178. The superbill includes which of the following?
    A. aging schedule
    B. truth-in-lending statement
    C. insurance claim
    D. deposit slip
    E. fee schedule

179. When reconciling the bank account, each of the following is correct EXCEPT
    A. deducting outstanding checks from the bank balance
    B. deducting bank charges from the checkbook
    C. deducting bank drafts from the checkbook
    D. adding outstanding deposits to the bank balance
    E. deducting deposits not in the checkbook

180. When computing personal income tax in an unincorporated business, each disbursement qualifies as the physician's personal deduction EXCEPT
    A. property taxes
    B. interest paid out on a mortgage
    C. contributions
    D. malpractice insurance
    E. interest paid out on a home equity loan

181. CHAMPUS requires prior authorization if
    A. the patient lives more than 40 miles from the military facility
    B. care is unavailable at the local military health care facility
    C. the civilian facility is closer in an emergency
    D. the eligible patient elects inpatient care in a civilian hospital
    E. the military hospital is temporarily unable to handle the case

182. BC/BS service benefit plan features include
    A. no copayments
    B. flat fees regardless of the amount of care
    C. no deductible
    D. direct payment considered payment-in-full
    E. payments directly to the patient

183. Each of the following is a true statement concerning coordination of benefits EXCEPT
    A. Private insurance is the secondary carrier for patients in workers' compensation cases.
    B. When both spouses carry insurance, the patient's plan will pay.
    C. When both spouses carry insurance, remaining expenses will be paid by the spouse's plan.
    D. A father's insurance is considered the primary carrier for a child.
    E. Medicare is the secondary carrier for patients with group insurance.

184. In which of the following situations is Medicare considered the primary carrier?
    A. a retired 65-year-old patient with group insurance
    B. a retired 68-year-old patient with CHAMPUS
    C. a retired 65-year-old patient with medigap supplemental
    D. a retired 68-year-old patient with Medicaid
    E. a semiretired 62-year-old patient with Medicaid

185. Incidents of child abuse and neglect should be suspected in each condition EXCEPT
    A. chronic infections of the ear
    B. malnutrition
    C. poor growth pattern
    D. poor hygiene
    E. gross dental problems

186. A mother calls and reports her child has ingested a poison. The mother states the child swallowed about 1 teaspoon of Ipecac syrup. The medical assistant should first
    A. reassure the mother that this amount is not harmful
    B. call poison control
    C. instruct the mother that nausea and vomiting will occur quickly
    D. instruct the mother to go to an emergency room
    E. ascertain the child's age and weight

187. Color-coded stickers are useful for each of the following EXCEPT
    A. identifying past-due accounts
    B. identifying allergies
    C. purging of records
    D. coding specific symptoms
    E. assigning specialty types

188. True statements about the medical record include each of the following EXCEPT
    A. The patient owns the information.
    B. The physician owns the information.
    C. Legally, if it is recorded, it was done.
    D. Legally, if it is not recorded, it was not done.
    E. The physician owns the record.

189. In the problem-oriented medical record you would chart a familial disease under
    A. subjective
    B. objective
    C. assessment
    D. plan
    E. inactive problems

190. The patient record is a legal document and therefore each of the following is required EXCEPT
    A. legible handwriting
    B. entries printed not longhand
    C. written in ink
    D. no erasures
    E. signature with every entry

191. If the physician is unable to be reached, the medical assistant should set a next available appointment for the incoming caller, if the patient is experiencing
    A. a nosebleed
    B. severe chest pain without shortness of breath or nausea
    C. severe difficulty breathing
    D. intermittent loss of consciousness
    E. severe vomiting and diarrhea with high fever

192. Calls that should be handled by the medical assistant include
    A. the physician's professional associate
    B. questions regarding illness treatment
    C. patient emergency
    D. call from a patient's family regarding a treatment plan
    E. patient progress report during an acute illness

193. Continuation sheets should
    A. be at least one paragraph long
    B. be at least two lines long
    C. begin with the writer's name, the date, and the page number
    D. begin four lines from the top of the paper
    E. begin one line below a 1-inch top margin

194. In a modified semiblock letter, which of the following parts of a letter must always be typed flush left?
    A. special mailing notations or on-arrival notations
    B. patient account number or policy number
    C. both A and B
    D. attention line
    E. both A and D

195. Which of the following letter parts may differ between the modified block letter and the modified semiblock letter?
    A. Date line
    B. Signature block
    C. Both A and B
    D. Paragraph indentations
    E. Both A and D

196. Telephone verification of a patient's entitlement to benefits is termed
    A. certification of eligibility
    B. assignment of insurance benefits
    C. explanation of benefits
    D. prior authorization
    E. precertification

197. The total number of ICD-9 codes allowed on the HCFA-1500 claim form is
    A. one
    B. two
    C. four
    D. five
    E. 10

198. Files and documents for which personalized file extensions can be used include
    A. WordPerfect
    B. Lotus 1-2-3
    C. Excel
    D. Data files DBase
    E. Fox Pro

199. The form (Fig. 5–1) is needed anytime
    A. a promise is needed from the patient that the bill will be paid
    B. credit is extended to a patient
    C. credit is extended to a patient for the first time
    D. patient payment schedules include four or more payments
    E. it is suspected that the patient is a poor credit risk

200. The form (Fig. 5–1) is not necessary if
    A. the patient signs a promissory note
    B. there is no interest
    C. the charges are not financed
    D. there is no down payment
    E. there is a down payment

LEONARD S. TAYLOR, M.D.
2100 WEST PARK AVENUE
CHAMPAIGN, ILLINOIS 61820

TELEPHONE 352-7658

FEDERAL TRUTH IN LENDING STATEMENT
For professional services rendered

Patient _____

Address _____

_____

Parent _____

1. Cash Price (fee for service) $ _____

2. Cash Down Payment $ _____

3. Unpaid Balance of Cash Price $ _____

4. Amount Financed $ _____

5. FINANCE CHARGE $ _____

6. Finance Charge Expressed As
   Annual Percentage Rate   _____

7. Total of Payments (4 plus 5) $ _____

8. Deferred Payment Price (1 plus 5) $ _____

"Total payment due" (7 above) is payable to _____
at above office address in _____ monthly installments of $ _____
The first installment is payable on _____ 19 ____, and
each subsequent payment is due on the same day of each consecutive month
until paid in full.

_____   _____
Date   Signature of Patient; Parent if Patient is a Minor

FORM 9402 COLWELL SYSTEMS. INC., CHAMPAIGN. ILLINOIS

Figure 5–1. Truth-in lending form. (Courtesy of Colwell Systems, Inc., Champaign, IL.)

Part 3—Clinical Procedures

Directions: *Each of the following questions or incomplete statements precedes five suggested answers or completions. Select the ONE answer or completion that is BEST in each case and fill in the circle containing the corresponding letter on the answer sheet.*

201. Oral glass thermometers soaking in a chemical solution should be rinsed and dried before using because the chemical solution
   A. harbors certain organisms
   B. obscures an accurate reading
   C. irritates the oral mucosa
   D. constricts the mercury column
   E. tastes bad

202. Tagamet decreases the acidity of the stomach by
   A. directly neutralizing stomach acidity
   B. blocking the action of histamine
   C. buffering the acid in the stomach
   D. absorbing stomach acid into a gel mass
   E. coating the lining of the stomach

203. One drug used to treat hypertension is
   A. Amoxil
   B. Tenormin
   C. Lanoxin
   D. Prozac
   E. Zantac

204. Which lead is placed at the fifth intercostal space at the junction of the left mid-clavicular line?
   A. V_2
   B. V_3
   C. V_4
   D. V_5
   E. V_6

205. The horizontal axis of the ECG measures
   A. time
   B. voltage
   C. amplification
   D. speed
   E. "gain" or output of the amplifier

206. A multichannel ECG instrument records 12 leads simultaneously, using how many sensors?
   A. 5
   B. 7
   C. 9
   D. 10
   E. 12

207. Muscle artifact voltages have an amplitude and frequency that can be described as
   A. consistent
   B. erratic
   C. violent shifting
   D. breaking up along complexes
   E. shifting along the baseline

208. Repolarization is the
   A. heart at rest
   B. discharge of electrical energy
   C. heart's contraction
   D. time interval between atrial contraction and ventricular contraction
   E. electrical recovery of the heart

209. During examination of the patient in the lithotomy position, she experiences cramping of the right calf. The medical assistant would
   A. assist the patient to the supine position
   B. press down the knee cap and push up on the ball of the foot
   C. A then B
   D. offer support to the right calf so that the patient can maintain the position until the examination is over
   E. B then D

210. The patient is supine with both feet flexed sharply at the knees. This position is
    A. dorsal recumbent
    B. Trendelenburg
    C. Sims'
    D. jackknife
    E. lithotomy

211. If a patient develops anaphylactic shock after receiving a dose of penicillin, which of the following symptoms will the patient most likely experience FIRST?
    A. blurred vision
    B. difficulty breathing
    C. projectile vomiting
    D. urinary retention
    E. decreasing levels of consciousness

212. In a phlebotomy "multidraw" using three tubes—red, lavender, and gray—the order of the draw is
    A. red stopper color first
    B. lavender stopper color first
    C. gray stopper color first
    D. red stopper color last
    E. lavender stopper color last

213. Emetics are used to induce vomiting if the
    A. patient is at least semiconscious
    B. poison is a petroleum distillate, such as kerosene
    C. poison is a convulsant, such as strychnine
    D. poison is a corrosive, such as a strong acid
    E. overdose is a brand of acetaminophen

214. Which of the following cardiac compressions per minute is recommended for adults needing cardiopulmonary resuscitation?
    A. 10–15
    B. 40
    C. 60
    D. 80–100
    E. 120–160

215. Which of the following drug therapies would be likely to decrease a patient's prothrombin time?
    A. coumarin
    B. heparin
    C. fibrinolysin
    D. vitamin K
    E. streptokinase

216. When one is using the hemacytometer, on which lines are cells counted?
    A. top
    B. right
    C. top and right
    D. left
    E. top and left

217. When administering a ventrogluteal injection, the palm of the medical assistant should be placed on the patient's
    A. greater trochanter
    B. anterior superior iliac spine
    C. iliac crest
    D. sacral spine
    E. posterior spine or the ilium

218. A technique used to relax muscle when giving a ventrogluteal intramuscular injection is to have the patient
    A. stretch the toes
    B. point the toes inward
    C. point the toes outward
    D. flex the knees
    E. lie with a pillow under the abdomen

219. If a medication label becomes illegible,
    A. relabel the container over the original label
    B. relabel the container but not cover the original label
    C. discard the container and medication
    D. transfer the medication to a new container and label
    E. return the container to the manufacturer for credit

220. The physician orders 20 units of insulin. The vial reads U-100/mL. Which syringe will be used?
    A. U-40
    B. U-80
    C. either U-40 or U-80
    D. 1.0 mL Tuberculin
    E. either U-40 or 1.0 mL Tuberculin

221. In an obese adult patient, the recommended needle length for a ventrogluteal intramuscular injection is
    A. ½ in
    B. ⅝ in
    C. 1 in
    D. 1½ in
    E. 2½ in

222. If a deltoid muscle is small, before injecting a needle
   A. grasp the muscle in your hand
   B. spread the muscle taut in your hand
   C. pull the muscle upward with your hand
   D. push the muscle to one side with your hand
   E. have the patient open and close the fist several times

223. Blood collected in Vacutainer tubes without anticoagulants are centrifuged
   A. immediately
   B. within 15 minutes
   C. after 20–30 minutes
   D. after 1 hour
   E. after refrigeration for 1 hour

224. Unless otherwise ordered, which of the following quantities is the maximum that should be given to an adult patient in any one intramuscular injection?
   A. 0.5 mL
   B. 1.0 mL
   C. 2.0 mL
   D. 2.5 mL
   E. 5.0 mL

225. Of the following, which is the quickest absorption route for a medication?
   A. subcutaneous
   B. intramuscular
   C. oral
   D. transdermal patch
   E. inhalation

226. Before withdrawing a medication from a multiuse vial, the medical assistant should be certain that
   A. no air is injected into the vial
   B. 1 mL of air is injected into the vial
   C. an amount of air equal to the medication to be withdrawn is injected
   D. 2 mL of air is injected into the vial
   E. 0.5 mL more than the amount of medication to be withdrawn is injected

227. Regular insulin peaks in the bloodstream in
   A. 30–60 minutes
   B. 2–5 hours
   C. 6–8 hours
   D. 12 hours
   E. 24 hours

228. How much diluent would you add to prepare 1 gal of 70% isopropyl alcohol from a 90% isopropyl alcohol stock solution?
   A. 28 oz
   B. 38 oz
   C. 70 oz
   D. 90 oz
   E. 100 oz

229. The antacid sodium bicarbonate (soda mint)
   A. works locally by absorbing acid
   B. may increase stomach acid secretion
   C. works locally by absorbing acid and may increase stomach acid secretion
   D. is a systemic antacid
   E. is a systemic antacid and may increase stomach acid secretion

230. For which of the following conditions does first aid include the application of cold?
   A. hypovolemic shock
   B. anaphylactic shock
   C. septic shock
   D. angioedema
   E. fainting

231. The type of diet most likely prescribed for a patient with hypertension is
   A. bland
   B. low fat
   C. low sodium
   D. high protein
   E. high carbohydrates

232. Of the following sexually transmitted diseases, which is considered to place a woman at a much higher risk of developing cervical cancer?
   A. herpes genitalis
   B. gonorrhea
   C. syphilis
   D. chlamydia
   E. *Haemophilus vaginalis*

233. A Pap smear showing atypical cytology but no evidence of cancer is reported as
   A. grade I
   B. grade II
   C. grade III
   D. grade IV
   E. grade V

234. Patient instructions for the administration of a rectal drug intended for a systemic effect include which?
    A. Remain lying for 20–30 minutes.
    B. Administer before a bowel movement.
    C. Administer before a bowel movement and remain lying for 20–30 minutes.
    D. Administer after a bowel movement.
    E. Administer after a bowel movement and remain lying for 20–30 minutes.

235. When instructing a patient to introduce cream into the vagina, the medical assistant would teach the patient to direct the applicator toward the patient's
    A. pubis symphysis
    B. base of the spine
    C. cervix
    D. umbilicus
    E. mons pubis

236. Medical assistants should instruct their patients to examine their breasts
    A. a few days before the menstruation period
    B. during the menstruation period
    C. 1 week after the menstruation period
    D. 2 weeks after the menstruation period
    E. 3 weeks after the menstruation period

237. The scalpel and blade choice for an incision and drainage of a carbuncle on the left lumbar region is
    A. no. 3 handle and no. 11 or 15 blade
    B. no. 3 handle and no. 12 blade
    C. no. 4 handle and no. 21 blade
    D. no. 4 handle and no. 22 blade
    E. no. 7 handle and no. 12 blade

238. An Allis tissue forceps can be recognized by which of the following parts?
    A. intermeshing teeth
    B. ratchets
    C. intermeshing teeth and ratchets
    D. spring-type handle
    E. intermeshing teeth and spring-type handle

239. Pregnancy tests that use immunologic methods to detect the presence of human chorionic gonadotropin (HCG) are based on
    A. reproductive tract changes in laboratory animals
    B. detection of serum antibodies specific to HCG antigens
    C. suppression of blood serum levels of HCG
    D. an increase of blood serum levels of HCG
    E. increased progesterone production during the first trimester

240. An infection that requires isolation for one week and strict isolation for children under 3 years of age is
    A. rubella
    B. dysentery, amebic
    C. influenza
    D. infectious mononucleosis
    E. measles (rubeola)

241. Following surgery to an extremity, the affected limb is elevated to help prevent
    A. edema to the part
    B. external wound drainage
    C. edema to the part and external wound drainage
    D. separation of the wound edges
    E. edema to the part and separation of the wound edges

242. During a minor surgical procedure, the primary reason for the surgical drape at the surgical site is to
    A. destroy all pathogenic organisms
    B. prevent contamination from unprepped patient skin surfaces
    C. limit contamination to nonpathogenic organisms
    D. ensure sterility of all materials and equipment
    E. protect health personnel from cross-infection

243. A patient's diabetic condition is being controlled by diet therapy. To monitor his disease at home, the medical assistant will need to teach him to
    A. calculate food exchange values
    B. inject insulin
    C. calculate food exchange values and inject insulin
    D. measure urine glucose levels
    E. calculate food exchange values and measure urine glucose levels

244. During a microscopic urine examination, yeast is differentiated from red blood cells by testing with
   A. acetic acid
   B. acetone
   C. KOH
   D. Benedict's solution
   E. sulfosalicyclic acid

245. Which of the following is viewed under a microscopic low-power field?
   A. red blood cells
   B. white blood cells
   C. epithelial cells
   D. casts
   E. crystals

246. Which of the following microscopic elements in urine can be reported as "few-moderate-many?"
   A. erythrocytes
   B. leukocytes
   C. both A and B
   D. bacteria
   E. both A and D

247. When filing three Vacutainer tubes, when is the correct time to remove the tourniquet?
   A. before pushing the first tube into the rear cannula of the holder
   B. while the first tube is filing
   C. during the second tube draw
   D. during the last tube draw
   E. after the needle is removed

248. Which of the following Vacutainer brand tubes are not inverted at the time of blood collection?
   A. red and black stopper color
   B. red stopper color
   C. gray stopper color
   D. green stopper color
   E. yellow stopper color

249. Capillary puncture blood flow is facilitated by doing which of the following before the puncture?
   A. make a tourniquet around the finger with your fingers.
   B. Tap the fingertip with your fingertips.
   C. Gently squeeze the finger.
   D. Place the finger in warm water or a warm towel.
   E. Have the patient shake the hand to increase blood flow.

250. When collecting blood for a hematocrit, correct equipment includes
   A. plain microhematocrit tubes for EDTA anticoagulated blood
   B. plain microhematocrit tubes for capillary blood
   C. both A and B
   D. heparinized microhematocrit tubes for capillary blood
   E. both A and D

251. The physician orders a complete blood count and differential. Which of the following Vacutainers would be required to obtain 5–7 mL of collected blood?
   A. lavender top
   B. blue top
   C. red top
   D. gray top
   E. black top

252. In the Vacutainer specimen, which of the following statements concerning the liquid portion (on top the cells) is true?
   A. The liquid portion in the lavender tube is called serum; in the red tube, it is called plasma.
   B. The liquid portion in the red tube is called plasma.
   C. The liquid portion in the lavender tube is called plasma; in the red tube, it is called serum.
   D. The liquid portion in both the lavender and red tubes is called plasma.
   E. The liquid portion in both the lavender and red tubes is called serum.

253. Sudden dizziness upon arising from a reclining position is a temporary condition called
   A. latent hypertension
   B. latent hypotension
   C. secondary hypertension
   D. orthostatic hypertension
   E. orthostatic hypotension

254. The number of heartbeats for every respiration is normally an average of
   A. 1–2
   B. 1–3
   C. 1–4
   D. 1–6
   E. 1–10

255. The presence of an ausculatory gap is common in
    A. all patients
    B. children
    C. after exercise
    D. patients with hypertension and heart disease
    E. pregnancy, if anemia is present

256. In a blood pressure reading of 140/96/70, the 96 represents when the medical assistant heard a
    A. first sharp sound
    B. temporary disappearance of sound
    C. distinct, sharp tapping sound
    D. muffled sound
    E. no sound

257. When determining a patient's blood pressure, before inflating the cuff for an auscultatory reading, the medical assistant would
    A. inflate the cuff 30 mm above the disappearance of the radial pulse
    B. inflate the cuff 30 mm above the disappearance of the brachial pulse
    C. inflate the cuff until the radial pulse disappears and mentally add 30 mm to it
    D. palpate the radial artery
    E. palpate the brachial artery

258. Each of the following analgesics is likely to complicate a patient-history of an increased bleeding time or an increased prothrombin time EXCEPT
    A. Motrin
    B. Aspirin
    C. Indocin
    D. Tylenol with Codeine
    E. Darvocet-N

259. In cardiopulmonary resuscitation, each of the following techniques for cardiac compressions is correct EXCEPT
    A. placing one hand directly over the other hand
    B. a second rescuer administering 60 cardiac compressions per minute
    C. interlocking fingers for cardiac compressions
    D. flexing elbows slightly
    E. bringing the shoulders directly over the hands as they are positioned on the chest

260. Reactions to adrenocorticosteroid injections include
    A. fainting
    B. anaphylaxis
    C. both A and B
    D. swelling at the injection site
    E. both A and D

261. Narcotic analgesics may be used to treat each of the following EXCEPT
    A. pain during the late stages of delivery
    B. cough
    C. postsurgical pain
    D. dysentery
    E. pain of acute coronary or pulmonary vascular occlusion

262. Each of the following statements concerning antacids is true EXCEPT
    A. Antacids are contraindicated in peptic ulcers.
    B. Antacids may have a laxative effect.
    C. Antacids may have a constipating effect.
    D. Antacids should be taken with water or milk.
    E. Antacids should not be used with tetracyclines.

263. Each of the following is an effect of a narcotic analgesic EXCEPT
    A. depressed respiration
    B. nausea and vomiting
    C. depressed cough reflex
    D. increased response to stress
    E. decreased intestinal motility

264. Under high power examination of urine, each of the following statements about red blood cells is true EXCEPT which?
    A. In hypotonic (dilute) urine, RBCs swell and burst.
    B. In hypertonic (concentrated) urine, RBCs may resemble WBCs.
    C. RBCs are easily confused with yeast cells.
    D. RBCs are easily confused with oil droplets.
    E. RBCs have a granular appearance and contain a multilobed nucleus.

265. Each of the following statements about urine crystals is true EXCEPT
 A. Crystals will precipitate if the urine is allowed to cool.
 B. Crystals are reported out using numerical ranges based on the average.
 C. Large amounts of crystals indicate imminent renal stone formation.
 D. Identification of crystals first begins with pH determination.
 E. The presence of most crystals is not clinically significant.

266. Each of the following statements about protein in the urine is true EXCEPT
 A. A small amount of protein is normally excreted in the urine every day.
 B. In some patients with proteinuria, first morning specimens may yield a negative result.
 C. Proteinuria is common in pregnancy.
 D. Proteinuria is almost always present after heavy exercise.
 E. Proteinuria is an indicator of phenylketonuria in infants.

267. Each of the following is a correct technique for a difficult venipuncture EXCEPT which?
 A. If a vein is not located, remove the tube from the needle before withdrawing the needle.
 B. If the vein is transfixed, slowly pull back the needle until blood flows.
 C. If blood does not flow, push the tube stopper once again slightly past the guideline.
 D. If blood flow is slow, leave the tourniquet in place.
 E. A slow filling or partially filled tube may be corrected by deeper vein entry.

268. For obtaining an adult blood pressure, each of the following is an accepted technique EXCEPT:
 A. placing the patient in the supine position
 B. using an aneroid sphygmomanometer
 C. using a cuff that is 9 cm (3.5 in)
 D. placing the cuff 2 in above the antecubital space
 E. placing the stethoscope diaphragm below the cuff

Using the Neubauer hemacytometer (Fig. 5–2), answer the following two questions:

(9 square millimeters)

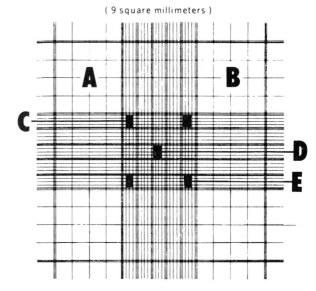

Figure 5–2. Neubauer hemacytometer.

269. What is the first white-blood cell counting area?

270. What is the fifth red-blood cell counting area?

Using the glucose tolerance test-times listed below answer the following three questions:

 A. fasting
 B. 0.5 hour
 C. 1 hour
 D. 2 hours
 E. 5 hours

271. The patient is given an oral drink before which test time?

272. The first blood is collected at which test time?

273. The test time at which the blood sugar should return to normal limits.

Using the capillary puncture site diagrams (Fig. 5–3), answer the following two questions:

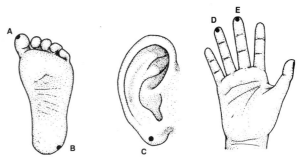

Figure 5–3. Capillary puncture sites.

274. The most common site for adult capillary puncture.

275. The most common site for capillary puncture of a 6-month-old infant.

276. Universal blood and body-fluid precaution barriers include
    A. gowns and aprons
    B. laboratory coats
    C. both A and B
    D. contact lenses
    E. both A and D

277. Situations in which the medical assistant should wear *sterile* gloves include
    A. administering an injection
    B. withdrawing blood by finger puncture
    C. withdrawing blood by venipuncture
    D. changing a dressing covering an infected wound
    E. employees with cuts, scratches, or breaks in their skin

278. Quaternary ammonium compounds should be relied on to achieve
    A. instrument disinfection
    B. sterilization
    C. skin disinfection
    D. inactivation of blood contaminants
    E. sanitization when combined with soap detergents

279. Procedures for which the patient needs to fast before a CT scan test include
    A. CT spine
    B. CT head
    C. both A and B
    D. CT bone densitometry
    E. both A and D

280. Laxatives are a necessary preparation for each of the following tests EXCEPT
    A. CT ABD/pelvis
    B. pelvic ultrasound
    C. abdominal ultrasound
    D. colonoscopy
    E. IVP

281. The ECG activity of lead II is the
    A. right arm
    B. left arm
    C. both A and B
    D. left leg
    E. both A and D

282. Instruments used to open a cavity for examination include each of the following EXCEPT
    A. a trocar
    B. a dilator
    C. a retractor
    D. a speculum
    E. a catheter

283. The otoscope is used to examine the
    A. optic blood vessels
    B. macula lutes (yellow spot)
    C. nasal passages
    D. central fovea
    E. optic disk (blink spot)

284. Do not induce vomiting in a patient, if the poison ingested is
    A. gasoline
    B. barbiturates
    C. both A and B
    D. poisonous shrubbery
    E. both A an D

285. As an antiemetic ipecac may be used in adults
    A. in severe inebriation
    B. in heart disease
    C. with activated charcoal
    D. with water
    E. with milk

286. Blood levels that will be increased in hyperthyroidism include:
    A. serum cholesterol
    B. potassium
    C. calcium
    D. sodium
    E. triglycerides

287. The physician orders morphine sulfate 6 mg prepared. The label reads grains ⅛ per mL. How much would the medical assistant prepare?
    A. 0.75 mL
    B. 12.5 grains
    C. ⅛ mL
    D. 1.0 mL
    E. 8.0 mg

288. When giving an intramuscular injection each is correct procedure EXCEPT
    A. inserting the needle quickly
    B. injecting the medication slowly
    C. injecting the medication into one place
    D. removing the needle slowly
    E. briskly massaging, when indicated

289. Patients who should NOT have M-M-R-II vaccine include those who
    A. are allergic to dairy products
    B. have had tetanus antitoxin
    C. are allergic to eggs
    D. are allergic to horse hair
    E. have had anaphylactic reactions to eggs

290. Which of the following is a neurologic examination of reflex?
    A. knee jerk
    B. Romberg test
    C. Weber test
    D. Rinne test
    E. visual acuity

291. Instructions to a patient 5–6 hours after a cervical biopsy may include
    A. to douche
    B. to insert a tampon
    C. to return to normal sexual activity
    D. to remove vaginal packing
    E. to begin antibiotic therapy

292. Directions to a patient for the collection of feces for a fecal occult blood include which of the following?
    A. Collect one specimen 4 hours before the appointment.
    B. No red meat should be ingested 48–72 hours before and during the test.
    C. both A and B
    D. Withhold all medications.
    E. both A and D

293. Which of the following urine findings may be associated with urinary tract infection, if they occur in increased numbers either individually or as a grouping?
    A. white blood cells
    B. presence of nitrate
    C. both A and B
    D. squamous epithelial cells
    E. both A and D

294. Which of the following microscopic urine findings are associated with kidney damage?
    A. white blood cells in the absence of other findings
    B. yeast in the specimen of a female patient without other findings
    C. mucous threads in the absence of red blood cells
    D. bacteria in the absence of white blood cells
    E. red blood cells in the presence of red blood cell casts.

295. When too little blood is collected in a Vacutainer EDTA (lavender) tube, misleading results may arise from
    A. hemolysis of the cells
    B. an inability to separate the serum from the clot
    C. the blood clotting in the tube
    D. too much additive adversely affecting the specimen
    E. any delays in processing

296. When using the Vacutainer system, hemoconcentration of the blood specimen will result from
    A. using a needle with too large a gauge
    B. removing the tube before complete filling of the specimen
    C. shaking the specimen
    D. failing to release the tourniquet as soon as the blood flows
    E. releasing the tourniquet too early

297. A wide pulse pressure is usually present in
    A. atherosclerosis
    B. edema
    C. both A and B
    D. cerebral vascular accident
    E. both A and D

600,000 units of long-acting penicillin IM is ordered for a 30-pound child. You have on hand procaine penicillin G 1,200,000 units in a pre-packaged Tubex unit.

298. Each of the following is a true statement concerning the administration of this drug EXCEPT which?
    A. Inject deep IM.
    B. The medication must be warmed.
    C. Roll the medication between your palms to mix.
    D. Expel 0.5 mL before administration.
    E. The patient may leave immediately after treatment.

299. In the situation above, true statements concerning the administration of this drug include:
    A. Massage the injection site.
    B. Do not allow the drug to remain in the needle or syringe for any length of time.
    C. both A and B
    D. The preferred site is the gluteal muscle.
    E. both A and B

300. In the same situation, immediate side effects and reactions include
    A. skin rashes
    B. respiratory distress within 20 minutes
    C. both A and B
    D. superinfections
    E. both A and D

ANSWER KEY FOR SIMULATION TEST 5

1. **E.** Pneumonia. *Tamparo & Lewis, p. 177.*

2. **D.** A closed reduction is the repair of a fracture or dislocation by manipulation, followed by the application of a sling or cast. *Gylys & Wedding, p. 223; Tamparo & Lewis, p. 297.*

3. **B.** Sickling of the cells increases when body oxygen content is low, with strenuous physical exertion, and on exposure to extremes of hot and cold. Because of the altitude, mountains are cold, there is less oxygen available, and activities are more strenuous. *Scanlon, pp. 55–56(b).*

4. **E.** A pulmonary embolism most likely will originate in a lower limb vein. Emboli easily travel away from vascular bifurcation (two smaller parts branching into one larger part) as the blood returns to the heart. Once the blood is pumped from the heart to the lungs, the clot travels toward bifurcation (one part branching into smaller parts) until it eventually gets caught and occludes a pulmonary artery. *Tamparo & Lewis, p. 191.*

5. **D.** Calculi are stonelike formations that may be found anywhere in the urinary tract. *Tamparo & Lewis, p. 89.*

6. **D.** Fractures of the neck of the femur commonly occur in older people from a slight fall or stumble. *Tamparo & Lewis, p. 298; Sheldon, pp. 552, 566.*

7. **C.** The presence of air in the pleural space is known as a pneumothorax. *Tamparo & Lewis, pp. 180–181.*

8. **E.** Vital capacity is the difference between total lung capacity and residual volume. It is the maximal volume of air that can be forcibly expelled from the lungs after a maximal inspiration. Forced expiratory volume in 1 second (FEV$_1$) is recorded on a spirometer and the test results provide an excellent index of pulmonary function. *Taber's, p. 723.*

9. **B.** The skin of the external ear canal is closely adherent to the surfaces of bone and cartilage; therefore, growths and boils in the external canal will produce extreme sensitivity and radiate severe pain. *Taber's, p. 598.*

10. **C.** Conditions associated with hyperthyroidism include an enlarged thyroid gland, goiters, and exophthalmos. Myxedema is associated with hypothyroidism. *Tamparo & Lewis, pp. 274–276.*

11. **D.** Mitral stenosis is the impeded blood flow from the left atrium to the left ventricle. *Tamparo & Lewis, pp. 209–210.*

12. **C.** The largest artery in the body is the aorta, which pumps blood to all the other arteries of the body. *Gylys & Wedding, p. 148.*

13. **A.** Cracking of joints is generally due to the sudden development of a partial vacuum in the joint cavity as the articular surfaces are pulled apart. The partial vacuum is occupied by water vapor and blood gases under reduced pressure. *Taber's, p. 1037.*

14. **D.** Electromyography is the study of muscle contraction as a result of electrical stimulation. It is used to detect the presence of muscle inflammation or degeneration and during neurosurgery to monitor nerve impulses intraoperatively. *Gylys & Wedding, p. 221.*

15. **B.** A concave curvature posteriorly (secondary curvature) is called lordosis, whereas a concave curvature anteriorly (primary curvature) is termed kyphosis. *Tamparo & Lewis, p. 288.*

16. **D.** If the sternocleidomastoid muscle is injured or shortened, the result is torticollis (wryneck). *Taber's, p. 2012.*

17. **B.** The protrusion of the stomach through the esophageal hiatus of the diaphragm is a type of diaphragmatic hernia, often termed a hiatal hernia. *Tamparo & Lewis, pp. 143–144.*

18. **A.** The hypothalamus regulates the autonomic and neuroendocrinological functions of the body, such as body temperature, appetite, fluid balance, and sex drives. *Gylys & Wedding, p. 323.*

19. **A.** Exacerbation means an increase in the severity of a disease or any of its symptoms. *Gylys & Wedding, p. 221.*

20. **B.** A fiber that carries impulses to the brain from a sensory fiber is termed a sensory (afferent) fiber. A fiber than stimulates or activates skeletal muscle is termed a motor (efferent) fiber. *Gylys & Wedding, p. 318.*

21. **C.** The supraspinatus holds the head of the humerus in place. A minor tear or a calcified deposit in the supraspinatus tendon may cause "painful arc" during the midrange abduction of the upper arm. *Taber's, p. 1409.*

22. **A.** Patients who have rheumatic fever often have chronic defects of the mitral valve later in life. *Tamparo & Lewis, p. 209.*

23. **E.** Most spores are difficult to destroy. They are especially resistant to light, heat, and cold. Special care has to be taken to autoclave for the specified amount of time in order to destroy spores. *Taber's, p. 1856.*

24. **E.** The mandible, or the lower jaw bone, and the temporal bone are involved in temporomandibular joint (TMJ) dysfunction. *Taber's, p. 1960.*

25. **C.** Proximal means nearest to the point of attachment or origin. *Gylys & Wedding, p. 52.*

26. **A.** A drop of an atropine-like drug placed on the eye annuls the actions of ciliary muscles and the sphincter pupillae, both of which are under parasympathetic control, and control the lens of the eye. *Gylys & Wedding, p. 356.*

27. **B.** Freely movable joint cavities are lined with synovial membranes. *Gylys & Wedding, p. 210.*

28. **C.** The perineum is the pelvic floor and the associated structures occupying the pelvic outlet. During childbirth the perineum may be torn. To avoid a tear, the obstetrician often cuts the perineum just before delivery and sutures the incision afterwards. The incision is called an episiotomy. *Gylys & Wedding, p. 270.*

29. **D.** A virus is unique because it will have either DNA or RNA but never both. Viruses have a complete set of hereditary factors in half the number of chromosomes and, therefore, can reproduce only within living cells. *Sheldon, pp. 190–192.*

30. **D.** An abnormal, tubelike passage leading from one internal organ to another or from an internal organ to the surface of the body is termed a fistula. Among the many types of fistulas, the anal type (fistula in ano) is one of the most common. *Tamparo & Lewis, p. 382.*

31. **D.** The ischium forms the posterior portion of the hip bone and supports the trunk in the sitting position. *Scanlon, p. 119.*

32. **B.** An artificial opening (stoma) of the small intestine, brought to the surface of the abdomen for the purpose of evacuating feces, is termed an ileostomy. *Gylys & Wedding, p. 104.*

33. **A.** The *Borrelia* genus includes the spirochete that transmits Lyme disease to humans through tick bites. *Frew, Lane, Frew, p. 774(t).*

34. **B.** The portal vein carries venous blood from the digestive organs and the spleen to the liver, supplying the liver with products of digestion so that the liver can perform its functions on foodstuffs. The blood carried to the liver by the portal vein is carbon dioxygenated blood on its way back to the heart. *Sheldon, pp. 387 (f), 389.*

35. **E.** Ligaments connect bone to bone; tendons connect bone to muscle; the bursa and synovium are contained within the joint capsule. *Gylys & Wedding, pp. 210, 213.*

36. **C.** Any circumstance that increases the myocardial oxygen demand or reduces the oxygen supply is capable of inducing angina. Angina pectoris is transient chest pain due to temporary and reversible ischemia of the myocardium. *Tamparo & Lewis, p. 214.*

37. **C.** Acute cholecystitis is the inflammation of the gallbladder, which may be either acute or chronic. Acute cholecystitis usually follows impaction of a gallstone in the cystic duct. The gallbladder becomes distended with bile, blood, and pus, and the ability of the gallbladder to concentrate bile is lost, resulting in fat intolerance, dyspepsia, and flatulence. *Tamparo & Lewis, p. 159.*

38. **D.** The crescent-shaped area of the nail is called the lunula. *Gylys & Wedding, p. 66.*

39. **A.** Abandonment is the failure to be available to patients in an emergency or over a period of time where injury results is abandonment. *Lewis & Tamparo, pp. 63–64.*

40. **C.** Certain regulations written by state boards of medicine governing medical assisting practice are addressed in medical practice acts and are called administrative laws. Statutory laws governing medical practice originate in state legislative bodies. *Lewis & Tamparo, p. 57.*

41. **C.** Have the patient sign a consent form stating he will not hold the physician responsible if his discontinuing the treatment has an adverse effect on him. *Lewis & Tamparo, p. 103.*

42. **B.** State laws are statutes written and passed by state legislatures. Common law is derived from court decisions; constitutional law is derived from the Constitution of the United States; federal law is national in scope and not written by the state; and administrative law is a regulation created for government agencies and written by the executive branches of state and federal government. *Lewis & Tamparo, p. 42.*

43. **E.** Ignorance, honest mistakes, and physical conditions do not relieve a person from his or her responsibility to persons whom he or she has injured. Under the law of negligence, each member of society is required to act in such a manner that it does not endanger another, and that personal conduct cannot be below accepted standards. The medical assistant has a personal responsibility to question an order if there is good reason, and not to make mistakes or perform illegal acts. *Lewis & Tamparo, p. 59–60.*

44. **C.** When the needs of the patient are not attended to with reasonable promptness, the medical assistant and the physician risk a law suit based on medical negligence. *Lewis & Tamparo, pp. 68–69.*

45. **B.** Vitamin B may turn the urine bright yellow to intense blue-green. *Lane, Keenon, Coleman (eds.), p. 565(t).*

46. **A.** Based on Maslow's hierarchy of needs, love and emotional security must precede the desire for and attainment of all other psychosocial needs, except for safety, food, and shelter. *Taber's, p. 1281.*

47. **A.** If the patient is unruly, it is best to talk to him or her. Too many people dealing with the patient may confuse or upset the patient more. The other selections imply punishment of one type or another and should not be considered. *Davis, p. 42.*

48. **D.** Being able to express feelings and fears is most helpful in coming to terms with death. *Davis, p. 168.*

49. **B.** When patients express that there is some mistake, they are most likely denying impending death. Anger statements are more likely to those such as "Why does this have to happen to me?" Expressions of bargaining include, "If I could have more time, I would . . ." Depression, a feeling of sadness; and acceptance, getting ready for death are later steps. *Davis, p. 170.*

50. **C.** Communication with seriously ill and dying patients may be especially difficult for office employees. Professionals and family members need to be understanding no matter how angry the patient becomes. Listening is important to allow patients to vent their own feelings. Do not try to gain control over the conversation or argue a point; increasing the patient's anxieties may make the situation worse. Although touch has a soothing effect, this patient appears to need expression as a diffuser more than physical comfort. *Davis, p. 173.*

51. **C.** Daydreaming is an example of fantasy. Fantasy is normal in healthy children and adults, unless it begins to occupy a large amount of time when no satisfaction can be found in reality or it becomes a substitute for seeking real goals in life. *Taber's, p. 494.*

52. **D.** It is generally agreed that the best attitude is that of hopefulness, as long as it is realistic. There could be remissions or medical advances that could help the patient. *Davis, p. 174.*

53. **A.** Pain is a subjective symptom based on perceptions. It most often occurs as a warning before tissues have been permanently damaged; sometimes there is no pain in a body part after permanent damage. Pain does not necessarily occur in proportion to the extent of damage or the size of the patient. People perceive or refuse to perceive pain, many times, based on environmental and cultural influences. *Tamparo & Lewis, pp. 354–355.*

54. **E.** In this procedure, pieces of the prostate gland are removed through a cystoscope, which is inserted into the prostate gland via the urethra. A suprapubic or retropubic prostatectomy incision is made on the lower abdominal wall. The perineal site is the site of entry for a radical prostatectomy. *Gylys & Wedding, p. 246.*

55. **D.** "rrhaphy" means suture repair; "perineo-" is the combining form for perineum. Perineotomy and episiotomy are terms for the surgical incision of the perineum. Perioneoplasty is plastic repair of the perineum; episioplasty, of the vulva. *Gylys & Wedding, pp. 12, 270.*

56. **E.** Exophthalmos. *Taber's, p. 691.*

57. **D.** Directions: one tablet, every day, one hour before bedtime. Refill when needed. *Lane, Medications, p. 3.*

58. **C.** Ischemia. *Taber's, p. 1024.*

59. **A.** Phlebitis. *Taber's, p. 1494.*

60. **C.** Bifurcate. *Taber's, p. 221.*

61. **B.** A synonym for tumor or growth is neoplasm. One that is not cancerous is said to be benign. *Gylys & Wedding, p. 72.*

62. **B.** The symbol +++ means moderate amount of reaction. The symbol ++ means trace or notable reaction; ++++, large amount or pronounced reaction; ↑ increase; and 2°, secondary. *Lane, Keenon, Coleman (eds.), p. 731.*

63. **A.** A condition characterized by a decreased number of platelets in the circulating blood is thrombocytopenia. *Tamparo & Lewis, p. 393.*

64. **C.** "Hyper" means excessive; "tropho," nourishment. *Gylys & Wedding, pp. 3, 15, 35, 70, 97, 301.*

65. **B.** "Dorsal" means in the back of an organ or the body. *Taber's, p. 570.*

66. **B.** Myxedema. *Taber's, p. 1268.*

67. **C.** Contraindication. *Frew, Lane, Frew, p. 554.*

68. **A.** Goiter. *Taber's, p. 816.*

69. **A.** Pharynx. *Taber's, pp. 1490.*

70. **E.** The central nervous system controls the functions associated with the special senses and the muscular activity of the head and part of the neck. *Gylys & Wedding, p. 318.*

71. **E.** This question is not appropriate because it is a closed-ended question; the patient will answer yes or no. In addition, the medical assistant will not want to suggest to the patient any medical solutions. *Frew, Lane, Frew, p. 58.*

72. **B.** Information regarding the clarity of the maxillary sinuses can be obtained in a dark room by means of a strong light placed inside the mouth with the sinuses being observed through the face. *Frew, Lane, Frew, p. 860.*

73. **D.** The dermis, or true skin, is made up of connective tissue. *Sheldon, p. 3.*

74. **D.** Common cross-infections from normal flora occur in the genitourinary tract. *Tamparo & Lewis, p. 90.*

75. **C.** The central nervous system functions to: mediate mental and behavioral activities, such as learning and language; control skeletal muscular activity; and allow for sensations from the body's sense organs. *Gylys & Wedding, pp. 322–324.*

76. **A.** Herpes zoster, also called shingles, produces inflammation and blistering of the nerve roots and the spinal ganglia. *Tamparo & Lewis, p. 326.*

77. **E.** Typhoid fever (*Salmonella* sp.) and amebic dysentery (*Endamoeba histolytica*) are both spread by fecal contamination of food and water. Typhus and malaria are spread by vectors (insects). *Lane, Keenon, Coleman, pp. 434, 436.*

78. **C.** The sternum is used as an anatomical landmark for cardiopulmonary resuscitation, electrocardiograms, and auscultation of the heart. *Gylys & Wedding, p. 206.*

79. **E.** Smooth muscle is regulated by the autonomic nervous system that supplies the motive power for the various activities of digestion, circulation, secretion, and excretion. *Sheldon, pp. 8, 30.*

80. **C.** Macule. *Tamparo & Lewis, p. 386.*

81. **E.** Varices refers to abnormally dilated and twisted veins, arteries, or lymph vessels. *Tamparo & Lewis, p. 394.*

82. **D.** Cerebrospinal fluid is a protein-free substance that protects the brain and serves to minimize damage from blows to the head and neck. *Sheldon, pp. 546–547.*

83. **B.** Pyelonephritis is the most common type of kidney disease and is far more common in women than in men. *Tamparo & Lewis, p. 85.*

84. **C.** *Monilia* is normally present in small and harmless quantities in the mouth, digestive tract, and vagina, as well as on the skin. It is not present in the urinary tract. *Taber's, p. 301.*

85. **C.** Radiographs are usually taken in the posterior and lateral views. The lateral view is from side to side. *Gylys & Wedding, p. 51.*

86. **B.** The iris is the eye's diaphragm that lies in front of the lens around the pupil. The contraction of the iris results in the constriction of the pupil (miosis). The iris contracts reflexively when light reaches the retina (light reflex) and during focusing on a near object (accommodation reaction). The light refractive apparatus of the eye is composed of the cornea, aqueous humor, the lens, and the vitreous body. *Gylys & Wedding, p. 345.*

87. **E.** The liver functions to synthesize and store glucose, produce (but not store) bile, store vitamins, produce blood proteins, such as prothrombin and fibrinogen, break down toxic substances, and destroy old red blood cells. *Gylys & Wedding, p. 92.*

88. **C.** A simple reflex arc involves two nerves and one synapse. The stimulus sends an impulse along a sensory nerve that is relayed to a motor nerve by synapse. The stimulus is a tap or stretch, and is not painful. This reflex occurs while the brain is just becoming aware of the tap and needs no thought for the motor response. *Gylys & Wedding, pp. 320–322.*

89. **E.** The peritoneal cavity is completely closed in the male; whereas in the female, the uterine tubes open into it. Therefore, air injected into the uterus to test for tubal patency eventually reaches the peritoneal cavity. The peritoneum exudes fluid and cells in the presence of injury or infection and tends to localize or wall off infections. *Sheldon, p. 378.*

90. **B.** Numerous small anatomoses can enlarge considerably during the course of a coronary artery occlusion that develops slowly. In such instances, individuals may later survive complete occlusion of one coronary artery (myocardial infarction), or even both. ***Sheldon, pp. 93–94.***

91. **C.** Even in cases with good results, the patient may sue the physician for trespass or assault and battery if the physician fails to explain the procedure verbally, note in the patient's medical record that the discussion took place and what the patient's decision was, and have the patient sign a consent form. Signed informed consent includes discussion of possible risks and expected results, alternate treatment and their risks, and results if no treatment is given. Informed consent does not guarantee results. ***Lewis & Tamparo, p. 65.***

92. **D.** Corporate physicians have certain increased tax benefits and a decrease in personal liability in case of lawsuit. ***Lewis & Tamparo, p. 20.***

93. **D.** The medical assistant most likely will be charged with a federal crime and privately sued for negligence by the person injured. Liability extends to physicians only when medical assistants act within the scope of their duties or employment and/or commit the act in a physician's presence. ***Lewis & Tamparo, pp. 47, 62.***

94. **C.** According to the AMA's Principles of Medical Ethics, a physician shall obtain consultation and use the talents of other health professionals when indicated. Additionally, a physician shall recognize a responsibility to voluntarily participate in service to the community. The AMA Principles of Medical Ethics state that a physician, except in an emergency, shall be free to choose whom to serve, with whom to associate, and the environment in which to provide medical services. ***Frew, Lane, Frew, p. 42.***

95. **A.** The elements of a tort include a breach of a duty for which the wrongdoer did not use due care and skill based on concepts of legal standards of conduct, and in that failure to use due care, caused damage to another. Torts are classified as either intentional (premeditated) or nonintentional, such as in negligence or strict liability. ***Lewis & Tamparo, p. 64.***

96. **E.** An autistic child is self-absorbed, inaccessible, unable to relate to others, and often mute. The child may play happily alone for hours. There is an obsessive desire to maintain the status quo; the child is extremely sensitive to change and to sensory stimulation. The autistic child is often above-average in intelligence, even gifted. ***Taber's, pp. 175–176.***

97. **C.** Nonverbal communications are delivered by body actions. Verbal communications are delivered by using words in speech or in writing. ***Frew, Lane, Frew, p. 56.***

98. **E.** The symbol "++" can be used to mean trace or notable reaction. ***Lane, Keenon, Coleman (eds.), p. 731.***

99. **B.** An agglutinogen is an antigen that stimulates the body to form agglutinins, which are also called antibodies. Toxins are poisons, pollens, or drugs that are considered antigens if the body reacts to them by producing antibodies, which are also called antitoxins. ***Lane, Medications, pp. 237–239.***

100. **C.** Candidiasis and moniliasis are terms used to refer to a *Monilia* infection. Candidiasis is an infection caused by the fungus, *Candida albicans*, most commonly affecting the skin, the oral mucosa (thrush), and the vagina. *Monilia* is the former name of the genus now called *Candida*. Yeast is the general term for fungi. ***Lane, Medications, p. 286.***

101. **C.** When the medical assistant determines that the patient is ill and needs to be examined on the same day, the appointment is scheduled in the first available block designed for acute illness. ***Frew, Lane, Frew, p. 193.***

102. **A.** ASCII is the acronym for American Standard Code for Information Interchanges and is a generic format that you can use to convert one type of word processing program to another program that accepts ASCII documents. ***Frew, Lane, Frew, p. 221.***

103. **C.** Each floppy disk has a write-protect notch on the right edge. When you cover this notch with an adhesive tab, the disk is protected from accidental erasure or overwriting. If you want to overwrite or otherwise change what is on the disk, first remove the tab, then proceed with your changes. ***Walter, p. 25.***

104. **C.** Default directories and settings are commands the computer program automatically returns to in documents, data bases, and other global (universal) options. ***Gylys, p. 372.***

105. **A.** The overpayment difference must be entered in the balance column as a credit: 0 charge; 178.00 payment; <8.00> balance. This credit balance is money owed to the patient. ***Lane, Keenon, Coleman (eds.), p. 92.***

106. **B.** A W4, the Employee Withholding Allowance Certificate, must be completed at the time of hire. W2 and 1099 forms are tax and wage statements that are given to employees and consultants annually. The 941 and 940 are, respectively, employer quarterly and annual tax returns. ***Lane, Keenon, Coleman (eds.), p. 133.***

107. **D.** When you want to find what percentage, decimal, or fraction one number is of another, you divide the first number by the second: 12/96 = 0.125. Move the decimal point two places to the right to change a decimal to a percentage: 0.125 = 12.5%. ***No reference needed.***

108. **B.** The ordinary method of calculating interest gives each month 30 days and the year 360 days. Principal ($5000) × Rate (13.5% = 0.135) × Time (12/360) = Interest ($22.50). ***Frew, Lane, Frew, p. 234.***

109. **C.** When reconciling the bank account, outstanding checks are deducted from the new bank balance and outstanding deposits are added to the new bank balance. ***Lane, Keenon, Coleman (eds.), p. 106.***

110. **D.** The total income less the total expense equals a $1510.00 net profit for the month. ***Lane, Keenon, Coleman (eds.), pp. 142–144.***

111. **D.** Since an adjustment is actually a subtraction from a charge, enter the charge as it is on your fee schedule, then deduct it as a negative figure enclosed in a circle or parentheses in the charge column with an explanation of the entry. ***Lane, Keenon, Coleman (eds.), p. 90.***

112. **C.** In addition to the judgment for the amount owned, the plaintiff (the physician) may also recover interest and the costs of filing the suit. Damages are not awarded at the small claim level. ***Lane, Keenon, Coleman (eds.), p. 120.***

113. **B.** The proper way to render a check nonnegotiable, write "VOID" across the check, then permanently store for audit purposes. ***Lane, Keenon, Coleman (eds.), p. 101.***

114. **B.** On the accrual basis, income is considered earned when services are rendered; on the cash basis, income is considered earned when payment is received. ***Lane, Keenon, Coleman (eds.), p. 124.***

115. **C.** The statement for services rendered should be mailed to the estate of the deceased, c/o the spouse or next of kin. If you do not know the name of the executor of the estate, you may request that information from the probate department of the Superior Court of your county or city. ***Frew, Lane, Frew, p. 258.***

116. **A.** The defendant may appeal to have the judgment set aside. The plaintiff may not appeal; the decision of the court is final. Parties to small claims actions may not be represented by the professional legal system. ***Lane, Keenon, Coleman (eds.), p. 119.***

117. **B.** A restrictive endorsement indicates the condition of endorsement and limits the negotiability of the check. ***Frew, Lane, Frew, p. 235.***

118. **C.** Dishonored checks may be returned to a depositor with a bank notice indicating the funds were nonsufficient to cover the check. ***Frew, Lane, Frew, pp. 240–241.***

119. **B.** Bankruptcy claims are handled by immediately ceasing all attempts to collect the account and completing a special form (obtainable from any stationery store) and sending the completed form to the referee of the bankruptcy case. ***Frew, Lane, Frew, p. 258.***

120. **C.** If a contact must be made at the patient's place of business, do not reveal to a third party the reason of the contact. The patient's privacy and reputation must be protected. ***Lane, Keenon, Coleman (eds.), p. 118.***

121. C. A physician must file a doctor's first report of occupational injury within 72 hours of the patient's initial visit. *Frew, Lane, Frew, p. 299.*

122. A. Without a prior authorization form (DD1251), CHAMPUS does not cover well-baby care and routine immunizations. A family deductible is $100; if CHAMPUS does cover the procedure, it would pay 80% of the allowable charge less a $50 deductible or, in other words still zero. *Frew, Lane, Frew, pp. 294–296.*

123. D. A patient may seek care from his or her own attending physician, but the medical assistant must establish a separate chart and ledger card to limit release of information to the case at hand, in case the records are required by the courts for the settlement of a claim. *Frew, Lane, Frew, p. 297.*

124. C. In the ICD-9-CM coding system, special "NEC" (not elsewhere classifiable) codes have been designated for reporting unlisted procedures. *Lane, Keenon, Coleman (eds.), p. 195.*

125. A. A copayment is the patient's portion of a service fee. This amount could be as low as $2 to $3 per visit or up to 20% of the total cost. *Frew, Lane, Frew, p. 286.*

126. D. Volume 2 of the ICD coding system lists diagnoses in an alphabetic sequence, using standard nomenclature. *Lane, Keenon, Coleman (eds.), p. 190.*

127. A. Bill Medicare first; the additional carrier is considered secondary. *Frew, Lane, Frew, p. 290.*

128. C. Workers' compensation covers medical expenses and partial income benefits for workers who are injured on the job or who become ill as a direct result of the job. *Frew, Lane, Frew, p. 297.*

129. D. If the physician "accepts assignment," then a claim is submitted directly to the insurance carrier. The patient is billed for 20% of the *allowable* charges. Although the physician will not receive less money than the 80% of the allowable charge, he or she may receive less than the actual charge and have to write off the difference. *Lane, Keenon, Coleman (eds.), p. 170.*

130. D. Never bill one fee to the insurance carrier and another to the patient. Always bill the physician's usual, customary, and reasonable fee, less any amounts already paid by the patient or another carrier. Attaching operative reports will secure better payment for the patient. Listing all preoperative and postoperative care may result in higher payment. *Lane, Keenon, Coleman (eds.), p. 181.*

131. E. To be considered for payment, Medicare claims must be filed by December 31 of the year after the year in which the services were rendered. *Lane, Keenon, Coleman (eds.), p. 179.*

132. D. IPAs and IPPs are based on the traditional fee-for-service concept, except when an insurer contracts with a group of physicians who agree on a predetermined list of charges for all services. The insurance company then pays that rate. The other selections are alternative prepayment plans and not based on reasonable, actual costs. *Frew, Lane, Frew, p. 301.*

133. A. A Form XIX-TPD-1-76 is the assignment authorization form. *Lane, Keenon, Coleman (eds.), p. 176.*

134. D. A denied Medicare or Medicaid charge can be reconsidered only within 6 months after denial. *Lane, Keenon, Coleman (eds.), p. 183.*

135. D. Jehovah's Witnesses will refuse blood transfusions based on religious grounds. *Lewis & Tamparo, p. 100.*

136. D. Discussion of a medical case is unethical if it involves the names of the patients, and it may result in court action for slander. Restrict discussion to general medical issues. *Lewis & Tamparo, pp. 65–66.*

137. C. TIA, transient ischemic attack. *Lane, Keenon, Coleman (eds.), p. 698.*

138. A. CHF, congestive heart failure. *Lane, Keenon, Coleman (eds.), p. 696.*

139. A. All files are first grouped together by the last two digits, then by their middle digits, and finally by the first two digits; so that 87 34 23 precedes 88 34 23. *Lane, Keenon, Coleman (eds.), p. 21.*

140. **D.** Para is used with numerals to designate the number of pregnancies that have resulted in the birth of viable offspring. *Lane, Keenon, Coleman (eds.), p. 467.*

141. **E.** Information on new purchases should be filed under "Purchases." After equipment is purchased, maintenance agreements and contracts are filed under "Maintenance and Repairs" or "Contracts." *Frew, Lane, Frew, pp. 100–101.*

142. **D.** The numbers are filed backward in groups from right to left, instead of from left to right. *Lane, Keenon, Coleman (eds.), p. 21.*

143. **D.** The medical history, as it is related by the patient, is subjective in nature. As the physician observes the patient during an examination, it is objective in nature. *Frew, Lane, Frew, p. 323.*

144. **D.** A tickler file is a card file system by day and month. The other selections are uses of the system. *Frew, Lane, Frew, p. 113.*

145. **E.** I&D—incision and drainage, or incision and debridement. *Lane, Keenon, Coleman (eds.), p. 697.*

146. **E.** United States government and foreign government names are indexed and subdivided by department, bureau, division, commission, and board. File this material: United States Government Health & Human Services Department Centers for Disease Control. If, however, the practice involves only limited contact with an organization, institution, agency or bureau, it may be best to use the descriptive method of indexing, which could likely be CDC rather than US Government. *Frew, Lane, Frew, pp. 110–111.*

147. **E.** Records subpoenaed may be released without the patient's consent. *Lewis & Tamparo, p. 64.*

148. **C.** Physicians who regularly engage in dispensing narcotic drugs are required by the DEA to keep dispensing and inventory records. A prescribed narcotic, to be filled by the pharmacist, is recorded only on the patient medical record. *Lewis & Tamparo, pp. 70–71.*

149. **E.** A few bacteria may be found in normal urine, but concentrations of bacteria greater than occasional or few indicate urinary tract infection. *Wedding and Toenjes, p. 119.*

150. **B.** UTI is urinary tract infection. *Lane, Keenon, Coleman (eds.), p. 698.*

151. **E.** Consulting physicians should always be transferred to the physician. The medical assistant takes personal call messages (unless otherwise directed) and calls concerning reports from staff nurses, pharmacy refills, and laboratory results. *Frew, Lane, Frew, p. 166.*

152. **B.** Depending on the situation, either the medical assistant or the physician may return calls concerning normal test results and medication refills. Abnormal test results are always handled by the physician, who will explain the meaning and consequence of the results. *Frew, Lane, Frew, p. 166.*

153. **A.** The medical assistant should record the message and have the physician return the call. The issue is not what type of insurance coverage or billing, but fees and services. Physicians should personally discuss fees and services with their patients. *Frew, Lane, Frew, p. 165.*

154. **E.** If available, ask the physician to listen and interpret for you. This will eliminate having to do the report a second time. If the physician is not available, it is preferred that the medical assistant leave the area blank, then ask the physician to fill in the word(s) on the draft. If you interpret it yourself, use similar reports, or ask another assistant to interpret, you must bring the interpreted area of dictation to the physician's attention for proofreading and confirmation. *Frew, Lane, Frew, p. 146.*

155. **E.** The block letter style is most often used when typing open punctuation correspondence. *Frew, Lane, Frew, p. 125.*

156. **C.** The subject line may be entirely capitalized and not underlined, or the first letters of the key words in the subject line may be capitalized and every word underlined. The subject line is positioned two lines beneath the salutation and should not be confused with the reference line or the attention line, each of which is positioned above the salutation. *Frew, Lane, Frew, p. 129.*

157. **B.** Microfilming reduces the space necessary for file storage. It is an added expense when used in conjunction with other systems. It is not practical for active patient records; it does not reduce time searching for files; it may increase time for those not accustomed to its use; and files may be lost or misfiled in the microfilming process, making some files almost impossible to find in the future. *Lane, Keenon, Coleman (eds.), pp. 23–24.*

158. **C.** Politely neutral complimentary closes include Sincerely or Cordially. *Frew, Lane, Frew, p. 129.*

159. **D.** Answering the phone must always begin with the name of the office, a courteous greeting of some design, then gathering at least the patient's name and phone number before placing the patient on hold. Then the patient should be given the choice to hold or call back. If the patient is disconnected, your information will enable you immediately to reach the patient, especially in cases of emergency. The reason for the call can be delayed until you return to the line unless, of course, the patient immediately states that there is an emergency. *Frew, Lane, Frew, p. 178.*

160. **E.** The system is indirect and requires extensive indexing, but once the system is mastered, fewer errors occur than in alphabetic filing and physical control over the system is easier. The other four selections are correct statements concerning numeric filing. *Frew, Lane, Frew, p. 106.*

161. **B.** Patient records are admissible in a court of law. Records are used for research purposes; reviewed for evaluating the quality of care; and often used for teaching and informational purposes for office staff and students. *Lewis & Tamparo, p. 112.*

162. **C.** The salutation may not be included, depending on the letter style chosen and the nature of the letter itself. *Lane, Keenon, Coleman (eds.), p. 39.*

163. **D.** Invasion of privacy is not the taking of a photograph of a patient but the unauthorized publicity of patient information, released without the patient's knowledge or permission. Photographs may be taken without written permission, if the photographs are used only by the physician for purposes of treatment progress. If photographs are to be published, however, permission must be obtained at least before the photographs are made public. *Frew, Lane, Frew, p. 32.*

164. **B.** The written permission must be signed by the patient's guardian. *Lewis & Tamparo, pp. 98–99.*

165. **C.** Storage options include disk drives that preserve data on floppy or hard disk media. *Gylys, p. 9.*

166. **C.** A macro is a programmed sequence of keystrokes assigned to a single key or to certain key combinations that allow you to go through a sequence of multiple commands with one command stroke, such as ALT-A or CONTROL-F8. *Walter, p. 136.*

167. **A.** The standard character that stands for a grouping of material to be retrieved is the asterisk. *Walter, p. 82.*

168. **C.** Creating a new document, rather than overwriting a retrieved document, can be accomplished with "Saving" the document with a new name or new extension or by pathing it to a separate directory. You cannot "Copy" a document until you have first saved it. *Walter, p. 126.*

169. **B.** C:\> copy template.ltr a:. *Walter, p. 89.*

170. **C.** Passport applications are available from post offices, passport offices (in larger US cities), or from travel agents. *Frew, Lane, Frew, p. 151.*

171. **C.** The theft of controlled substances is immediately reported to the DEA and the local law. *Lewis & Tamparo, p. 71.*

172. **D.** Social security taxes and federal income tax withheld are deposited monthly. Federal unemployment tax is deposited quarterly. *Lane, Keenon, Coleman (eds.), p. 152.*

173. **D.** A refund for a patient overpayment is a credit adjustment. Correcting a charge by increasing it and reentering a patient charge after a returned check are debit adjustments. *Lane, Keenon, Coleman (eds.), p. 91.*

174. **E.** The pegboard system provides the patient with a total of the office visit, as well as a total statement of account and the notation of a next appointment. The one-write system eliminates unnecessary duplication of clerical work known as posting and therefore minimizes the possibility of clerical errors. *Frew, Lane, Frew, p. 251.*

175. **A.** The physician is considered an employee if the practice is a corporation or a health maintenance organization. *Lewis & Tamparo, p. 23.*

176. **C.** The preprinted "MICR" number includes the ABA bank number, the account number, and the check number. Although the bank may imprint the check amount at the bottom of the check with magnetic ink at the time of deposit, amounts, of course, cannot be printed on the checks at the time checks are ordered. *Lane, Keenon, Coleman (eds.), p. 98.*

177. **A.** A credit balance occurs when a patient has paid in advance or has overpaid for a service. A professional discount and an insurance disallowance are examples of credit adjustments. *Frew, Lane, Frew, p. 254.*

178. **C.** The superbill is a one-write charge slip, patient statement, and insurance form. *Frew, Lane, Frew, p. 251.*

179. **E.** Outstanding checks are deducted from the bank balance; outstanding deposits, added to the bank balance. Bank charges and automatic drafts must be deducted from your checkbook, and deposits not in the register are added to bring it in balance with the bank statement. *Lane, Keenon, Coleman (eds.), p. 107.*

180. **D.** Property taxes, interest paid out on a mortgage or home equity loan, and contributions qualify as personal deductions in computing personal income tax. Malpractice insurance is a business expense and is deductible when determining the taxable net income of the practice. *Lane, Keenon, Coleman (eds.), pp. 138–139.*

181. **D.** Care is covered without prior authorization in the case of an emergency, if the patient lives more than 40 miles from the military facility, or if the care needed is not available at the military facility. With prior authorization, a patient may elect to use a civilian hospital, even in nonemergency situations and when the patient lives near the military facility. *Frew, Lane, Frew, pp. 294–295.*

182. **D.** BC/BS service plans are fee-for-service plans. Patients are responsible for any copayment and deductible amount required by their certificate of membership. The member physician receives payment directly from BS and agrees in advance to accept payment from BS as payment in full. *Gylys, p. 201.*

183. **A.** Medical insurance companies are not billed for workers' compensation coverage. *Frew, Lane, Frew, p. 297.*

184. **C.** Medicare is billed as a primary payer when the patient's only other coverage is a Medigap plan. *Gylys, p. 210; Frew, Lane, Frew, p. 290.*

185. **A.** Recurrent otitis is common in children under 6 years of age. Malnutrition, poor growth pattern, poor hygiene, gross dental problems, and unattended medical needs may indicate neglect and/or abuse. *Tamparo & Lewis, p. 349; Lewis & Tamparo, p. 89.*

186. **E.** Important information includes: is the child okay; what was taken; how much was taken; when was the poison ingested; and the age and weight of the child. Whether or not treatment is necessary, and where, should be the decision of either the physician or poison control. *Frew, Lane, Frew, p. 682.*

187. **D.** There are too many different symptoms to match to colors without a cross-reference. Color-coding is intended for faster recognition of items. *Lane, Keenon, Coleman, p. 19.*

188. **B.** The patient owns the medical information; the physician owns the physical record. Omissions are as important in litigation as what is included in a medical record. The courts consider procedures omitted from the medical record not performed and what is written on the medical record as being done. *Lewis & Tamparo, p. 111.*

189. **C.** Assessment includes the physician's evaluation based on subjective and objective data which includes items in the family history that may impact on the patient's health. *Lewis & Tamparo, pp. 109–110.*

190. **B.** As a legal document that may be presented in a court of law as evidence, the record must be legible, complete, written in ink, and contain no erasures. Corrections are made by crossing a single line through material, writing in the correction, then initialing the correction. Each entry must be signed. Entries may be written in long hand. *Frew, Lane, Frew, pp. 87–88.*

191. **A.** Although the experience can be frightening, nosebleeds rarely cause severe blood loss. The medical assistant should arrange for emergency transportation to a hospital if the patient has severe chest pain, whether or not there is shortness of breath or nausea, severe difficulty breathing, loss of consciousness, severe vomiting and diarrhea, hemorrhage, and high fever, either in adults or in children. *Frew, Lane, Frew, pp. 165, 674.*

192. **D.** Always put through calls regarding emergencies and illness progress reports and treatments to the physician, as well as the physician's professional associates. For calls from the patient's family, the medical assistant takes the message. The medical assistant or the physician may then return the call. *Frew, Lane, Frew, pp. 166–167.*

193. **B.** A second sheet should be more than two lines in length and begin with the addressee's name, the date of the correspondence, and the page number. The heading for a continuation sheet should be seven lines from the top edge of the paper. *Frew, Lane, Frew, pp. 130–131.*

194. **E.** Special mailing notations, on-arrival notations, and the attention line are always typed flush left. An account or policy number, if needed, is blocked with the date, one line above or below it. A subject line may be typed in all capitals two lines below the salutation and is typically centered on the page. *Lane, Keenon, Coleman, p. 38.*

195. **D.** Paragraphs are not indented in the modified block style but are indented in the modified semiblock style. For both styles, the date line and the signature block are the same. *Frew, Lane, Frew, pp. 128–129.*

196. **A.** A certification of eligibility verifies that a patient is a policy holder entitled to benefits and what type of plan the patient has. *Frew, Lane, Frew, p. 892.*

197. **C.** The HCFA-1500 claim form will allow for submission of up to four codes. *Lane, Keenon, Coleman (eds.), p. 196.*

198. **A.** Database programs use their own extensions for their internal filing systems. Be sure not to use your own extensions with purchased database programs. *Walter, p. 80.*

199. **D.** A truth-in-lending form is required by law anytime a patient payment schedule equals four or more payments. *Gylys, pp. 104–105.*

200. **C.** This form is not needed if the patient charges are not financed and the patient pays for the services in less than four payments. If, with or without a down payment, four or more payments are required, a truth-in-lending form must be completed, whether or not interest is charged. *Gylys, pp. 104–105.*

201. **C.** Although it is true that chemical solutions taste bad, it is for safety reasons that thermometers must be rinsed and dried before human use, because chemical disinfectants are irritating to the oral mucosa. *Frew, Lane, Frew, p. 599.*

202. **B.** Histamine secretion triggers the secretion of gastric acid. Tagamet is a histamine receptor blocking agent, which inhibits the release of gastric acid. *Lane, Medications, p. 292.*

203. **B.** Tenormin is used to treat hypertension. Amoxil is an antibiotic; Lanoxin, a cardiac glycoside used to treat disorders of heartbeat and to strengthen heart contraction; Prozac, an antidepressant; Zantac, an ulcer medication. *Lane, Medications, p. 292.*

204. **C.** V_4 is placed at the fifth intercostal space at the junction of the left midclavicular line. *Lane, Keenon, Coleman (eds.), p. 500.*

205. **A.** The horizontal axis of the ECG measures time; the vertical axis, voltage. *Lane, Keenon, Coleman (eds.), p. 502.*

206. **D.** Multichannel instruments record 12 leads simultaneously, using 10 sensors. *Lane, Keenon, Coleman (eds.), p. 500.*

207. **B.** AC artifact voltage is generally consistent, whereas muscular artifact voltage is generally erratic. Improper sensor application is usually distinguished by wandering, drifting, or instability of the tracing. Broken or loose lead wires usually cause a breaking up along the complexes. *Frew, Lane, Frew, pp. 843–844.*

208. **E.** Repolarization refers to the electrical recovery of the heart, when the cells recharge themselves. Polarization refers to the heart at rest; depolarization is the term for the discharge of electrical energy; and the time interval between atrial and ventricular contractions is the P-R segment and is part of the depolarization process. *Lane, Keenon, Coleman (eds.), p. 501.*

209. **C.** If cramping occurs, the patient is assisted out of the lithotomy position. The patient can be assisted in treating the cramping by pressing down on the knee cap while pushing up on the ball of the foot. Any position should be modified to alleviate patient discomfort or to accommodate a weakened or painful body part. *Frew, Lane, Frew, p. 390.*

210. **A.** The patient lying on her back with knees flexed and feet on the table is in the dorsal recumbent position. *Frew, Lane, Frew, p. 388.*

211. **B.** Both local and systemic anaphylaxis may quickly progress to respiratory swelling, bronchospasm, and laryngeal edema. If not reversed, the patient will die of respiratory failure. Another less common series of events is vascular collapse resulting from a shift in body fluid and manifested by hypotension, decreasing levels of consciousness, blurred vision, tachycardia, and diminished production of urine. *Lane, Medications, p. 236.*

212. **A.** In a "multidraw," the red stoppered tubes contain no additives and must be filled first. *Wedding & Toenjes, p. 143.*

213. **E.** In cases of acetaminophen (such as Tylenol) vomiting may be induced. *Frew, Lane, Frew, p. 683.*

214. **D.** Cardiac compressions should be 80 to 120 per minute. *Frew, Lane, Frew, p. 700.*

215. **D.** Vitamin K would decrease the time required for blood to clot. The function of vitamin K is prothrombin formation and maintenance of normal blood coagulation. Coumarin and heparin are anticoagulants, and will increase the time required for blood to clot. Fibrinolysin and streptokinase are thrombolytic agents, used to dissolve or split up a thrombus (clot). *Lane, Keenon, Coleman (eds.), p. 754.*

216. **E.** All cells within the squares are counted. Only cells touching top and left boundary lines are counted. *Lane, Keenon, Coleman (eds.), p. 587.*

217. **A.** To locate the site, place the palm of the hand on the greater trochanter of the femur, then put the index finger on the anterior iliac spine and spread the middle finger over to the crest of the ilium. The center of the triangle formed by the index and middle fingers forms the site for the injection. *Lane, Medications, p. 206.*

218. **B.** Pointing the toes inward helps relax the muscles of the buttock and makes the injection less painful. *Lane, Medications, p. 208.*

219. **C.** Once the original label of a medication becomes illegible, the entire container and its contents must be destroyed. *Lane, Medications, p. 101.*

220. **D.** In the absence of U-100 insulin syringe, the Tuberculin syringe is the only syringe that should be used to measure 20 units of U-100 insulin. *Lane, Medications, pp. 248–249.*

221. **E.** In the obese adult patient, a 2.5-inch needle will be most likely necessary to reach the proper depth of the muscle. *Lane, Medications, pp. 133, 202.*

222. **A.** If the muscular area of an injection site is small, bunch the muscle in your hand to create more room for the needle. *Lane, Medications, p. 209.*

223. **C.** Blood collected in tubes without anticoagulants must rest in a vertical position for 20–30 minutes before centrifuging and be centrifuged within 1 hour. *Wedding & Toenjes, p. 150.*

224. **E.** As a general rule, not more than 5 mL is given in a single injection. If more drug must be injected, more than one site is recommended. *Lane, Medications, p. 202.*

225. **E.** Because of the large surface area and rich vascular supply of the lungs, inhaled drugs are of the fastest absorbed, usually within minutes. Intramuscular drugs may be absorbed within 20–30 minutes or may be absorbed over long periods, depending on the type of solution. Oral drugs must be absorbed in the stomach or small intestine and then pass through the liver before reaching systemic circulation. Transdermal patches are used for prolonged release because the drugs are slowly absorbed over a period of time. *Lane, Medications, p. 189.*

226. **C.** To maintain the correct vacuum in the vial, you must replace any liquid withdrawn with an equal amount of air. *Lane, Medications, p. 208.*

227. **B.** Regular insulin is fast-acting. The onset is usually within 30–60 minutes and reaches its peak effect in 2–5 hours. Its duration of action is usually 6–8 hours. More frequent injections are required than for the longer acting insulins. *Lane, Medications, p. 249.*

228. **A.** 70% is to 90% alcohol as x is to 1 gal; 70/90 = x/128 oz (1 gal); 90x = 70 × 128 = 8960; x = 8960/90 = 99.555 oz (round this off to 100 oz of alcohol). To prepare 1 gal of 70% alcohol, then, you would add 100 oz of alcohol and 28 oz of (diluent) water. *Lane, Medications, p. 171.*

229. **E.** Sodium bicarbonate is a systemic antacid, which neutralizes HCl and provides temporary relief of peptic ulcer pain or indigestion within a short duration. Because of its high sodium content, patients should be discouraged from using it. It may cause "acid rebound"—increased acid secretion by the stomach; and because it is readily absorbed into the bloodstream, it may cause systemic alkalosis. *Lane, Medications, p. 43.*

230. **D.** Angioedema, temporary edema of blood vessels and hives, is treated with cold application. *Lane, Medications, p. 235.*

231. **C.** A low-sodium diet is prescribed because the patient with hypertension has a tendency to retain sodium and fluids. *Frew, Lane, Frew, p. 534.*

232. **A.** Studies have shown a relationship between the incidence of herpes genitalis and the incidence of cervical cancer. *Lane, Keenon, Coleman (eds.), p. 447.*

233. **B.** A grade II report represents atypical cytology but no evidence of cancer. *Gylys & Wedding, p. 384.*

234. **E.** Instructions include administering after a bowel movement and cautioning the patient to remain lying for 20–30 minutes to prevent accidental evacuation. *Lane, Medications, pp. 194–195.*

235. **B.** A vaginal applicator should be inserted by tilting it downward and backward, toward the base of the patient's spine. *Lane, Medications, p. 194.*

236. **C.** The best time to examine the breasts is a little more than 1 week after the menstruation period, when breasts are usually not tender or swollen. Some masses may be palpated at this time that may be obscured during other times in the cycle. *Frew, Lane, Frew, p. 486.*

237. **A.** The No. 3 handle with a No. 11 or 15 blade is the most commonly used scalpel in the medical office. It is used for an I&D. *Frew, Lane, Frew, p. 640.*

238. **C.** The Allis tissue forceps is a ring-handled instrument with ratchets and delicate intermeshing teeth at the tip. *Lane, Keenon, Coleman (eds.), p. 384.*

239. **B.** HCG is produced by the placenta and is present in the blood stream 8–10 days after fertilization and in the urine 10–14 days after the first missed period. Immunologic tests detect the presence of HCG in blood and urine based on the fact that HCG is an antigen, and it can be detected by serum containing antibodies specific for this antigen. Although the corpus luteum continues to secrete progesterone for about 3 months, it is the HCG hormone that indicates a pregnancy. *Wedding & Toenjes, pp. 317–318.*

240. **E.** Measles (rubeola). *Frew, Lane, Frew, p. 498.*

241. **A.** Elevation of a part helps to increase circulation and reduce edema to the part. Bandaging and immobilization prevents separation of wound edges. Elevation of a part is not a treatment for external wound drainage, with or without a drain. *Frew, Lane, Frew, p. 453.*

242. **B.** The primary purpose of the surgical drape is to protect the incisional site from bacteria on the unprepped patient skin surfaces. It limits both pathogenic and nonpathogenic organisms around the surgical site. *Frew, Lane, Frew, p. 636.*

243. **E.** The medical assistant will teach the patient to measure urine glucose levels and calculate food exchanges values, if he is to monitor his own disease. Insulin is treatment not monitoring, and not a part of this patient's therapy. *Frew, Lane, Frew, pp. 536–538, 817–819.*

244. **A.** Diluted acetic acid added to urine sediment will dissolve the red blood cells but leave the yeast intact. *Wedding & Toenjes, p. 117.*

245. **D.** The microscopic examination of urine begins with locating casts under the low-power objective. *Wedding & Toenjes, p. 127.*

246. **D.** The report of "moderate" is used to describe urinary sediment elements. *Wedding & Toenjes, p. 119.*

247. **B.** Multiple specimens may be taken with one venipuncture and without loss of blood by releasing the tourniquet while the first tube is filling, and switching tubes while the needle remains in the vein. *Wedding & Toenjes, pp. 147, 152.*

248. **B.** The red stopper contains no additives and is used for serum determinations in chemistry, serology, and blood banking. It requires no inversion at collection time. *Frew, Lane, Frew, p. 723.*

249. **D.** The finger is warmed to increase blood flow. The other selections may either cause hemolysis or not be effective at all. *Wedding & Toenjes, p. 204.*

250. **E.** Blood must be anticoagulated. Venous blood may be anticoagulated in an EDTA Vacutainer tube. Blood from a skin puncture must be anticoagulated by heparin in the microhemotocrit capillary tube. *Lane, Keenon, Coleman (eds.), p. 578.*

251. **A.** The Vacutainer choice for a CBC and differential would be a lavender-top. *Frew, Lane, Frew, p. 724.*

252. **C.** The liquid portion on top of cells in the lavender-stopper Vacutainer tube is plasma; the liquid portion on top of cells in the red-stopper Vacutainer tube is serum. *Frew, Lane, Frew, pp. 723–724.*

253. **E.** Sudden dizziness caused by the decrease of blood flow to the brain upon sudden standing from a reclining position is called orthostatic hypotension. *Frew, Lane, Frew, p. 357.*

254. **C.** There are usually four to five heartbeats to every respiration. *Frew, Lane, Frew, p. 354.*

255. **D.** Auscultatory gaps (phase II sound disappearance) occur particularly in patients with hypertension and heart disease. In children, after exercise, and in the anemic pregnant patient, phase IV sounds may be affected by continuing to zero. *Frew, Lane, Frew, p. 359.*

256. **D.** The "fading sound" is the change from the sharp, tapping sound of phase III to the sounds of phase IV, when there is a softer tapping, which becomes muffled and begins to grow fainter. *Frew, Lane, Frew, p. 359.*

257. **C.** Before determining a patient's blood pressure by the auscultatory method, determine the maximum inflation by palpating the radial artery, inflating the cuff until the artery feels obliterated, and then mentally adding 30 mm to the reading at obliteration. Next, deflate the cuff and wait at least 1 minute before reinflation. Reinflate to the mental number and begin the auscultatory determination. *Lane, Keenon, Coleman (eds.), p. 318.*

258. **E.** Darvocet-N is not known to increase bleeding and prothrombin times. Motrin, aspirin, and Indocin may increase the effects of anticoagulants and limit platelet function, leading to bleeding tendencies. When Tylenol is used with anticoagulants, anticoagulants must be reduced to avoid possible hemorrhage. *Lane, Medications, pp. 242–244, 279.*

259. **D.** The rescuer's elbows should be extended during cardiac compressions to apply pressure straight down to depress the sternum. *Frew, Lane, Frew, p. 700.*

260. **C.** Common untoward reactions include fainting, anaphylaxis, flushing, and dizziness. *Lane, Medications, p. 205.*

261. **A.** Narcotic analgesics pass the placental barrier and depress the respiration of the newborn. *Lane, Medications, p. 242.*

262. **A.** Antacids are an important part of ulcer treatment. Antacids containing magnesium have a laxative effect; those containing aluminum or calcium, a constipating effect. Liquids act as a vehicle transporting the antacid to the stomach. Magnesium salts inhibit tetracyclines. *Lane, Medications, p. 83.*

263. **D.** Narcotic analgesics decrease the capacity of the patient to respond to stress. *Lane, Medications, pp. 241–242.*

264. **E.** RBCs are pale and nongranular, and contain no nuclei. *Frew, Lane, Frew, p. 765.*

265. **B.** Crystals are reported out using the system of none, occasional, few, moderate, many. *Wedding & Toenjes, p. 119.*

266. **E.** Although phenylketonuria is a congenitally caused protein deficiency, the disease is not detectable by testing for protein in the urine. A special screening test with Phenistix is necessary to detect the presence of phenylketones in the urine. *Frew, Lane, Frew, pp. 763, 761.*

267. **C.** Push the top of the stopper until it meets the guide line then leave it there. The tube stopper will retract below the guide line with the full point of the needle embedded in the stopper. Pushing the stopper in further will result in either blood leakage once the vein is found or in premature loss of vacuum. *Frew, Lane, Frew, p. 727f.*

268. **C.** A 9-cm (3.5-inch) cuff is a pediatric cuff and should not be used with adult patients. *Frew, Lane, Frew, p. 359.*

269. **A.** The upper left large corner section is used for the first white blood cell counting area. *Lane, Keenon, Coleman (eds.), p. 587.*

270. **D.** The middle black square is the fifth red blood cell counting area. *Lane, Keenon, Coleman (eds.), p. 587.*

271. **B.** An oral carbohydrate drink is given after the fasting blood and urine measurements. After the drink, blood and urine are first collected at the 0.5-hour interval. *Wedding & Toenjes, p. 176.*

272. **A.** For an oral glucose tolerance test, blood and urine are first measured with the patient in a fasting state. *Wedding & Toenjes, p. 176.*

273. **D.** Two hours after receiving the loading dose of carbohydrate, the blood sugar should be within normal limits. *Lane, Keenon, Coleman (eds.), p. 606.*

274. **D.** The ring finger is the most common site for adult capillary puncture. *Wedding & Toenjes, p. 202.*

275. **B.** The lateral heel is the most common site for pediatric capillary puncture on a non-walking infant. *Lane, Keenon, Coleman (eds.), p. 534.*

276. **C.** During invasive procedures that may splash or soil clothing, gowns, aprons, or laboratory coats should be worn. *Frew, Lane, Frew, pp. 750–751.*

277. **D.** Although new CDC Universal Blood and Body-Fluid Precautions recommend wearing nonsterile gloves in any situation the medical assistant may come in contact with the patient's blood or body fluids, sterile gloves should be worn when surgical asepsis is important. *Frew, Lane, Frew, p. 345.*

278. **A.** QAC disinfectants are bactericidal and effective against fungi and pseudomonas. They are not considered a sterilant or effective against the tubercle bacillus, hydrophilic viruses, or spores. They are not for skin antiseptic use. They are inactivated in the presence of blood, serum, mucus, or soap. *Frew, Lane, Frew, p. 600.*

279. **B.** The patient must fast for four hours before a computerized tomography of the head and chest. *Frew, Lane, Frew, p. 862.*

280. **A.** The gastrografin preparation designed to outline the intestines and colon is NOT meant to produce a laxative effect and should not provide any discomfort. *Frew, Lane, Frew, p. 862.*

281. **E.** The ECG activity "picture" from lead II is in the direction of the right arm to the left leg. *Frew, Lane, Frew, p. 843.*

282. **E.** A catheter is a tube through which air can be blown, an obstruction can be cleared, or the patency of a canal can be tested. *Frew, Lane, Frew, p. 607.*

283. **C.** The otoscope is used to examine the nasal passages. The physician uses an ophthalmoscope to examine the retina, which contains the macula lutea (the yellowish irregular depression of the retina), the central fovea (the small pit in the center of the macula lutea), the optic disc, and the vessels of the eyeball. *Frew, Lane, Frew, pp. 403–405.*

284. **A.** Do NOT induce vomiting if the poison is a petroleum product. Vomiting may cause inhaled fumes or aspiration of the substance into the lungs, which would cause chemical pneumonia. *Frew, Lane, Frew, pp. 682, 687; Lane, Keenon, Coleman (eds.), p. 741.*

285. **D.** Ipecac works both locally and systemically. In adults, ipecac should be followed by 200–300 mL of water. *Lane, Medications, pp. 257–258.*

286. **C.** In hyperthyroidism, calcium blood levels will be increased. *Lane, Keenon, Coleman (eds.), pp. 598–600.*

287. **A.** ⅛ gr = 8 mg
$$\frac{6 \text{ mg}}{8 \text{ mg}} = \frac{x}{1 \text{ mL}}$$
$$8x = 6$$
$$x = \frac{6}{8} = 0.75 \text{ mL}$$

Lane, Medications, pp. 160–161.

288. **D.** The needle should be injected and removed quickly, with one single motion. Medication should be injected slowly so as not to damage tissues, and should be deposited in one place—the place where you have aspirated before injecting and determined that the needle is not in a blood vessel. *Lane, Medications, p. 209.*

289. **E.** A patient who previously had anaphylactic reactions to eggs may suffer an immediate anaphylactoid reaction. Patients who have egg allergies not characterized by anaphylactic-type reactions do not appear to be at increased risk. *Lane, Medications, p. 262.*

290. **A.** The neurologic examination includes the simplex reflex arc (e.g., knee jerk), passive stretching of long muscles to test stretch reflexes, nociceptive reflexes (e.g., gag reflexes), and certain conditioned reflexes (learned), such as walking. *Frew, Lane, Frew, pp. 416–417.*

291. **D.** If the patient has had vaginal packing inserted, she may remove the packing after 6–8 hours. Because of the possibility of infection, the patient should not douche, use tampons, or have sexual intercourse for about 1 week. Antibiotics are not indicated. *Lane, Keenon, Coleman (eds.), p. 456.*

292. **B.** The patient should not eat red meat before or during the test and should withhold only medications containing iron, iodines, salicylates, steroids, and ascorbic acid. *Lane, Keenon, Coleman (eds.), pp. 630–631.*

293. **A.** White blood cells in the presence of nitrite in a fresh sample supports the diagnosis of UTI. Squamous epithelial cells present in large numbers usually indicate vaginal contamination in the female patient. *Wedding & Toenjes, p. 116.*

294. **E.** Casts almost always indicate damage to the kidney. WBCs, yeast, and mucous threads without any additional findings usually indicate contamination with vaginal contents during collection of the specimen. Heavy bacterial concentrations in the absence of white blood cells usually indicate the specimen has been allowed to sit at room temperature too long before testing. *Frew, Lane, Frew, pp. 765–767.*

295. **D.** Tests involving any anticoagulant are based on a certain ratio of anticoagulant to blood volume. If an inadequate volume is drawn, this ratio will be affected and result in inaccurate results. *Frew, Lane, Frew, p. 742.*

296. **D.** Hemoconcentration results from a slowed blood flow. Hemolysis of the cells will occur from using too small a lumen to draw blood; removing the tube before it is full, which results in air rushing in; and shaking rather than gently inverting the specimen. Although a prolonged tourniquet application may result in hemoconcentration, it will not hemolyze the cells. *Frew, Lane, Frew, pp. 741–743.*

297. **E.** A wide differential between the systolic and diastolic pressures usually occurs in disease and trauma of the neurological system, especially the brain (such as shock or CVA), or in diseases of the arteries (such as arteriosclerosis and atherosclerosis). *Frew, Lane, Frew, p. 357.*

298. **E.** Patients should remain under observation for 20–30 minutes. Keep the drug under refrigeration until just before use. Before injecting, roll the syringe in your hands to warm, then roll in your palms to entirely mix just before injection. If you do not intend to use all of a prepackaged medication, eject the amount not to be used before administration. Inject deep IM. *Lane, Medications, p. 256.*

299. **B.** This medication is irritating to the skin and should be injected deeply. Do not massage long-acting penicillins after injection. This medication is thick and tends to clump on standing. After expelling part of the medication, do not let the drug remain in the needle for long. The preferred infant site for deep intramuscular injections is the vastus lateralis. *Lane, Medications, pp. 209, 256.*

300. **C.** Penicillins are potent sensitizing agents, and it is estimated that 15% of the American population is presently allergic to penicillin. Hypersensitivity reactions are reported to be on the increase in pediatric practice, and include rashes and anaphylaxis. Digestive and vaginal superinfections may occur with the use of penicillin, but these new infections are not immediate. *Lane, Medications, pp. 245, 256.*

APPENDIX A $\quad$ *Reference and Study Aid Listing*

1. American Medical Association: Physician's Current Procedural Terminology. AMA, Chicago, 1994.

2. Davis, Carol M: Patient Practitioner Interaction: An Experimental Manual for Developing the Art of Health Care, 2nd ed. Slack, Thorofare, NJ, 1994.

3. Fordney, Marilyn Takahashi, and Diehl, Marcy Otis: Medical Transcription Guide Do's and Don'ts. WB Saunders, Philadelphia, 1990.

4. Frew, Mary Ann, Lane, Karen, and Frew, David R: Comprehensive Medical Assisting: Competencies for Administrative and Clinical Practice, 3rd ed. FA Davis, Philadelphia, 1995.

5. Gylys, Barbara, A: Medical Terminology Simplified: A Programmed Learning Approach by Body Systems. FA Davis, Philadelphia, 1993.

6. Gylys, Barbara A: Computer Applications for the Medical Office: Medical Care Basic Management System. FA Davis, Philadelphia, 1991.

7. Gylys, Barbara A, and Wedding, Mary Ellen. Medical Terminology: A Systems Approach, 3rd ed. FA Davis, Philadelphia, 1995.

8. Haverty, John R (ed): Webster's Medical Secretaries Handbook. Springfield, Massachusetts, Merriam-Webster, 1979.

9. Lane, Karen: Medications: A Guide for the Health Professions. FA Davis, Philadelphia, 1992.

10. Lane, Karen, Keenon, Jean, and Coleman, Crystal (eds): The Saunders Manual of Medical Assisting Practice. WB Saunders, Philadelphia, 1994.

11. Lewis, Marcia A, and Tamparo, Carol D: Medical Law, Ethics, and Bioethics in the Medical Office, 3rd ed. FA Davis, Philadelphia, 1993.

12. Scanlon, Valerie C., Sanders, Tina: Essentials of Anatomy and Physiology, 2nd ed. FA Davis, Philadelphia, 1995.

13. Sheldon, Huntington: Boyd's Introduction to the Study of Disease, 11th ed. Lea and Febiger, Philadelphia, 1992.

14. Strunk, William, Jr, and White, EB: The Elements of Style, 3rd ed. Macmillan, New York, 1979.

15. Tamparo, Carol, and Lewis, Marcia A: Diseases of the Human Body, 2nd ed. FA Davis, Philadelphia, 1995.

16. Thomas, Clayton L (ed): Taber's Cyclopedic Medical Dictionary, 17th ed. FA Davis, Philadelphia, 1993.

17. U.S. Department of Labor; Occupational Safety and Health Administration: OSHA Hazard Communication Rule (29 CFR 1910.1200). OSHA Publications, Washington, DC, 1987.

18. U.S. Department of Labor/Department of Health and Human Services: Joint Advisory Notice—Protection Against Occupational Exposure to Hepatitis B Virus and Human Deficiency Virus (HIV). OSHA Publications, Washington, DC, 1987.

19. Walter, Russ: The Secret Guide to Computers, 16th ed. Russ Walter, Publisher, Somerville, MA,1992.

20. Wedding, Mary Ellen, and Toenjes, Sally A: Medical Laboratory Procedures. FA Davis, Philadelphia, 1992.

CMA Application Sample

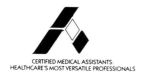

CERTIFIED MEDICAL ASSISTANTS:
HEALTHCARE'S MOST VERSATILE PROFESSIONALS

```
┌────────────────────────────────────┐
│        FOR OFFICE USE ONLY          │
│  Date Received _____    │
│  Fee Received _____    │
│  Date Guide Sent _____    │
└────────────────────────────────────┘
```

Application
for the Certification Examination Conducted by
the Certifying Board of the
American Association of Medical Assistants, Inc.
DO NOT USE THIS FORM TO APPLY FOR THE RECERTIFICATION EXAMINATION

Complete this form using BLACK INK. Both sides of this form must be completed.

All applicants must submit: (1) A completed form; (2) all verification required on the form; and (3) appropriate fee by certified check or money order, made payable to the AAMA Certification Fund, or complete credit card information in full.

PLEASE REFER TO PAMPHLET "INSTRUCTIONS FOR COMPLETION OF APPLICATION" BEFORE PREPARING THIS APPLICATION FORM. DIRECT QUESTIONS TO THE AAMA CHICAGO OFFICE.

1. SOCIAL SECURITY NUMBER: [ ][ ][ ]—[ ][ ]—[ ][ ][ ][ ]   2. DATE OF BIRTH: [ ][ ][ ]
                                                                         Month   Day   Year

3. NAME: [ ][ ][ ]... [ ][ ][ ]... [ ]
        Last   First   Middle initial

   Previous last name: [ ][ ][ ]...
                     Last

4. ADDRESS to be used for communications from AAMA about this application:
   [ ][ ][ ]...
   Number and Street
   [ ][ ][ ]... [ ][ ][ ]...
   City and State or Province   Zip Code

5. TELEPHONE NUMBERS: Day [ ][ ][ ]—[ ][ ][ ]—[ ][ ][ ][ ]   Eve [ ][ ][ ]—[ ][ ][ ]—[ ][ ][ ][ ]
                                 Area Code   Area Code

6. EXAMINATION LOCATION (refer to list of examination locations and make three selections): Do not list any unrealistic alternatives.

   First Choice
   Second Choice
   Third Choice
       Center Code No.   City   State

7. STATUS (previous examination experience):

   ☐ New applicant   ☐ Repeating applicant (indicate past exam experience below)

8. EXAMINATION CYCLE (indicate administration desired):

   ☐ Summer examination (last Friday in June) ☐ Winter examination (last Friday in January)

9. FEES (circle appropriate fee and enclose certified check or money order with application):

	Student (CAHEA)	AAMA Member	Nonmember
Examination			
Certification	current fee	current fee	current fee

   All examination fees include a nonrefundable $25 administrative fee.

10. AAMA MEMBERSHIP:

   ☐ AAMA member, _____   ☐ Not a member of AAMA
                              Chapter

Visa _____ MasterCard _____
(check one)

Expiration Date _____

Credit Card # _____

Interbank #(4 digits above name) __ __ __ __

Signature _____

11. ELIGIBILITY STATUS. Complete one section only (I, II or III) and enclose any requested documentation.

☐ I. Student or Recent Graduate in CAHEA-Accredited Program. Student or recent graduate applications must be signed by the medical assisting program director to verify enrollment and anticipated graduation date or prior graduation date. *If the student fails to graduate by the required date, the examination will be considered invalid, no scores will be released, and no refund of fees will be made.* Applicants completing this section are eligible for student rates.

☐☐☐☐ School code (obtain from program director)

School _____ Address _____

City _____ State _____ Zip Code _____

I verify that this student is enrolled in the medical assisting program at the school noted above. I further verify that the entire course, including externship, will be completed by, and that the student will graduate by: _____/_____/_____
                  mo. day yr.

_____   _____
Print name of program director   Signature of program director

II. Practicing Medical Assistant/Allied Health Practitioner (see *note below)

☐   A. Graduate of a CAHEA-accredited program. Enclose verification of graduation.

     School _____ Address _____

     City _____ State _____ Zip Code _____

     Graduation date _____ ☐☐☐☐ School code (obtain from program director)

     Name, if different at time of graduation _____

☐   B. Graduate of other formal non-CAHEA medical assisting program with a minimum of 12 months full-time or 24 months part-time work experience. A list of the names, addresses and telephone numbers of your employers, length of service and dates of employment *must* be attached to the application. A list or resume is adequate. We do *NOT* require letter(s) or signature(s) of employers. You must answer the question below.

☐   C. Graduate of other allied health profession program with a minimum of 12 months full-time or 24 months part-time work experience. A list of the names, addresses and telephone numbers of your employers, length of service and dates of employment *must* be attached to the application. A list or resume is adequate. We do *NOT* require letter(s) or signature(s) of employers. You must answer the question below.

☐   D. On-the-job trained with a minimum of 12 months full-time or 24 months part-time work experience. A list of the names, addresses and telephone numbers of your employers, length of service and dates of employment *must* be attached to the application. A list or resume is adequate. We do *NOT* require letter(s) or signature(s) of employers. You must answer the question below.

☐ III. Medical Assisting Instructor. Verification of teaching position must be attached.

     School _____ Address _____

     City _____ State _____ Zip Code _____

*NOTE: ALL CANDIDATES IN CATEGORY II *MUST* ANSWER THE FOLLOWING QUESTION:

How would you describe your work experience?

a. less than 1 year

b. 1-3 years (at least 1 but less than 3)

c. 3-5 years (at least 3 but less than 5)

d. more than 5 years

12. AFFIDAVIT (all applicants must sign):

I hereby certify that I have not served as a proctor or assistant proctor for a certification examination nor served on an AAMA/NBME Test Construction Task Force within the last 23 months. I certify that the information supplied in this application is true and accurate to the best of my knowledge. I acknowledge that the AAMA may refuse to accept this application, may decline to permit me to take the examination, or may invalidate my scores on this examination if it receives evidence satisfactory to AAMA that the statements I have made are not true and accurate.

I also acknowledge that I have read and I understand the eligibility requirements and fees and refund policy, as stated in the "Instructions for Completion of Application." I understand that the information on this form and the examination results may be used for statistical and research purposes, and that access thereto will be under the direction of the Certifying Board of the American Association of Medical Assistants, Inc.

Signature _____ Date _____
                                   Month/Day/Year

Have You:

☐ Enclosed payment   ☐ Signed Affidavit

☐ Completed <u>all</u> items   ☐ Retained copies

☐ Double-checked test center choices

Eligibility Requirements

Eligibility for the certification examination conducted by the AAMA requires any *one* of the following:

A. STUDENT IN OR RECENT GRADUATE FROM CAHEA ACCREDITED PROGRAM. Formal training in a medical assisting program accredited by the Committee on Allied Health Education and Accreditation.

Students must have completed their formal training, including externship, by the end of the month in which they wish to be examined (January 31 for the Winter cycle, and June 30 for the Summer examination.) Recent graduates must have graduated no more than 11 months before the date of the examination.

Student applications must be signed by the Program Director to verify enrollment and anticipated completion date.

If the student applicant fails to graduate by the required date, the examination will be considered invalid, no scores will be released, and no refund of fees will be made.

Applicants qualifying under this eligibility status are eligible for student rates.

B. GRADUATE OF A CAHEA ACCREDITED PROGRAM. Individuals who hold an associate degree, certificate or diploma from a medical assisting program accredited by the Committee on Allied Health Education and Accreditation are eligible to sit for the basic certification examination, even if they have no work experience. If the program was not accredited at the time of graduation, but was accredited within one year of the gradu-

ation date, candidates may apply under this eligibility status. Questions on this should be directed to the AAMA Chicago Office. **Verification of graduation must accompany application.**

C. MEDICAL ASSISTING INSTRUCTOR. Individuals qualifying under this eligibility status must be instructors in post-secondary institutions that are approved by a nationally-recognized accrediting agency. Candidates must provide the name and address of the institution in which they are teaching and submit documentation of their current teaching position with the application form.

D. EXPERIENCED MEDICAL ASSISTANT/EXPERIENCED ALLIED HEALTH PROFESSIONAL. To qualify on the basis of employment experience, applicants must have completed at least 12 months of full-time or 24 months of part-time employment at the time of application for the examination.

Medical assisting or allied health work experience must have been under the supervision of a *licensed health care practitioner*. The name and address of each employer, length of service, and dates of employment must be included in the application.

You are not eligible to take the certification examination if you have served as a proctor or assistant proctor for the Certification Examination or have served on an AAMA/NBME Test Construction Task Force within the 23 months preceding the administration for which you are applying.

Candidate's Guide

A guide for the certification examination has been developed by the AAMA Certifying Board to help you prepare for the examination. It provides explanations of how to approach the types of questions used on the examination, and tips on how to study for the content that will be tested.

A sample 120-question examination is also provided. Questions

on this examination are drawn from the item pool used for actual examinations, and should help you evaluate your knowledge of the categories and content tested on the examination.

The *Candidate's Guide* will be forwarded to you upon receipt of a completed examination application and examination fee. Please allow four weeks for delivery.

- -

Order Form*

Please send: _____ AAMA membership information

I am planning to apply for the examination in:
_____ January   _____ June

Name _____

Address _____

City _____ State _____ Zip _____

☐ AAMA member, _____ Chapter.

☐ Not a member of AAMA.

Social Security Number _____

*Please retain a copy of the reverse side of this page.

Content of the Certification Examination

The Certification Examination is designed to identify a medical assistant who has the knowledge and skills to perform competently the routine* clinical and administrative duties in the office of a primary care physician. An individual who is able to successfully demonstrate competence will be designated as a Certified Medical Assistant.

I. **General**
   A. Medical Terminology
   B. Anatomy and Physiology
   C. Behavioral Science
   D. Mediocolegal Issues and Ethics
II. **Basic Administrative Procedures**
   A. Oral communication

B. Written communication
C. Bookkeeping, credits and collections
D. Records management
E. Office facilities
F. Patient insurance
G. Nonpatient insurance

III. **Perform Clinical Duties**
   A. Examination room techniques
   B. Laboratory procedures
   C. Administer specified medications
   D. Emergencies

Routine refers to duties that are frequent, important and/or critical. (Definitions adopted by the AAMA Certifying Board in March 1978.)

How to Complete the Application Form

The following instructions correspond to those items on the Application that may cause processing problems if they are not completed correctly. Please read carefully. Both the ACKNOWLEDGEMENT CARD and the APPLICATION FORM must be completed entirely. We suggest you keep a copy of everything you submit.

Acknowledgement Card. Do not remove the card from the application form. Print your name and address on the reverse side of the card, as directed.

Application Form. Type or print all requested data; sign and date form.

3. NAME. Print your last name, first name and middle initial, one letter to a box, in the spaces provided. Give your name in exactly this way on all correspondence with the Certifying Board.

4. ADDRESS TO BE USED FOR ALL COMMUNICATIONS FROM THE CERTIFYING BOARD. Your admission card will be sent to this address approximately two weeks prior to the examination. Enter your address, printing only one number or letter in each box. Be sure to enter your zip code.

6. EXAMINATION LOCATIONS. Refer to the examination center code list on the last page of this flyer. Some centers are not available for all examinations.

   Enter your center selection, with second and third choices to be used in the event space is not available in your first choice, or in the event that a test center may not be available for a given examination. **Do not list second or third choices to which you could not travel.**

   Center changes will be made, if space is available, in response to *written* requests providing that the request is *received at least eight weeks in advance of the examination,* and is accompanied by a certified check or money order for the $25 test center change fee.

   The Certifying Board reserves the right to close a test center if the number of examinees requesting it does not reach the required minimum, or if circumstances arise which, in the judgment of the Board, indicate that administration of the test at that center would jeopardize the security of the examination material or the integrity of scores derived from the examination.

9. FEES. Indicate the amount enclosed (your certified check or money order must cover the full cost of the examination) by circling the appropriate fee. Keep your receipt for the certified check or money order.

10. AAMA MEMBERSHIP. Membership in AAMA is not required for certification.

11. ELIGIBILITY STATUS. Complete only one section concerning eligibility — I, II or III. If you complete section II, you must answer questions concerning your work experience and other education you may have.

   I. STUDENT OR RECENT GRADUATE IN CAHEA-ACCREDITED PROGRAM. The Program Director must provide the school code, indicate the graduation date of recent graduates or the date a current student is expected to graduate, and sign the form.

   II. PRACTICING MEDICAL ASSISTANT/PRACTICING ALLIED HEALTH PROFESSIONAL

      A. GRADUATE OF A CAHEA-ACCREDITED PROGRAM. Complete as requested, and enclose with the application verification of graduation signed by a school official or a photostatic copy of a diploma, certificate or transcript which shows the date of graduation. Student rate does not apply.

         If you do not know the school code, check with the Medical Assisting Program Director.

      B. GRADUATE OF OTHER FORMAL NON-CAHEA MEDICAL ASSISTING PROGRAM WITH A MINIMUM OF 12 MONTHS OF FULL-TIME OR 24 MONTHS OF PART-TIME WORK EXPERIENCE. Attach employment history and answer question.

      C. GRADUATE OF OTHER ALLIED HEALTH PROFESSION PROGRAM WITH A MINIMUM OF 12 MONTHS OF FULL-TIME OR 24 MONTHS OF PART-TIME WORK EXPERIENCE. Attach employment history and answer question.

      D. ON-THE-JOB TRAINED FOR A MINIMUM OF 12 MONTHS OF FULL-TIME OR 24 MONTHS OF PART-TIME WORK EXPERIENCE. Attach employment history and answer question.

   III. MEDICAL ASSISTING INSTRUCTOR. Complete as requested and attach verification.

12. SIGNATURE AND DATE. Read the affidavit carefully before signing.

13. Provided your application is in order, your admission card informing you exactly where to report will be sent to you approximately two weeks before the examination. It is the candidate's responsibility to call the Certifying Board if the admission card is not received or if the card shows any errors.

Address all correspondence about cancellation, test center changes or address changes to:

AAMA Certifying Board
20 North Wacker Drive, Suite 1575
Chicago, IL 60606   312/899-1500

Score Report

A report of scores achieved and certification status (pass/fail) will be mailed approximately twelve weeks after the examination date.

Candidates who pass the certification examination will receive the credential Certified Medical Assistant (CMA).

Examination Locations

Select your examination location from this list and record the appropriate numeric code in section 6 on your application. "S" designates a summer location. "W" designates a winter location. "S/W" designates a summer and winter location. Please make your selections according to your examination cycle choice. Please transfer the code numbers with care since you will be registered by test center number. It is each candidate's responsibility to list realistic alternatives and transfer the code numbers accurately.

ALABAMA
S/W   0101   Birmingham
S   0102   Decatur
W   0103   Enterprise
S   0104   Mobile

ALASKA
S/W   0201   Anchorage
S/W   0202   Fairbanks

ARIZONA
S   0301   Phoenix
W   0302   Tucson
W   0303   Prescott

ARKANSAS
S/W   0401   Russellville
S/W   0402   Little Rock

CALIFORNIA
S/W   0501   Los Angeles Area
S/W   0502   San Diego
S/W   0503   Sacramento
S/W   0504   San Francisco Bay Area
S   0505   Redding
S   0506   Bakersfield
W   0507   San Bernardino
S/W   0508   Fresno
S/W   0526   San Jose

COLORADO
S/W   0701   Denver

CONNECTICUT
S/W   0802   Hartford
S/W   0801   Norwich

DELAWARE
S/W   0901   Wilmington

FLORIDA
S/W   1101   Ft. Lauderdale
S/W   1102   Jacksonville
S/W   1103   Winter Park
S/W   1104   Sarasota
S   1105   Panama City

GEORGIA
S/W   1201   Atlanta
S/W   1202   Augusta
W   1203   Rome
S   1204   Columbus
S   1205   Albany
W   1206   Valdosta
S/W   1207   Savannah

HAWAII
S/W   1401   Honolulu

IDAHO
S/W   1301   Boise

ILLINOIS
S/W   1602   Chicago Area
W   1604   Danville
S/W   1605   River Grove
S/W   1606   Bloomington

INDIANA
S   1701   Ft. Wayne/Muncie
S/W   1702   Indianapolis
W   1703   Lafayette
W   1704   South Bend
W   1705   Terre Haute
W   1706   Evansville

IOWA
W   1801   Cedar Rapids
W   1802   Ft. Dodge
S/W   1803   Ankeny
W   1804   W. Burlington

KANSAS
S   1901   Wichita
W   1902   Topeka

KENTUCKY
S/W   2001   Louisville
W   2002   Lexington
S/W   2003   Richmond
S   2004   Morehead
S   2005   Paducah

LOUISIANA
S/W   2101   Baton Rouge
S   2102   New Orleans
W   2103   Shreveport

MAINE
S/W   2201   Portland
S/W   2202   Bangor

MARYLAND
S/W   2301   Baltimore

MASSACHUSETTS
W   2401   Long Meadow
S/W   2402   Springfield
S/W   2403   Boston Area

MICHIGAN
S/W   2500   Dearborn Heights
W   2501   Troy
S   2502   Kalamazoo
W   2503   Flint
S   2504   Traverse City

MINNESOTA
S/W   2601   Minneapolis
S/W   2604   E. Grand Forks
S/W   2605   Rochester

MISSISSIPPI
S   2701   Jackson
W   2702   Booneville

MISSOURI
S   2801   Kansas City
S/W   2802   St. Louis

MONTANA
W   2901   Helena
S/W   2902   Bozeman
S/W   2903   Billings

NEBRASKA
S/W   3001   Omaha Area
S/W   3002   Lincoln

NEVADA
S/W   3201   Las Vegas

**N E W
HAMPSHIRE**
S/W   3101   Claremont

**N E W
JERSEY**
S   3301   East Brunswick
S/W   3302   Jersey City
S/W   3303   Paramus

NEW MEXICO
W   3401   Albuquerque
S/W   3402   Roswell

NEW YORK
S/W   3501   Binghamton
S/W   3502   Syracuse
S   3503   Albany
S/W   3504   Buffalo
W   3505   Garden City
W   3506   Rochester
S   3507   Hauppauge

NORTH CAROLINA
S/W   3601   Charlotte
S/W   3602   Greenville
S/W   3603   Fayetteville
S   3604   Jamestown

NORTH DAKOTA
S/W   3701   Bismarck

OHIO
S/W   3801   Cincinnati
S/W   3802   Cleveland
S   3803   Dayton
S   3804   Nelsonville
S/W   3806   Toledo
S   3807   Canton

OKLAHOMA
S   3901   Norman
S/W   3902   Tulsa

OREGON
S/W   4001   Portland
W   4002   Eugene

PENNSYLVANIA
S/W   4101   Philadelphia
S/W   4102   Pittsburgh
S/W   4103   Summerdale
S   4108   Schnecksville

RHODE ISLAND
S/W   4201   Warwick

SOUTH CAROLINA
S/W   4503   Charleston
S/W   4504   Georgetown

SOUTH DAKOTA
S/W   4601   Rapid City

TENNESSEE
S   4701   Nashville
S/W   4702   Jackson
S/W   4703   Johnson City

TEXAS
S/W   4801   Dallas
S   4802   Bryan
S   4803   San Antonio
W   4804   Abilene
W   4805   Beaumont
S/W   4806   Corpus Christi
S/W   4807   El Paso
S   4808   Lubbock
W   4809   Odessa
W   4812   Waco
S   4813   Edinburg
S/W   4814   Houston Area

UTAH
S/W   4901   Salt Lake City

VERMONT
S/W   5002   Burlington

VIRGINIA
S/W   5101   Richmond
W   5102   Danville
S/W   5104   Virginia Beach

WASHINGTON
S/W   5401   Seattle
S/W   5402   Spokane

WISCONSIN
W   5601   Milwaukee
S/W   5602   Green Bay
S   5603   LaCrosse
S/W   5605   Madison
W   5607   Marshfield
S   5609   Racine

A minimum of ten (10) candidates is required to activate a location.

If a center is closed or at capacity, candidates will be assigned to their next available choice.

DO NOT LIST TEST CENTERS TO WHICH YOU WOULD NOT TRAVEL SHOULD YOUR FIRST CHOICE BE UNAVAILABLE.

AMERICAN MEDICAL TECHNOLOGISTS

710 Higgins Road

Park Ridge, Illinois 60068-5765

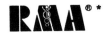

APPLICATION FOR CERTIFICATION
AS A
REGISTERED MEDICAL ASSISTANT — RMA(AMT)*

(Print or type)

Last name	First name	Middle initial

Permanent or mailing address

City	State	Zip + 4

IMPORTANT NOTICE TO APPLICANT

Read requirements for certification and follow instructions printed on page 2 of this application before completing.

Qualified applicants are considered for certification without regard to race, color, religion, sex, national origin, age, marital status, medical condition or handicap.

To help us comply with Federal/State equal opportunity record keeping, reporting, and other legal requirements, please answer all questions.

Do not write in space below

Date Application Received _____   Date Completed _____/_____/_____ Approved by _____

Application rejected by _____ Reason _____ Date Notified _____/_____/_____

Exam Date	Test Series	Exam ID	Exam Site/Proctor	Exam Score (or DNT)	Fee Paid
____/____/____					
____/____/____					
____/____/____					

Birthdate _____   GRANTED: Certificate # _____

Soc. Sec.# _____   Issue Date _____/_____/_____

*Registered Service Mark in the U.S. Patent and Trademark Office

MEDICAL ASSISTANT

A medical assistant is an integral member of the health care delivery team, qualified by education and experience to work in the administrative office, the examining room and the physician's office laboratory. The medical assistant, also a liaison between doctor and patient, is of vital importance to the success of the medical practice.

REQUIREMENTS FOR CERTIFICATION AS A
REGISTERED MEDICAL ASSISTANT — RMA(AMT)

1. **Applicant shall be of good moral character.**

2. **Applicant shall be a graduate of an accredited high school or acceptable equivalent.**

3. **Applicant must meet one of the following requirements** *(check one box only):*

   A. **Applicant shall be a graduate of a**

   ☐ _____ **1) medical assistant program or institution accredited by the Accrediting Bureau of Health Education School (ABHES).**

   ☐ _____ **2) medical assistant program accredited by a Regional Accrediting Commission.**

   ☐ _____ **3) formal medical services training program of the United States Armed Forces.**

   ☐ B. **Applicant shall have been employed in the profession of Medical Assisting for a minimum of five (5) years, no more than two (2) years of which may have been as an instructor in a postsecondary medical assistant program.**

   ☐ C. **The AMT Board of Directors has further determined that an applicant may qualify for certification on the basis of having completed a medical assistant course in a school holding national accreditation recognized by the Council on Postsecondary Accreditation (COPA) and acceptable to the AMT Board of Directors, and, in addition, shall have been employed as a medical assistant for a minimum of one (1) year.***

   *This requirement of an additional year employment does **not** apply to ABHES graduates. See 3.A.1) above.

4. **All applicants *must* take and pass the AMT certification examination for Registered Medical Assistant (RMA.)**

SPECIAL INSTRUCTIONS TO APPLICANT

1. Please type or print all information **except** where signatures are required.

2. Please check the Requirement above under which you are applying.

3. Before submitting this application, make sure you have provided the following:

   _____ $59.00 application fee
   _____ Proof of high school graduation or equivalent
   _____ Official final transcript stating graduation from medical assistant school, college or training program (with school seal affixed or notarized)
   _____ All solid line areas completed by applicant
   _____ Relevant dotted line areas completed by designated person
   _____ Complete names and addresses of employers for experience verification
   _____ Application signed and dated by applicant on back page

4. You will be notified upon approval of this application and informed of examination schedules. (ABHES students/graduates to be included in an examination administered at their school will receive confirmation of scheduling from the school.)

5. An applicant who does not appear at his/her scheduled examination will be assessed a $10.00 fee for subsequent rescheduling.

6. **Applicant must present photo identification at time of testing.**

PART I.
PERSONAL INFORMATION

Full Name_____Social Security Number_____

Street Address _____ City _____ State _____ Zip + 4 _____

Daytime Phone Number ( )_____ Date of Birth _____
                              Area

Maiden and/or any former names_____

Name and address of nearest relative (do not list spouse) _____

Marital Status: Single ☐ Married ☐ Divorced ☐ Widowed ☐	Sex: Female ☐ Male ☐

Race/Ethnic Group: White ☐   Black ☐   Hispanic ☐   American Indian/Alaskan Native ☐   Asian/Pacific Islander ☐

Are you a Veteran? Yes ☐ No ☐	Vietnam Era? Yes ☐ No ☐	Are you a disabled Veteran? Yes ☐ No ☐

Have you ever been convicted of a felony? Yes ☐   No ☐   If yes, when, what felony, and what court?_____

PERSONAL REFERENCES (Other than relatives)

	Name	Street Address	City and State	Zip
(1)				
(2)				
(3)				

PART II.
MEDICAL ASSISTANT EMPLOYMENT

Employer Name	Street Address	City/State/Zip	Dates of Employment (month and year)

Please indicate if any of the above employment was as a medical assisting instructor.

PART III.
EDUCATION AND TRAINING

A. SECONDARY
Proof of high school graduation or equivalent must be enclosed.

SENIOR
HIGH
SCHOOL:

Name/Complete Address	Dates Attended	Graduation Date

G.E.D.:

Date of Certificate/City/State

B. COLLEGE OR UNIVERSITY

Name/Complete Address	Dates Attended	Hours Completed	Degree Awarded

PART III.   EDUCATION AND TRAINING (continued)

C. MEDICAL ASSISTANT TRAINING

This section must be completed by a proper school or training program official to verify training in medical assisting and graduation from a course wherein the curriculum is acceptable to this organization. The applicant's final transcript must also be provided.

Applicant Name . . . .

School/Program Name . . . .

School/Program Address . . . .

Course Dates: From . . . ./. . . . ./. . . . .   To . . . ./. . . . ./. . . . .

I hereby certify that the applicant named above did (or will) satisfactorily complete the entire prescribed medical assisting course and is recommended as a qualified candidate for certification as a Registered Medical Assistant of American Medical Technologists.

Date . . . .   School Official's Signature . . . .

Title/Position . . . .

PART IV.   RECOMMENDATION FOR CERTIFICATION

In order for this application to be processed, it must be signed by either a physician or an AMT member in good standing. (This section does **not** apply to ABHES graduates.)

☐ Physician   Signature . . . .

☐ AMT Member   Address . . . .

(If member) AMT Registry # . . . .

PART V.   OPTIONAL SCORE RELEASE

Some educational institutions request their graduates' examination results. To grant permission for your results to be eligible for release if requested, sign the release authorization below. Signing this release is VOLUNTARY, and will not affect the outcome of your examination in any way. If you do NOT want your results released, DO NOT sign the authorization.

I hereby authorize American Medical Technologists to release my examination results to:

_____   _____
Name of School   Address

_____
City   State   Zip

_____
Signature of Examinee

PART VI.   AGREEMENT

I consent to give AMT the authority to request the necessary information from individuals, institutions, and/or organizations named herein in order to validate credentials for certification.

I certify that the statements made herein are true and correct, to my knowledge and belief, and realize that certification is subject to revocation for misrepresentation. If accepted as a certificant, I agree to uphold and abide by the Standards of Practice and Bylaws of the AMERICAN MEDICAL TECHNOLOGISTS.

ENCLOSED HEREWITH IS MY APPLICATION FEE OF FIFTY-NINE DOLLARS ($59.00). *

Date _____ Applicant's Signature _____

*NOT REFUNDABLE. Applicant may take the examination two times within two years on this application. A retesting fee of $30.00 will be required for a second administration. If applicant fails the second administration, he/she must file a new application with a new fee of $59.00 and proof of further education and/or training to be tested a third time. Applicant may take the examination two more times within two years on the second application. A retesting fee of $30.00 will be required for a fourth administration. The applicant will not be considered for certification by AMT if he/she fails the examination the fourth time. If applicant fails to honor any application within two years of submitting, a new application must be filed.

Make all checks or money orders payable to

AMERICAN MEDICAL TECHNOLOGISTS
710 Higgins Road • Park Ridge, Illinois 60068-5765 • Phone: (708) 823-5169

September, 1994

Top 50 Prescription Drugs

Based on National Prescription Audit Plus, IMS America, Ltd.*

1996 Rank	Drug	Company
1	Premarin	Wyeth-Ayerst
2	Trimox	Apothecon
3	Synthroid	Knoll
4	Lanoxin	Allen & Hanburys
5	Zantac	Glaxo
6	Vasotec	Merck & Co.
7	Prozac	Dista
8	Procardia XL	Pratt
9	Hydrocodone/APAP	Watson
10	Coumadin Sodium	Du Pont Pharm
11	Zoloft	Roerig
12	Prilosec	Astra/Merck
13	Norvasc	Pfizer
14	Cardizem CD	Hoechst-Marion-Roussel
15	Albuterol	Warrick
16	Biaxin	Abbott
17	Amoxil	SmithKline Beecham
18	Triamterene/HCTZ	Geneva
19	Zestril	Zeneca
20	Claritin	Schering
21	Zocor	Merck & Co.
22	Furosemide	Mylan
23	Augmentin	SmithKline Beecham
24	Paxil	SmithKline Beecham
25	Cipro	Bayer Pharm
26	Amoxicillin Trihydrate	Biocraft
27	K-Dur	Key Pharm
28	Acetaminophen/Codeine	Lemmon
29	Veetids	Apothecon
30	Dilantin	Parke-Davis
31	Hytrin	Abbott
32	Mevacor	Merck & Co.
33	Ultram	McNeil
34	Propacet 100	Lemmon
35	Propoxyphene N/APAP	Mylan
36	Humulin N	Lilly
37	Proventil Inhaler	Key Pharm
38	Pepcid	Merck & Co.
39	Glucophage	Bristol-Myers Squibb
40	Cephalexin	Biocraft
41	Pravachol	Bristol-Myers Squibb
42	Relafen	SmithKline Beecham
43	Alprazolam	Geneva
44	Prinivil	Merck & Co.
45	Ambien	Searle
46	Atrovent	Boehringer Ingelheim
47	Ortho-Novum 7/7/7-28	Ortho Pharm
48	Prempro	Wyeth-Ayerst
49	Zithromax Z-Pak	Pfizer
50	Levoxyl	Daniels

*Extracted from "Top 200 Drugs of 1996." *Pharmacy Times*, April 1997.

Directions for Marking Answers

- Use a black lead pencil (No. 2 or softer). Do NOT use pen or a pencil with hard lead.
- Make each mark heavy and black enough to completely obliterate the letter within the circle. Marks should fill the circles.
- Erase clearly any answer you wish to change.
- Make no stray marks on this answer sheet.
- Mark one and only one answer for each question. Multiple answers will be counted as wrong.

Example

WRONG Ⓐ Ⓑ Ⓒ Ⓓ Ⓔ
WRONG Ⓐ Ⓑ Ⓒ Ⓓ Ⓔ
WRONG Ⓐ Ⓑ Ⓒ Ⓓ Ⓔ
RIGHT Ⓐ Ⓑ Ⓒ ● Ⓔ

1 Ⓐ Ⓑ Ⓒ Ⓓ Ⓔ	26 Ⓐ Ⓑ Ⓒ Ⓓ Ⓔ	51 Ⓐ Ⓑ Ⓒ Ⓓ Ⓔ	76 Ⓐ Ⓑ Ⓒ Ⓓ Ⓔ
2 Ⓐ Ⓑ Ⓒ Ⓓ Ⓔ	27 Ⓐ Ⓑ Ⓒ Ⓓ Ⓔ	52 Ⓐ Ⓑ Ⓒ Ⓓ Ⓔ	77 Ⓐ Ⓑ Ⓒ Ⓓ Ⓔ
3 Ⓐ Ⓑ Ⓒ Ⓓ Ⓔ	28 Ⓐ Ⓑ Ⓒ Ⓓ Ⓔ	53 Ⓐ Ⓑ Ⓒ Ⓓ Ⓔ	78 Ⓐ Ⓑ Ⓒ Ⓓ Ⓔ
4 Ⓐ Ⓑ Ⓒ Ⓓ Ⓔ	29 Ⓐ Ⓑ Ⓒ Ⓓ Ⓔ	54 Ⓐ Ⓑ Ⓒ Ⓓ Ⓔ	79 Ⓐ Ⓑ Ⓒ Ⓓ Ⓔ
5 Ⓐ Ⓑ Ⓒ Ⓓ Ⓔ	30 Ⓐ Ⓑ Ⓒ Ⓓ Ⓔ	55 Ⓐ Ⓑ Ⓒ Ⓓ Ⓔ	80 Ⓐ Ⓑ Ⓒ Ⓓ Ⓔ
6 Ⓐ Ⓑ Ⓒ Ⓓ Ⓔ	31 Ⓐ Ⓑ Ⓒ Ⓓ Ⓔ	56 Ⓐ Ⓑ Ⓒ Ⓓ Ⓔ	81 Ⓐ Ⓑ Ⓒ Ⓓ Ⓔ
7 Ⓐ Ⓑ Ⓒ Ⓓ Ⓔ	32 Ⓐ Ⓑ Ⓒ Ⓓ Ⓔ	57 Ⓐ Ⓑ Ⓒ Ⓓ Ⓔ	82 Ⓐ Ⓑ Ⓒ Ⓓ Ⓔ
8 Ⓐ Ⓑ Ⓒ Ⓓ Ⓔ	33 Ⓐ Ⓑ Ⓒ Ⓓ Ⓔ	58 Ⓐ Ⓑ Ⓒ Ⓓ Ⓔ	83 Ⓐ Ⓑ Ⓒ Ⓓ Ⓔ
9 Ⓐ Ⓑ Ⓒ Ⓓ Ⓔ	34 Ⓐ Ⓑ Ⓒ Ⓓ Ⓔ	59 Ⓐ Ⓑ Ⓒ Ⓓ Ⓔ	84 Ⓐ Ⓑ Ⓒ Ⓓ Ⓔ
10 Ⓐ Ⓑ Ⓒ Ⓓ Ⓔ	35 Ⓐ Ⓑ Ⓒ Ⓓ Ⓔ	60 Ⓐ Ⓑ Ⓒ Ⓓ Ⓔ	85 Ⓐ Ⓑ Ⓒ Ⓓ Ⓔ
11 Ⓐ Ⓑ Ⓒ Ⓓ Ⓔ	36 Ⓐ Ⓑ Ⓒ Ⓓ Ⓔ	61 Ⓐ Ⓑ Ⓒ Ⓓ Ⓔ	86 Ⓐ Ⓑ Ⓒ Ⓓ Ⓔ
12 Ⓐ Ⓑ Ⓒ Ⓓ Ⓔ	37 Ⓐ Ⓑ Ⓒ Ⓓ Ⓔ	62 Ⓐ Ⓑ Ⓒ Ⓓ Ⓔ	87 Ⓐ Ⓑ Ⓒ Ⓓ Ⓔ
13 Ⓐ Ⓑ Ⓒ Ⓓ Ⓔ	38 Ⓐ Ⓑ Ⓒ Ⓓ Ⓔ	63 Ⓐ Ⓑ Ⓒ Ⓓ Ⓔ	88 Ⓐ Ⓑ Ⓒ Ⓓ Ⓔ
14 Ⓐ Ⓑ Ⓒ Ⓓ Ⓔ	39 Ⓐ Ⓑ Ⓒ Ⓓ Ⓔ	64 Ⓐ Ⓑ Ⓒ Ⓓ Ⓔ	89 Ⓐ Ⓑ Ⓒ Ⓓ Ⓔ
15 Ⓐ Ⓑ Ⓒ Ⓓ Ⓔ	40 Ⓐ Ⓑ Ⓒ Ⓓ Ⓔ	65 Ⓐ Ⓑ Ⓒ Ⓓ Ⓔ	90 Ⓐ Ⓑ Ⓒ Ⓓ Ⓔ
16 Ⓐ Ⓑ Ⓒ Ⓓ Ⓔ	41 Ⓐ Ⓑ Ⓒ Ⓓ Ⓔ	66 Ⓐ Ⓑ Ⓒ Ⓓ Ⓔ	91 Ⓐ Ⓑ Ⓒ Ⓓ Ⓔ
17 Ⓐ Ⓑ Ⓒ Ⓓ Ⓔ	42 Ⓐ Ⓑ Ⓒ Ⓓ Ⓔ	67 Ⓐ Ⓑ Ⓒ Ⓓ Ⓔ	92 Ⓐ Ⓑ Ⓒ Ⓓ Ⓔ
18 Ⓐ Ⓑ Ⓒ Ⓓ Ⓔ	43 Ⓐ Ⓑ Ⓒ Ⓓ Ⓔ	68 Ⓐ Ⓑ Ⓒ Ⓓ Ⓔ	93 Ⓐ Ⓑ Ⓒ Ⓓ Ⓔ
19 Ⓐ Ⓑ Ⓒ Ⓓ Ⓔ	44 Ⓐ Ⓑ Ⓒ Ⓓ Ⓔ	69 Ⓐ Ⓑ Ⓒ Ⓓ Ⓔ	94 Ⓐ Ⓑ Ⓒ Ⓓ Ⓔ
20 Ⓐ Ⓑ Ⓒ Ⓓ Ⓔ	45 Ⓐ Ⓑ Ⓒ Ⓓ Ⓔ	70 Ⓐ Ⓑ Ⓒ Ⓓ Ⓔ	95 Ⓐ Ⓑ Ⓒ Ⓓ Ⓔ
21 Ⓐ Ⓑ Ⓒ Ⓓ Ⓔ	46 Ⓐ Ⓑ Ⓒ Ⓓ Ⓔ	71 Ⓐ Ⓑ Ⓒ Ⓓ Ⓔ	96 Ⓐ Ⓑ Ⓒ Ⓓ Ⓔ
22 Ⓐ Ⓑ Ⓒ Ⓓ Ⓔ	47 Ⓐ Ⓑ Ⓒ Ⓓ Ⓔ	72 Ⓐ Ⓑ Ⓒ Ⓓ Ⓔ	97 Ⓐ Ⓑ Ⓒ Ⓓ Ⓔ
23 Ⓐ Ⓑ Ⓒ Ⓓ Ⓔ	48 Ⓐ Ⓑ Ⓒ Ⓓ Ⓔ	73 Ⓐ Ⓑ Ⓒ Ⓓ Ⓔ	98 Ⓐ Ⓑ Ⓒ Ⓓ Ⓔ
24 Ⓐ Ⓑ Ⓒ Ⓓ Ⓔ	49 Ⓐ Ⓑ Ⓒ Ⓓ Ⓔ	74 Ⓐ Ⓑ Ⓒ Ⓓ Ⓔ	99 Ⓐ Ⓑ Ⓒ Ⓓ Ⓔ
25 Ⓐ Ⓑ Ⓒ Ⓓ Ⓔ	50 Ⓐ Ⓑ Ⓒ Ⓓ Ⓔ	75 Ⓐ Ⓑ Ⓒ Ⓓ Ⓔ	100 Ⓐ Ⓑ Ⓒ Ⓓ Ⓔ

Name _____ Meg _____ **Date** _____
Last   Test 1   First   Middle

Directions for Marking Answers

- Use a black lead pencil (No. 2 or softer). Do NOT use pen or a pencil with hard lead.
- Make each mark heavy and black enough to completely obliterate the letter within the circle. Marks should fill the circles.
- Erase clearly any answer you wish to change.
- Make no stray marks on this answer sheet.
- Mark one and only one answer for each question. Multiple answers will be counted as wrong.

Example

WRONG   Ⓐ Ⓑ Ⓒ Ⓓ Ⓔ
WRONG   Ⓐ Ⓑ Ⓒ Ⓓ Ⓔ
WRONG   Ⓐ Ⓑ Ⓒ Ⓓ Ⓔ
RIGHT   Ⓐ Ⓑ Ⓒ ● Ⓔ

101 Ⓐ Ⓑ Ⓒ Ⓓ Ⓔ	126 Ⓐ Ⓑ Ⓒ Ⓓ Ⓔ	151 Ⓐ Ⓑ Ⓒ Ⓓ Ⓔ	176 Ⓐ Ⓑ Ⓒ Ⓓ Ⓔ
102 Ⓐ Ⓑ Ⓒ Ⓓ Ⓔ	127 Ⓐ Ⓑ Ⓒ Ⓓ Ⓔ	152 Ⓐ Ⓑ Ⓒ Ⓓ Ⓔ	177 Ⓐ Ⓑ Ⓒ Ⓓ Ⓔ
103 Ⓐ Ⓑ Ⓒ Ⓓ Ⓔ	128 Ⓐ Ⓑ Ⓒ Ⓓ Ⓔ	153 Ⓐ Ⓑ Ⓒ Ⓓ Ⓔ	178 Ⓐ Ⓑ Ⓒ Ⓓ Ⓔ
104 Ⓐ Ⓑ Ⓒ Ⓓ Ⓔ	129 Ⓐ Ⓑ Ⓒ Ⓓ Ⓔ	154 Ⓐ Ⓑ Ⓒ Ⓓ Ⓔ	179 Ⓐ Ⓑ Ⓒ Ⓓ Ⓔ
105 Ⓐ Ⓑ Ⓒ Ⓓ Ⓔ	130 Ⓐ Ⓑ Ⓒ Ⓓ Ⓔ	155 Ⓐ Ⓑ Ⓒ Ⓓ Ⓔ	180 Ⓐ Ⓑ Ⓒ Ⓓ Ⓔ
106 Ⓐ Ⓑ Ⓒ Ⓓ Ⓔ	131 Ⓐ Ⓑ Ⓒ Ⓓ Ⓔ	156 Ⓐ Ⓑ Ⓒ Ⓓ Ⓔ	181 Ⓐ Ⓑ Ⓒ Ⓓ Ⓔ
107 Ⓐ Ⓑ Ⓒ Ⓓ Ⓔ	132 Ⓐ Ⓑ Ⓒ Ⓓ Ⓔ	157 Ⓐ Ⓑ Ⓒ Ⓓ Ⓔ	182 Ⓐ Ⓑ Ⓒ Ⓓ Ⓔ
108 Ⓐ Ⓑ Ⓒ Ⓓ Ⓔ	133 Ⓐ Ⓑ Ⓒ Ⓓ Ⓔ	158 Ⓐ Ⓑ Ⓒ Ⓓ Ⓔ	183 Ⓐ Ⓑ Ⓒ Ⓓ Ⓔ
109 Ⓐ Ⓑ Ⓒ Ⓓ Ⓔ	134 Ⓐ Ⓑ Ⓒ Ⓓ Ⓔ	159 Ⓐ Ⓑ Ⓒ Ⓓ Ⓔ	184 Ⓐ Ⓑ Ⓒ Ⓓ Ⓔ
110 Ⓐ Ⓑ Ⓒ Ⓓ Ⓔ	135 Ⓐ Ⓑ Ⓒ Ⓓ Ⓔ	160 Ⓐ Ⓑ Ⓒ Ⓓ Ⓔ	185 Ⓐ Ⓑ Ⓒ Ⓓ Ⓔ
111 Ⓐ Ⓑ Ⓒ Ⓓ Ⓔ	136 Ⓐ Ⓑ Ⓒ Ⓓ Ⓔ	161 Ⓐ Ⓑ Ⓒ Ⓓ Ⓔ	186 Ⓐ Ⓑ Ⓒ Ⓓ Ⓔ
112 Ⓐ Ⓑ Ⓒ Ⓓ Ⓔ	137 Ⓐ Ⓑ Ⓒ Ⓓ Ⓔ	162 Ⓐ Ⓑ Ⓒ Ⓓ Ⓔ	187 Ⓐ Ⓑ Ⓒ Ⓓ Ⓔ
113 Ⓐ Ⓑ Ⓒ Ⓓ Ⓔ	138 Ⓐ Ⓑ Ⓒ Ⓓ Ⓔ	163 Ⓐ Ⓑ Ⓒ Ⓓ Ⓔ	188 Ⓐ Ⓑ Ⓒ Ⓓ Ⓔ
114 Ⓐ Ⓑ Ⓒ Ⓓ Ⓔ	139 Ⓐ Ⓑ Ⓒ Ⓓ Ⓔ	164 Ⓐ Ⓑ Ⓒ Ⓓ Ⓔ	189 Ⓐ Ⓑ Ⓒ Ⓓ Ⓔ
115 Ⓐ Ⓑ Ⓒ Ⓓ Ⓔ	140 Ⓐ Ⓑ Ⓒ Ⓓ Ⓔ	165 Ⓐ Ⓑ Ⓒ Ⓓ Ⓔ	190 Ⓐ Ⓑ Ⓒ Ⓓ Ⓔ
116 Ⓐ Ⓑ Ⓒ Ⓓ Ⓔ	141 Ⓐ Ⓑ Ⓒ Ⓓ Ⓔ	166 Ⓐ Ⓑ Ⓒ Ⓓ Ⓔ	191 Ⓐ Ⓑ Ⓒ Ⓓ Ⓔ
117 Ⓐ Ⓑ Ⓒ Ⓓ Ⓔ	142 Ⓐ Ⓑ Ⓒ Ⓓ Ⓔ	167 Ⓐ Ⓑ Ⓒ Ⓓ Ⓔ	192 Ⓐ Ⓑ Ⓒ Ⓓ Ⓔ
118 Ⓐ Ⓑ Ⓒ Ⓓ Ⓔ	143 Ⓐ Ⓑ Ⓒ Ⓓ Ⓔ	168 Ⓐ Ⓑ Ⓒ Ⓓ Ⓔ	193 Ⓐ Ⓑ Ⓒ Ⓓ Ⓔ
119 Ⓐ Ⓑ Ⓒ Ⓓ Ⓔ	144 Ⓐ Ⓑ Ⓒ Ⓓ Ⓔ	169 Ⓐ Ⓑ Ⓒ Ⓓ Ⓔ	194 Ⓐ Ⓑ Ⓒ Ⓓ Ⓔ
120 Ⓐ Ⓑ Ⓒ Ⓓ Ⓔ	145 Ⓐ Ⓑ Ⓒ Ⓓ Ⓔ	170 Ⓐ Ⓑ Ⓒ Ⓓ Ⓔ	195 Ⓐ Ⓑ Ⓒ Ⓓ Ⓔ
121 Ⓐ Ⓑ Ⓒ Ⓓ Ⓔ	146 Ⓐ Ⓑ Ⓒ Ⓓ Ⓔ	171 Ⓐ Ⓑ Ⓒ Ⓓ Ⓔ	196 Ⓐ Ⓑ Ⓒ Ⓓ Ⓔ
122 Ⓐ Ⓑ Ⓒ Ⓓ Ⓔ	147 Ⓐ Ⓑ Ⓒ Ⓓ Ⓔ	172 Ⓐ Ⓑ Ⓒ Ⓓ Ⓔ	197 Ⓐ Ⓑ Ⓒ Ⓓ Ⓔ
123 Ⓐ Ⓑ Ⓒ Ⓓ Ⓔ	148 Ⓐ Ⓑ Ⓒ Ⓓ Ⓔ	173 Ⓐ Ⓑ Ⓒ Ⓓ Ⓔ	198 Ⓐ Ⓑ Ⓒ Ⓓ Ⓔ
124 Ⓐ Ⓑ Ⓒ Ⓓ Ⓔ	149 Ⓐ Ⓑ Ⓒ Ⓓ Ⓔ	174 Ⓐ Ⓑ Ⓒ Ⓓ Ⓔ	199 Ⓐ Ⓑ Ⓒ Ⓓ Ⓔ
125 Ⓐ Ⓑ Ⓒ Ⓓ Ⓔ	150 Ⓐ Ⓑ Ⓒ Ⓓ Ⓔ	175 Ⓐ Ⓑ Ⓒ Ⓓ Ⓔ	200 Ⓐ Ⓑ Ⓒ Ⓓ Ⓔ

Name _____ **Date** _____

Last   _Test_ First   Middle

Directions for Marking Answers

Example

- Use a black lead pencil (No. 2 or softer). Do NOT use pen or a pencil with hard lead.
- Make each mark heavy and black enough to completely obliterate the letter within the circle. Marks should fill the circles.
- Erase clearly any answer you wish to change.
- Make no stray marks on this answer sheet.
- Mark one and only one answer for each question. Multiple answers will be counted as wrong.

WRONG   Ⓐ Ⓑ Ⓒ Ⓓ Ⓔ
WRONG   Ⓐ Ⓑ Ⓒ Ⓓ Ⓔ
WRONG   Ⓐ Ⓑ Ⓒ Ⓓ Ⓔ
RIGHT   Ⓐ Ⓑ Ⓒ ● Ⓔ

201 Ⓐ Ⓑ Ⓒ Ⓓ Ⓔ	226 Ⓐ Ⓑ Ⓒ Ⓓ Ⓔ	251 Ⓐ Ⓑ Ⓒ Ⓓ Ⓔ	276 Ⓐ Ⓑ Ⓒ Ⓓ Ⓔ
202 Ⓐ Ⓑ Ⓒ Ⓓ Ⓔ	227 Ⓐ Ⓑ Ⓒ Ⓓ Ⓔ	252 Ⓐ Ⓑ Ⓒ Ⓓ Ⓔ	277 Ⓐ Ⓑ Ⓒ Ⓓ Ⓔ
203 Ⓐ Ⓑ Ⓒ Ⓓ Ⓔ	228 Ⓐ Ⓑ Ⓒ Ⓓ Ⓔ	253 Ⓐ Ⓑ Ⓒ Ⓓ Ⓔ	278 Ⓐ Ⓑ Ⓒ Ⓓ Ⓔ
204 Ⓐ Ⓑ Ⓒ Ⓓ Ⓔ	229 Ⓐ Ⓑ Ⓒ Ⓓ Ⓔ	254 Ⓐ Ⓑ Ⓒ Ⓓ Ⓔ	279 Ⓐ Ⓑ Ⓒ Ⓓ Ⓔ
205 Ⓐ Ⓑ Ⓒ Ⓓ Ⓔ	230 Ⓐ Ⓑ Ⓒ Ⓓ Ⓔ	255 Ⓐ Ⓑ Ⓒ Ⓓ Ⓔ	280 Ⓐ Ⓑ Ⓒ Ⓓ Ⓔ
206 Ⓐ Ⓑ Ⓒ Ⓓ Ⓔ	231 Ⓐ Ⓑ Ⓒ Ⓓ Ⓔ	256 Ⓐ Ⓑ Ⓒ Ⓓ Ⓔ	281 Ⓐ Ⓑ Ⓒ Ⓓ Ⓔ
207 Ⓐ Ⓑ Ⓒ Ⓓ Ⓔ	232 Ⓐ Ⓑ Ⓒ Ⓓ Ⓔ	257 Ⓐ Ⓑ Ⓒ Ⓓ Ⓔ	282 Ⓐ Ⓑ Ⓒ Ⓓ Ⓔ
208 Ⓐ Ⓑ Ⓒ Ⓓ Ⓔ	233 Ⓐ Ⓑ Ⓒ Ⓓ Ⓔ	258 Ⓐ Ⓑ Ⓒ Ⓓ Ⓔ	283 Ⓐ Ⓑ Ⓒ Ⓓ Ⓔ
209 Ⓐ Ⓑ Ⓒ Ⓓ Ⓔ	234 Ⓐ Ⓑ Ⓒ Ⓓ Ⓔ	259 Ⓐ Ⓑ Ⓒ Ⓓ Ⓔ	284 Ⓐ Ⓑ Ⓒ Ⓓ Ⓔ
210 Ⓐ Ⓑ Ⓒ Ⓓ Ⓔ	235 Ⓐ Ⓑ Ⓒ Ⓓ Ⓔ	260 Ⓐ Ⓑ Ⓒ Ⓓ Ⓔ	285 Ⓐ Ⓑ Ⓒ Ⓓ Ⓔ
211 Ⓐ Ⓑ Ⓒ Ⓓ Ⓔ	236 Ⓐ Ⓑ Ⓒ Ⓓ Ⓔ	261 Ⓐ Ⓑ Ⓒ Ⓓ Ⓔ	286 Ⓐ Ⓑ Ⓒ Ⓓ Ⓔ
212 Ⓐ Ⓑ Ⓒ Ⓓ Ⓔ	237 Ⓐ Ⓑ Ⓒ Ⓓ Ⓔ	262 Ⓐ Ⓑ Ⓒ Ⓓ Ⓔ	287 Ⓐ Ⓑ Ⓒ Ⓓ Ⓔ
213 Ⓐ Ⓑ Ⓒ Ⓓ Ⓔ	238 Ⓐ Ⓑ Ⓒ Ⓓ Ⓔ	263 Ⓐ Ⓑ Ⓒ Ⓓ Ⓔ	288 Ⓐ Ⓑ Ⓒ Ⓓ Ⓔ
214 Ⓐ Ⓑ Ⓒ Ⓓ Ⓔ	239 Ⓐ Ⓑ Ⓒ Ⓓ Ⓔ	264 Ⓐ Ⓑ Ⓒ Ⓓ Ⓔ	289 Ⓐ Ⓑ Ⓒ Ⓓ Ⓔ
215 Ⓐ Ⓑ Ⓒ Ⓓ Ⓔ	240 Ⓐ Ⓑ Ⓒ Ⓓ Ⓔ	265 Ⓐ Ⓑ Ⓒ Ⓓ Ⓔ	290 Ⓐ Ⓑ Ⓒ Ⓓ Ⓔ
216 Ⓐ Ⓑ Ⓒ Ⓓ Ⓔ	241 Ⓐ Ⓑ Ⓒ Ⓓ Ⓔ	266 Ⓐ Ⓑ Ⓒ Ⓓ Ⓔ	291 Ⓐ Ⓑ Ⓒ Ⓓ Ⓔ
217 Ⓐ Ⓑ Ⓒ Ⓓ Ⓔ	242 Ⓐ Ⓑ Ⓒ Ⓓ Ⓔ	267 Ⓐ Ⓑ Ⓒ Ⓓ Ⓔ	292 Ⓐ Ⓑ Ⓒ Ⓓ Ⓔ
218 Ⓐ Ⓑ Ⓒ Ⓓ Ⓔ	243 Ⓐ Ⓑ Ⓒ Ⓓ Ⓔ	268 Ⓐ Ⓑ Ⓒ Ⓓ Ⓔ	293 Ⓐ Ⓑ Ⓒ Ⓓ Ⓔ
219 Ⓐ Ⓑ Ⓒ Ⓓ Ⓔ	244 Ⓐ Ⓑ Ⓒ Ⓓ Ⓔ	269 Ⓐ Ⓑ Ⓒ Ⓓ Ⓔ	294 Ⓐ Ⓑ Ⓒ Ⓓ Ⓔ
220 Ⓐ Ⓑ Ⓒ Ⓓ Ⓔ	245 Ⓐ Ⓑ Ⓒ Ⓓ Ⓔ	270 Ⓐ Ⓑ Ⓒ Ⓓ Ⓔ	295 Ⓐ Ⓑ Ⓒ Ⓓ Ⓔ
221 Ⓐ Ⓑ Ⓒ Ⓓ Ⓔ	246 Ⓐ Ⓑ Ⓒ Ⓓ Ⓔ	271 Ⓐ Ⓑ Ⓒ Ⓓ Ⓔ	296 Ⓐ Ⓑ Ⓒ Ⓓ Ⓔ
222 Ⓐ Ⓑ Ⓒ Ⓓ Ⓔ	247 Ⓐ Ⓑ Ⓒ Ⓓ Ⓔ	272 Ⓐ Ⓑ Ⓒ Ⓓ Ⓔ	297 Ⓐ Ⓑ Ⓒ Ⓓ Ⓔ
223 Ⓐ Ⓑ Ⓒ Ⓓ Ⓔ	248 Ⓐ Ⓑ Ⓒ Ⓓ Ⓔ	273 Ⓐ Ⓑ Ⓒ Ⓓ Ⓔ	298 Ⓐ Ⓑ Ⓒ Ⓓ Ⓔ
224 Ⓐ Ⓑ Ⓒ Ⓓ Ⓔ	249 Ⓐ Ⓑ Ⓒ Ⓓ Ⓔ	274 Ⓐ Ⓑ Ⓒ Ⓓ Ⓔ	299 Ⓐ Ⓑ Ⓒ Ⓓ Ⓔ
225 Ⓐ Ⓑ Ⓒ Ⓓ Ⓔ	250 Ⓐ Ⓑ Ⓒ Ⓓ Ⓔ	275 Ⓐ Ⓑ Ⓒ Ⓓ Ⓔ	300 Ⓐ Ⓑ Ⓒ Ⓓ Ⓔ